ANTIMICROBIAL
CHEMOTHERAPY

ANTIMICROBIAL CHEMOTHERAPY

Edited by
DAVID GREENWOOD
University Hospital, Queen's Medical Centre
Nottingham

OXFORD   NEW YORK   TOKYO
OXFORD UNIVERSITY PRESS
1995

Oxford University Press, Walton Street, Oxford OX2 6DP
Oxford   New York
Athens   Auckland   Bangkok   Bombay
Calcutta   Cape Town   Dar es Salaam   Delhi
Florence   Hong Kong   Istanbul   Karachi
Kuala Lumpur   Madras   Madrid   Melbourne
Mexico City   Nairobi   Paris   Singapore
Taipei   Tokyo   Toronto
and associated companies in
Berlin   Ibadan

Oxford is a trade mark of Oxford University Press

Published in the United States
by Oxford University Press Inc., New York

©Oxford University Press, 1995

A catalogue record for this book is available from the British Library

Library of Congress Cataloging-in-Publication Data
Antimicrobial chemotherapy / edited by David Greenwood.—3rd ed.
Includes bibliographical references and index.
1. Anti-infective agents.   2. Communicable diseases—Chemotherapy.
I. Greenwood ,David, 1935-.
[DNLM: 1. Anti-Infective Agents—therapeutic use.   2. Anti-Infective
Agents—pharmacology.   3. Infection—drug therapy.
QV 250 A629 1995]
RM267.A55   1995   616.9'0461—dc20   94-49516
ISBN 0-19-854944-X (pbk)
ISBN 0-19-854839-7 (hbk)

Typeset by Light Technology Ltd, Fife

Printed in Great Britain by
St Edmundsbury Press, Bury St Edmunds

Preface to the third edition

A great deal has been written in recent years about the rise of multi-resistant bacteria. There have been alarming reports of outbreaks of infection, generally caused by staphylococci, enterococci, mycobacteria or certain Gram-negative bacilli, that were resistant to nearly all available antimicrobial agents. Penicillin-resistant pneumococci, antibiotic-resistant salmonellae and shigellae, and chloroquine-resistant malaria parasites continue to proliferate in some parts of the world. There has even been talk of an impending 'post-antibiotic era'.

Such talk is premature. With more than 200 antibacterial agents on the world market, and an increasing number of antifungal, antiviral, and antiparasitic agents slowly becoming available, most common infections in and out of hospitals remain readily treatable, often with old and well-tried compounds. None the less, there is no room for complacency: the boundless versatility of microbes in finding ways to evade the antimicrobial onslaught is there for all to see; the flow of novel agents from the pharmaceutical houses has slowed to a trickle and shows few signs of increasing. Quite simply, we have to learn to use the valuable resources presently available with circumspection and common sense.

To a certain extent, microbial drug resistance is inevitable; microbes will always respond to the selective pressures of drug use. But multidrug resistance of the kind that makes successful treatment virtually impossible is not inevitable and can be avoided by the discriminating use of antimicrobial agents and by the thoughtful application of control of infection policies, particularly in hospitals. It is essential that all prescribers should understand the benefits and limitations of antimicrobial chemotherapy and that medical students and young doctors should learn good prescribing habits during their years of training. We sincerely hope that this book will go some way towards promoting sensible use of antimicrobial agents.

For the third edition the book has been given a thorough overhaul. Several new authors have been recruited and most of the chapters, including all those in Part III (*Resistance to Antimicrobial Agents*), have been extensively revised or rewritten. Antiviral agents and their use have been given greater prominence and there is a new chapter on *Infection in Immunocompromised Patients*. Chapters on the important topics of *Bacteraemia and Endocarditis* and *Meningitis and Brain Abscess* have been considerably expanded.

Once again our grateful thanks are due to our secretaries, in particular to Louise Spry who undertook the task of putting a large part of the text on to disk, and to the staff of Oxford University Press, who have seen the manuscript through to publication with their usual efficiency.

Nottingham   D.G.
September 1994

Preface to the first edition

Antimicrobial agents are among the most commonly prescribed of all drugs. An enormous profusion of them (often bearing confusingly similar names) is available to the practitioner and they continue to proliferate. They vary immensely in potency, spectrum of activity, and toxicity as well as in their pharmacokinetic behaviour in the patient. Moreover, they come in all shapes, sizes, and formulations. Two or more may be mixed in a single preparation; even alone they are frequently administered with other drugs with which they may interact.

Given this huge diversity, it is perhaps not surprising that a number of surveys have revealed that antimicrobial drugs are often prescribed inappropriately, irrationally, and inefficiently. The cost of such wasteful prescribing in terms of unnecessary adverse reactions in the patient, or simply in terms of cash, can only be guessed at.

A thorough knowledge of the properties of antimicrobial agents should be part of every doctor's stock-in-trade. It is puzzling to find, therefore, that the subject of antimicrobial chemotherapy seldom occupies a prominent place in the medical student's curriculum. It is particularly surprising that no introductory textbook devoted to the basic principles of antimicrobial therapy exists. In general, the student is expected to glean his information on antimicrobial agents from specialized textbooks of microbiology, pharmacology, or infectious disease.

Books abound that tabulate dosages, treatment regimens, and minimum inhibitory concentration values of antimicrobial drugs, or deal in depth with their chemistry and mechanism of action; some of these books are extremely good and are recommended to the student for reference at the end of the present volume.

However, our aims have been more modest: we have specifically avoided unnecessary attention to chemistry, inhibitory concentrations, and dosages. Instead, we have concentrated on introducing the student to the general properties of antibiotics; to the role of the microbiology laboratory; and to the basic principles underlying the choice of treatment. The question of how much microbiological and clinical background to include has exercised us considerably. In the event we have tried to err on the side of generosity, especially in those areas where the student's knowledge might be anticipated to be shaky. However, it must be stressed that this is not a textbook of microbiology or infectious disease, and students who feel that their background knowledge is lacking are advised to supplement their reading appropriately.

Our use of two terms needs clarification: 'antibiotic' and 'microbe'.

Antibiotic strictly refers to antimicrobial substances produced by micro-organisms. However, except in the Historical Introduction, where the distinction has some relevance, we have sometimes used the word more loosely to include those synthetic drugs that may be used systemically to treat microbial disease. Use of the word *microbe* has been arbitrarily extended to include helminths (worms); while it may be difficult to view a 5-m tapeworm as a microbe, the study of such beasts falls within the province of the microbiologist and treatment of such infections within the scope of chemotherapy.

The basic framework of this book is taken from the formal didactic component of a 6-week course that is offered to students at Nottingham during their third year, which at this Medical School is a specialized 'honours' year. We have been gratified to find that the course has proved extremely popular and has been explicitly commended by the students as being of practical value in their subsequent clinical studies.

We strongly believe that there is a need for a book of this description in Medical Schools, and it is at the trainee doctor that this work is primarily aimed. We hope that it will have relevance beyond the shores of this country and we have been particularly concerned to try to remember the needs of the less developed nations.

No book can be all things to all men, but it has not escaped our attention that a book pitched at the introductory level we have aimed at might also serve to fill a gap for groups other than medical students who are required in their training to have a basic knowledge of the properties and uses of antimicrobial drugs. Such groups would include trainee nurses, pharmacists, and medical laboratory scientific officers (particularly those specializing in microbiology) as well as those often-forgotten employees of the pharmaceutical houses who develop, test, manufacture, and sell most of the agents with which this book is concerned. Nor would the book be out of place in the hands of the newly qualified houseman, who may feel that his crowded curriculum has left him little time to study the principles of chemotherapy that he is now expected to practise daily.

It is our sincere hope that this book will respond to the needs of all these groups of people.

November 1982   D.G.

Contents

Contributors

Professor A. M. Emmerson, MBBS, FRC Path, FRCP(G)
Head of Department of Microbiology,
University Hospital,
Queen's Medical Centre,
Nottingham NG7 2UH

Professor R. G. Finch, FRCP, FRC Path, FFPM
Professor of Infectious Diseases,
Department of Microbiology and PHLS Laboratory,
University Hospital,
Queen's Medical Centre,
Nottingham NG7 2UH

Professor D. Greenwood, PhD, DSc, FRC Path
Professor of Antimicrobial Science,
Department of Microbiology and PHLS Laboratory,
University Hospital,
Queen's Medical Centre,
Nottingham NG7 2UH

Dr W. L. Irving, MA, MB, B Chir, MRCP, PhD, MRC Path
Senior Lecturer (Honorary Consultant) in Clinical Virology,
Department of Microbiology and PHLS Laboratory,
University Hospital,
Queen's Medical Centre,
Nottingham NG7 2UH

Dr P. Ispahani, Dip Bact, DCP, FRC Path
Consultant Microbiologist,
Department of Microbiology and PHLS Laboratory,
University Hospital,
Queen's Medical Centre,
Nottingham NG7 2UH

Dr R. C. B. Slack, MA, MB, B Chir, MRC Path, D Obst RCOG
Senior Lecturer (Honorary Consultant) in Communicable Disease Control,
Department of Microbiology and PHLS Laboratory,
University Hospital,
Queen's Medical Centre,
Nottingham NG7 2UH

Dr K. J. Towner, BSc, PhD
Consultant Clinical Scientist
Department of Microbiology and PHLS Laboratory,
University Hospital,
Queen's Medical Centre,
Nottingham NG7 2UH

Dr P. J. Wilkinson, MA, MB, FRC PATH
Director of Public Health Laboratory and Senior Lecturer,
Department of Microbiology and PHLS Laboratory,
University Hospital,
Queen's Medical Centre,
Nottingham NG7 2UH

Historical introduction

D. Greenwood

Although the 'antibiotic revolution' can be accurately dated to the early 1940s when Howard Florey and his colleagues in Oxford seized upon Alexander Fleming's penicillin and turned it into a major therapeutic compound and Selman Waksman in the United States began his systematic pursuit of antibiotics from soil micro-organisms, the quest for chemotherapeutic agents active against pathogenic microbes began much earlier. Indeed, hopes of discovering specific antimicrobial drugs were kindled almost as soon as the microbial enemy was definitively identified by Louis Pasteur, Robert Koch, and others during the second half of the nineteenth century. By the end of that century Paul Ehrlich, often called the 'father of chemotherapy', had started the work which was to put the quest on a sound scientific footing.

Of course, man's search for effective remedies is as old as mankind itself but, before the aetiological agents of infectious disease were identified and made amenable to laboratory investigation, progress had to rely entirely on the vagaries of chance and empirical observation.

Not surprisingly, therefore, mankind's earliest therapeutic successes against infecting organisms came in the form of plant extracts that expelled worms visible to the naked eye. Herbal anthelminthics known since antiquity include extract of male fern (*Dryopteris filix-mas*), an effective vermifuge for tapeworms, santonin (obtained from the seed-heads of *Artemisia cina*: wormseed), and oil of chenopodium (*Chenopodium ambrosioides*: American wormseed), both of which expel intestinal roundworms.

Observations that natural substances controlled the spectacular symptoms of certain diseases no doubt led to the initial recognition of two other ancient remedies: quinine, obtained from the bark of the cinchona tree, and emetine, an alkaloid obtained from ipecacuanha root. Curiously, both these compounds originated in South America, from where they were introduced into European medicine in the seventeenth century, both are active against protozoa (the parasites of malaria and amoebic dysentery respectively), and both have survived into present-day use.

So far as antibacterial remedies were concerned, little had been achieved when Ehrlich began his work. Mercury had been used for the treatment of syphilis since the sixteenth century (giving rise to the aphorism 'one night with Venus—a lifetime with Mercury'), and chaulmoogra oil from the seeds of various species of *Hydnocarpus* had been used since ancient times in India for the treatment of leprosy, but apart from these the only antibacterial compounds known were a few antiseptics—chiefly phenolic substances and mercury salts, which were far too toxic for systemic use. In addition, right at the end of the nineteenth century a compound called hexamine, which spontaneously decomposes in acid conditions to release formaldehyde, was described as being useful in urinary tract infection.

THE FOUNDATIONS OF MODERN CHEMOTHERAPY

Oddly, in view of later developments, the foundations of twentieth-century chemotherapy were built on a search for antiprotozoal agents, since it was to the newly discovered parasites of malaria and African sleeping sickness (trypanosomiasis) that Paul Ehrlich first turned his attention. He reasoned that, since these parasites could be differentiated from the tissues of infected patients by various dyes in the laboratory, such substances might display a preferential affinity for the parasites in the body as well. In a phrase, such dyes might exhibit *selective toxicity*.

Early tests of this hypothesis employed the aniline dyes methylene blue and trypan red. Neither compound proved to be of much value, but the idea was pursued by the French workers, F. Mesnil and M. Nicolle, who found that two related dyes, trypan blue and afridol violet, had some useful effects in trypanosomiasis of animals. Interest in dyes as chemotherapeutic agents continued, and was later to pay off in several directions (see below); however, Ehrlich was deflected from the study of dyes and turned to arsenicals.

ARSENICALS

The event that caught Ehrlich's interest appears to have been a report of the work of H. W. Thomas and A. Breinl from the Liverpool School of Tropical Medicine, who in 1905 demonstrated that an arsenical compound, atoxyl, protected mice from infection with trypanosomes. Arsenicals, in common with other metallic compounds, had been used in medicine at least since the time of the sixteenth-century Swiss physician, Paracelsus (Theophrastus Bombastus von Hohenheim). Atoxyl itself had been described 40 years before its antitrypanosomal activity was investigated.

Despite its name, atoxyl was anything but atoxic and Ehrlich, together with his Japanese assistant Sahachiro Hata and his chemist Alfred Bertheim, set about trying to modify the molecule to produce derivatives with a better *therapeutic index*: the ratio of the toxic to the effective dose. As the work developed, the spirochaetes of syphilis, relapsing fever, and chicken spirillosis were included in the screening programme. Success came in 1909, when the 606th derivative of atoxyl that Ehrlich's team tested was shown to cure animals infected with each of the three spirochaetes and, equally importantly, to display an acceptable therapeutic index. Compound 606, later known as arsphenamine and marketed as Salvarsan, was the first really efficacious antibacterial agent, although its activity was restricted to spirochaetes, which are scarcely typical bacteria. An improved derivative, neoarsphenamine (Neosalvarsan), was produced in Ehrlich's laboratory in 1912.

Interest in arsenicals and other metals was also pursued elsewhere. Hopes of finding a drug to replace atoxyl for the treatment of trypanosomiasis remained alive and a variety of arsenicals were tried, of which tryparsamide and (much later) melarsoprol (Mel B) have emerged as drugs of value. In some other parasitic diseases of the tropics, another ancient metallic remedy, tartar emetic (potassium antimony tartrate) was discovered to exhibit useful activity. Tartar emetic was a familiar nostrum of Victorian medicine; its chief value was judged to lie in its emetic properties. However, Ehrlich's success with arsenicals and their use in trypanosomiasis prompted doctors working in the tropics to try other metallic compounds empirically in previously untreatable conditions. This led to the discovery of the efficacy of tartar emetic in two very different tropical diseases: kala azar (a protozoal disease of the reticuloendothelial system) and bilharzia (a worm infection of the blood). Antimonials are still used for the treatment of kala-azar, but safer drugs have been developed with which to treat bilharzia.

DYES

Paul Ehrlich's optimistic hope of exploiting the differential affinities of dyes therapeutically came to nothing. However, the idea was to bear fruit eventually in a wide variety of therapeutically useful antimicrobial compounds which, though uncoloured themselves, were derived, directly or indirectly, from dyes.

Suramin

The most direct link with Ehrlich's ideas is provided by suramin (Germanin), a colourless derivative of trypan blue developed by scientists of the Bayer organization in Germany. Like tartar emetic, suramin has proved useful in two quite unrelated parasitic diseases, in this case trypanosomiasis and onchocerciasis (a worm disease of the skin).

Antimalarials

By a remarkable coincidence, the very discovery of aniline dyes was sparked off by an antimalarial compound: it was during an investigation into the possible synthesis of quinine from coal tar in 1856 that the 18-year-old William Perkin, a student at the Royal College of Chemistry, stumbled upon mauve purple, the first aniline dye.

The progression from dye to antimalarial was finally accomplished indirectly through attempts, again by scientists at Bayer, to improve the activity of Ehrlich's methylene blue. Modification of the dye produced nothing of value, but information gained on the effects of various substitutions prompted the chemists to try similar substitutions on other heterocyclic compounds. In this way the 8-aminoquinoline drug, pamaquine (originally called plasmochin), and the acridine derivative, mepacrine, were produced. In turn these compounds led to the synthesis of primaquine (another 8-aminoquinoline) and the 4-aminoquinoline, chloroquine, which are still in use today.

Sulphonamides

The German obsession with dyes also paid off with the discovery of the first broad-spectrum antibacterial agents, the sulphonamides. In the event, this discovery came about by another of those happy accidents with which the history of chemotherapy is littered. In 1932 Gerhard Domagk, a bacteriologist working in the laboratories of the Bayer wing of the I. G. Farbenindustrie consortium, tested a number of dyes synthesized by his colleagues, Fritz Mietzsch and Josef Klarer, in experimental streptococcal infection in mice. Remarkably, mice treated with one such dye, prontosil red, survived the otherwise fatal infection. However, when prontosil was tested against streptococci *in vitro* it was found to have no antibacterial activity whatsoever. This paradox was explained when it was discovered by the Tréfouëls and their colleagues in France that in the experimental animal the dye was split into two components, one of which was sulphanilamide—a colourless compound hitherto unsuspected of possessing any antimicrobial activity.

Sulphanilamide was already well known to the chemist and, since the compound lay in the public domain, Bayer were unable to protect the discovery by patent. Naturally, many other firms seized the opportunity to market the drug so that by 1940 sulphanilamide itself was available under at least thirty-three different trade names and a start had been made on producing the numerous sulphonamide derivatives that subsequently became available.

Such was the situation when penicillin appeared on the scene as a potential therapeutic agent in 1940 (see Table 1).

ANTIBIOTICS

Penicillin

When Howard Florey and his team at the Sir William Dunn School of Pathology in Oxford first took an interest in penicillin in the late 1930s, the concept of antibiosis and its therapeutic potential was not new. In fact, moulds had been used empirically in folk remedies for infected wounds for centuries and the observation that organisms, including fungi, sometimes produced substances capable of preventing the growth of others was as old as bacteriology itself. One antibiotic substance, pyocyanase, produced by the bacterium *Pseudomonas aeruginosa*, had actually been used therapeutically by instillation into wounds, at the turn of the century.

Thus, when Alexander Fleming returned from holiday to his laboratory in St Mary's Hospital in early September 1928 to make his famous observation on an old contaminated culture plate of staphylococci, he was merely one in a long line of workers who had noticed similar phenomena. However, it was Fleming's observation that was to spark off the events that led to the development of penicillin as the first non-toxic antibiotic in the strict sense of the term.

The actual circumstances of Fleming's discovery have become interwoven with myth and legend. Attempts to reproduce the phenomenon have led to the conclusion that the lysis of staphylococci in the area surrounding a contaminant *Penicillium* colony on Fleming's original plate could have arisen only by an extraordinary concatenation of accidental events, including the vagaries of temperature of an English summer.

Fleming was hopeful about the possible therapeutic value of his discovery and he made desultory attempts to use culture filtrates in superficial infections. There is, moreover, documentary evidence of the successful treatment of gonococcal ophthalmia in babies with filtrates of *Penicillium* cultures, as early as 1930. This was achieved in Sheffield by C. G. Paine, a former student of Fleming's. Curiously, Florey was Professor of Pathology in Sheffield at the time of Paine's successful use of penicillin, but this does not seem to have influenced subsequent events.

Early attempts to exploit penicillin foundered on a failure to purify and concentrate the substance. It was left to Ernst Chain, a German biochemist who had sought refuge in England from Nazi persecution, and who had been set the task by Florey of investigating naturally occurring antibacterial substances (including lysozyme, another of Fleming's discoveries), to obtain a crude, but stable extract of penicillin. It was with these crude extracts, which were subsequently shown to

Table 1. Some of the chemotherapeutic agents (and the indications for their use) that predate the introduction of penicillin in 1941

	extract of male fern	: tapeworm
	santonin	: intestinal roundworm
	oil of chenopodium	: intestinal roundworm
Pre-1890	cinchona bark (quinine)*	: malaria
	ipecacuanha root (emetine)*	: amoebic dysentery
	mercury	: syphilis
	chaulmoogra oil	: leprosy

Arsenicals and antimonials		Dyes and dye derivatives		Other substances	
1905 atoxyl	: trypanosomiasis	1891 methylene blue	: malaria	1895 hexamine*	: urinary infection
1909 arsphenamine	: syphilis	1904 trypan red	: trypanosomiasis	1899 pyocyanase	: bacteria (topically)
1912 neoarsphenamine	: syphilis	1906 trypan blue	: trypanosomiasis	1925 tetrachloroethylene*	: hookworm
1912 tartar emetic	: leishmaniasis	1906 afridol violet	: trypanosomiasis	1939 tyrothricin*	: bacteria (topically)
1917 tartar emetic	: schistosomiasis	1916 suramin*	: trypanosomiasis onchocerciasis		
1919 tryparsamide*	: trypanosomiasis	1926 plasmoquine	: malaria		
		1932 mepacrine*	: malaria (etc)		
		1932 prontosil red	: bacteria		
		1934 chloroquine*†	: malaria		

* Still in use (mepacrine is no longer in use as an antimalarial, but is still occasionally used in the treatment of giardiasis. Prontosil is no longer used, but has given rise to the large sulphonamide family).

† Chloroquine was discovered in 1934, but not used in malaria until 1945.

contain less than 1 per cent pure penicillin, that the first therapeutic experiments were performed in mice and men. In view of the impurity of the substances used, it is indeed fortunate that problems of serious toxicity were not encountered in these early trials.

Further development of penicillin was beyond the means of wartime Britain, and Florey visited the USA in 1941 with his assistant, Norman Heatley, to enlist the support of the American authorities and drug firms. Once Florey had convinced them of the potential of penicillin, progress was rapid and by the end of the Second World War bulk production of penicillin was in progress and the drug was beginning to become readily available.

Cephalosporins

The discovery of the first of the cephalosporins (sister compounds to the penicillins, which share many features of structure and activity) is, in its way, equally extraordinary. Between 1945 and 1948, Giuseppe Brotzu, former Rector of the University of Cagliari, Sardinia, investigated the microbial flora of a sewage outflow in the hope of discovering naturally occurring antibiotic substances. One of the organisms recovered from the sewage was a *Cephalosporium* mould which displayed striking inhibitory activity against several bacterial species, including *Salmonella typhi*—the causative organism of typhoid—that were beyond the reach of penicillin at that time. Brotzu carried out some preliminary bacteriological and clinical studies, and obtained some encouraging results. However, he lacked the facilities to develop the compound further, so through a British acquaintance the mould was sent to the Sir William Dunn School in Oxford.

The first thing to be discovered by the Oxford scientists was that Brotzu's mould produced two antibiotics, which they called cephalosporin P and cephalosporin N, because the former inhibited Gram-positive organisms (e.g. staphylococci and streptococci) while the later was active against Gram-negative organisms (e.g. *Escherichia coli* and *S. typhi*). As chance would have it, neither of these substances is a cephalosporin in the sense that the term is used today: cephalosporin P proved to be an antibiotic with a steroid-like structure; cephalosporin N turned out to be a penicillin (adicillin). The forerunner of the cephalosporins now in use, cephalosporin C, was detected later as a minor component on fractionation of cephalosporin N.

Antibiotics from soil

The development of penicillin, cephalosporin C, and, subsequently, their numerous derivatives represents only one branch of the anti-biotic story. The other main route to present-day antibiotics came through an investigation into antimicrobial substances produced by micro-organisms in soil. The chief moving spirit in this investigation was Selman A. Waksman, an emigré from the Russian Ukraine, who had taken up the study of soil microbiology in the USA as a young man. In 1940, Waksman initiated a systematic search for non-toxic antibiotics produced by soil micro-organisms, notably actinomycetes, a group that includes the *Streptomyces* spp. which were to yield many therapeutically useful compounds. Waksman was probably influenced in his decision to undertake this study by the then recent discovery by an ex-pupil, René Dubos, of the antibiotic complex tyrothricin in culture filtrates of *Bacillus brevis*.

Waksman's first discoveries were, like Dubos's tyrothricin, too toxic for systemic use, although they included actinomycin, a compound later used in cancer chemotherapy. The first real breakthrough came in 1943 with the discovery by Waksman's research student Albert Schatz of streptomycin, the first aminoglycoside antibiotic, which was found to have a spectrum of activity that neatly complemented penicillin by inhibiting many Gram-negative bacilli and—very importantly at that time—*Mycobacterium tuberculosis*.

The appearance of streptomycin triggered a more general hunt for naturally occurring antibiotics and, when the pharmaceutical houses joined in the chase, soil samples by the hundred thousand from all over the world were screened for antibiotic-producing micro-organisms. Thousands of antibiotic substances were discovered and rediscovered by this means and, although most failed preliminary toxicity tests, by the mid-1950s representatives of most of the major families of antibiotics, including aminoglycosides, chloramphenicol, tetracyclines, and macrolides, had been discovered.

Naturally occurring substances that inhibit pathogenic fungi were also found. The first of those was nystatin, named after the New York State Department of Health in whose laboratories it was discovered in 1949 by Elizabeth Hazen and her colleague Rachel Brown. The related polyene antibiotic, amphotericin B, was developed by scientists at Squibb in 1960. Another antifungal antibiotic, griseofulvin, was first described in 1939, but not used in human medicine until 1958, following the work by J. C. Gentles on dermatophyte infections in experimental animals.

FURTHER DEVELOPMENTS

Since 1960 only a very few truly novel antibiotic substances have been discovered, although a surprising number of naturally occurring substances displaying fundamental molecular variations on the penicillin structure have emerged. A more fruitful line of approach has been to modify existing agents chemically in an attempt to derive compounds with enhanced properties. This has been most successful in the penicillin and cephalosporin field, where numerous semi-synthetic derivatives are now available.

Chemists and microbiologists have been active, too, in exploiting the antibacterial potential of non-antibiotic substances, although none has arisen by premeditated attack on known biochemical pathways. In fact, all the synthetic antimicrobial drugs presently used therapeutically, including the diaminopyrimidines, nitrofurans, imidazoles, quinolones, and most antituberculous drugs, have emerged through an indefinable mixture of serendipity, biochemical know-how, inspired hunch, and luck.

THE SCOPE OF ANTIMICROBIAL CHEMOTHERAPY

Without question, the appearance in the late 1930s and early 1940s of potent, non-toxic chemotherapeutic agents selectively active against bacteria revolutionized the treatment of infection. Indeed, the discovery of these first 'miracle drugs'—sulphonamides, penicillin, and streptomycin—was sanguinely declared by some to herald the disappearance of bacterial infection as a disease entity of any importance. With more than 50 years' hindsight and hundreds of new agents at our disposal, we are now able to take a more dispassionate view of the benefits and limitations of antimicrobial therapy.

Many things have happened to modify our views of the capabilities of antimicrobial drugs, but four things stand out particularly.

1. Microbes have displayed a truly amazing versatility in terms of their ability to avoid, withstand, or repel the antibiotic onslaught.

2. The pattern of bacterial disease, particularly hospital-acquired infection, has altered considerably, most significantly in the wake of new operation procedures, instrumentation techniques, and treatment regimens which severely compromise the patient's own capacity to withstand infection.

3. The use of antibiotics often disturbs the delicate bacterial ecology of the body, allowing the proliferation of resistant species and sometimes initiating new infections that are worse than the one originally treated.

4. It turns out that no antimicrobial drug is entirely free from toxic side-effects so that use of any of these agents has its attendant risks.

Finally, it should not be forgotten that most of the spectacular therapeutic triumphs have been achieved in the treatment of bacterial disease.

Those numerous infections caused by viruses, protozoa, helminths, and fungi are, with some notable exceptions, less amenable to chemotherapy. Indeed some non-bacterial infections are treatable only by toxic agents of restricted potency, and a few lie beyond the scope of systemic therapy altogether.

Part I

General properties of antimicrobial agents

1

Inhibitors of bacterial cell wall synthesis

D. Greenwood

The essence of antimicrobial chemotherapy is selective toxicity—to kill or inhibit the microbe without harming the patient. So far as bacteria are concerned, a prime target for such an attack is the cell wall, since practically all bacteria (with the exception of mycoplasmas) possess a cell wall, whilst mammalian cells lack this feature.

Not all bacterial cell walls are the same. Indeed, of the many species that have been investigated, no two have been found to be identical. However, in general they conform to two basic patterns which may readily be distinguished by that most familiar of all microbiological techniques, the Gram stain.

The cell walls of Gram-positive and Gram-negative bacteria differ in many fundamental respects, but both groups possess a cross-linked chain of peptidoglycan (also called mucopeptide or murein), which gives the cell wall its strength. Cell-wall-active antibiotics act by interfering with the biosynthesis of this structure. Peptidoglycan consists of a backbone of alternating *N*-acetylglucosamine (NAG) and *N*-acetylmuramic acid (NAMA) units. The NAMA molecules are substituted with short peptides made up of five amino acids which cross-link (via an interpeptide bridge composed of further amino acids in most Gram-positive organisms) to provide the characteristic rigidity.

In Gram-positive organisms the peptidoglycan is thick (c. 30 nm), tightly cross-linked, and interspersed with polysugarphosphate residues (teichoic acids), some of which have a lipophilic tail buried in the cell membrane (lipoteichoic acids). Gram-negative bacteria, in contrast, have a relatively thin peptidoglycan layer (2–3 nm) which is loosely cross-linked.

External to the Gram-negative peptidoglycan is a membrane-like structure, composed chiefly of lipopolysaccharide and lipoprotein, which may prevent large hydrophilic molecules from reaching an otherwise susceptible cellular target. Small hydrophilic molecules gain access to Gram-negative bacilli by passing through aqueous channels, *porins*, within the outer membrane. Differential activity among some groups of antibiotics, notably the penicillins and cephalosporins, depends to a large extent on their ability to negotiate these porin channels and this, in turn, reflects the size and ionic change of substituent groups carried by the individual agents.

PEPTIDOGLYCAN SYNTHESIS

The bacterial peptidoglycan in both Gram-positive and Gram-negative organisms is assembled from units of NAG, initially linked to uridine-diphosphate (UDP). UDP–NAMA units are manufactured from UDP–NAG by the addition of a lactic acid moiety derived from phospho-enolpyruvate. The NAMA then receives, one by one, three amino acids which are usually L-alanine, D-glutamic acid, and either L-lysine (in Gram-positive organisms) or meso-diaminopimelic acid (in Gram-negative organisms). Meanwhile, two D-alanine residues, produced from L-alanine by an enzyme called alanine racemase, are joined together by another enzyme, D-alanine synthetase. The linked unit, D-ala–D-ala is added to the tripeptide side-chain of NAMA and the NAMA-pentapeptide thus formed is passed to a lipid carrier in the cell membrane. Here a UDP–NAG unit transfers its NAG to the NAMA-pentapeptide and any amino acids needed for interpeptide bridges are added to the L-lysine of the pentapeptide side-chain. The lipid carrier transports the whole building block across the cell membrane and the unit is added to the end of the growing peptidoglycan chain of the existing cell wall, where the final cross-linking reaction takes place. The process is illustrated in outline in Fig. 1.1.

The most important groups of antibiotics that interfere with cell wall synthesis are the glycopeptides and the β-lactam agents, but bacitracin, cycloserine, and fosfomycin also act at this level.

BACITRACIN

Bacitracin is one of a group of antibiotics, also including gramicidin and tyrocidine (Chapter 3), which exhibit a cyclic structure made up of about ten amino acids. Bacitracin itself (actually a mixture of three closely related compounds, bacitracin A, B, and C, of which bacitracin A is the major component) was first obtained from a strain of *Bacillus subtilis* grown from the infected wound of a 7-year-old girl called Margaret Tracy, in whose honour the antibiotic was named.

The spectrum of activity of bacitracin and the related cyclic peptides is virtually restricted to Gram-positive organisms. They are too toxic for systemic use but are found in topical preparations. Bacitracin itself is used as a growth promoter in animal feedstuffs and also finds a place in microbiology laboratories in the presumptive identification of *Streptococcus pyogenes*, which is exquisitely susceptible to its action.

The antibacterial activity of bacitracin appears to reside in its ability to prevent regeneration of the lipid carrier in the cell membrane, which is left in an unusable phosphorylated form (Fig. 1.1). Gramicidin and

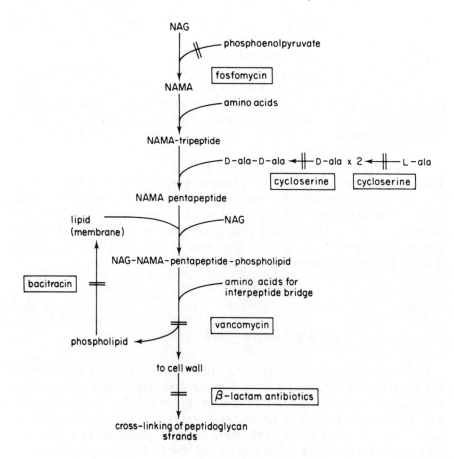

Fig. 1.1. Simplified scheme of bacterial cell wall synthesis showing site of action of cell-wall-active antibiotics.

tyrocidine have a different mechanism of action, interfering with the integrity of the cell membrane.

CYCLOSERINE

Cycloserine bears a structural resemblance to the D-isomer of alanine. Because of this, cycloserine interferes with alanine racemase (the enzyme that converts the natural form, L-alanine, into D-alanine) and also blocks the synthetase enzyme used to link two D-ala molecules together before they are inserted into the cell wall (Fig. 1.1).

Cycloserine has broad-spectrum, but rather feeble, antibacterial activity and has not found much use. Its chief attraction lies in its activity against *Mycobacterium tuberculosis*, but even against this important pathogen it is used only as a second-line drug, mainly because of toxicity problems.

FOSFOMYCIN

Fosfomycin (formerly known as phosphonomycin) is a naturally occurring antibiotic originally obtained from a species of *Streptomyces* isolated in Spain. Structurally, it is the simplest of all antibiotics (Fig.1.2). The molecule inhibits the pyruvyl transferase enzyme which brings about the condensation of phosphoenolpyruvate and N-acetylglucosamine in the formation of N-acetylmuramic acid (Fig. 1.1).

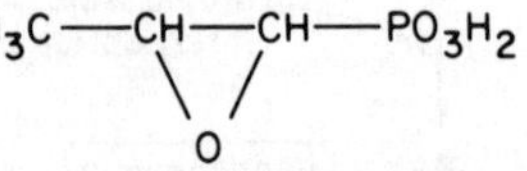

$$H_3C-CH-CH-PO_3H_2$$

Fig. 1.2. Structure of fosfomycin.

Although fosfomycin is available in the UK only as the trometamol salt, marketed for the single-dose treatment of cystitis, it has been more extensively used in some other parts of the world. It is well tolerated, and the ready emergence of bacterial resistance that is observed *in vitro* does not appear to have been a major problem in treatment. Gram-positive cocci are rather less susceptible than Gram-negative rods. The precise level of activity is a matter of dispute, since the *in vitro* activity can be manipulated by altering the test medium: the presence of glucose-6-phosphate potentiates the activity, whereas glucose and phosphate individually have an adverse effect. The potentiating effect of glucose-6-phosphate appears to be due to the fact that fosfomycin can enter bacteria by an active transport process that is inducible by glucose-6-phosphate but not by fosfomycin itself.

Fosfomycin is formulated as the sodium salt for parenteral use, but this is unsuitable for oral administration. The calcium salt, which has been widely used for oral therapy, is rather poorly and erratically absorbed, but the trometamol salt is highly soluble, well absorbed, and excreted in high concentration in urine.

GLYCOPEPTIDES

The glycopeptides, vancomycin and teicoplanin, are complex hetero-cyclic molecules consisting of a heptapeptide backbone to which are attached various substituted sugars. They act by binding to acyl-D-alanyl-D-alanine of peptidoglycan units, thereby preventing the addition of new building blocks to the growing cell wall (Fig. 1.1). Glycopeptides are too bulky to penetrate the external membrane of Gram-negative bacteria, so the spectrum of activity is generally restricted to Gram-positive organisms. Acquired resistance is uncommon, although resistant strains of enterococci are becoming more prevalent and coagulase-negative staphylococci exhibiting reduced susceptibility have also been described. Some Gram-positive genera, including *Lactobacillus* spp., *Pediococcus* spp., and *Leuconostoc* spp. are inherently resistant to glycopeptides, but these organisms are seldom implicated in disease.

Vancomycin

This compound has been particularly favoured for the treatment of bacterial endocarditis in patients who are hypersensitive to penicillin and for infections caused by staphylococci that are resistant to methicillin and other β-lactam antibiotics. Vancomycin is also useful in the treatment of antibiotic-associated diarrhoea caused by toxigenic strains of *Clostridium difficile* (see Chapter 22).

Early preparations of vancomycin contained impurities that gave the drug a reputation for toxicity. New, highly purified preparations are said to be much safer, but renal and ototoxicity still occur. The drug is given by slow intravenous infusion to avoid 'red man' syndrome (p. 209).

Teicoplanin

This is a naturally occurring mixture of several closely related compounds with a spectrum of activity similar to that of vancomycin, although some coagulase-negative staphylococci are less susceptible to teicoplanin. Unlike vancomycin, teicoplanin can be administered by intramuscular injection; it also has a much longer plasma half-life than vancomycin and appears to have a reduced propensity to give rise to adverse reactions.

PENICILLINS, CEPHALOSPORINS, AND OTHER β-LACTAM ANTIBIOTICS

The penicillins and cephalosporins are closely related families of compounds which share the structural feature of a β-lactam ring (Fig. 1.3);

such compounds are collectively known as *β-lactam antibiotics*. The β-lactam ring is the Achilles' heel of this group of antibiotics because many bacteria possess enzymes (β-lactamases; see Chapter 12) that are capable of breaking open the ring and rendering the molecule antibacterially inactive.

In the penicillins the β-lactam ring is fused to a five-membered thiazolidine ring, whereas the cephalosporins display a fused β-lactam/dihydrothiazine ring structure.

The original penicillin used in therapy, benzylpenicillin, contains a phenylacetamido side-chain at the 6-position of the fused-ring system (Fig. 1.3). Early attempts to modify this structure relied on presenting the *Penicillium* mould used to produce penicillin with different side-chain precursors during the manufacturing process. Later a method was discovered of removing the acyl side-chain of benzylpenicillin to liberate the penicillin nucleus, 6-aminopenicillanic acid (6-APA). Various chemical groupings could then be added to 6-APA according to the ingenuity of the chemist; a large number of compounds, collectively called *semi-synthetic penicillins*, have been prepared in this way.

Semi-synthetic cephalosporins can be prepared from cephalosporin C (Fig. 1.3) in an analogous way, the nucleus remaining after removal of the side-chain being, in this case, 7-aminocephalosporanic acid.

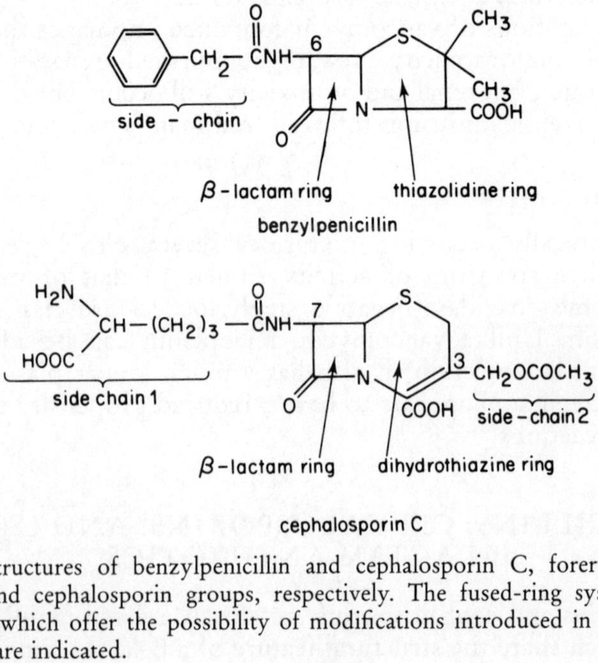

Fig. 1.3. Structures of benzylpenicillin and cephalosporin C, forerunners of the penicillin and cephalosporin groups, respectively. The fused-ring systems and the side-chains which offer the possibility of modifications introduced in semi-synthetic derivatives are indicated.

However, the extra carbon atom in the dihydrothiazine ring of cephalosporins offers the possibility of additional modifications at the C-3 position. Alterations at either end of the molecule may profoundly affect the antibacterial activity but, as a generalization, substituents at the C-3 position have more effect on pharmacokinetic properties. Cephalosporin C itself and some of its semi-synthetic derivatives (including cephalothin, cephapirin, cephacetrile, and cefotaxime) bear an acetoxymethyl group at the C-3 position. Cephalosporins exhibiting this feature are slowly metabolized in the body by liver enzymes which deacetylate the molecule to produce the corresponding hydroxymethyl cephalosporin. In general, the antibacterial activity of these derivatives is inferior to that of the parent compound and they may also display altered pharmacokinetic behaviour.

A number of cephalosporins, including cephamandole, cefotetan, cefmenoxime, cefoperazone and the oxa-cephem latamoxef possess a methyltetrazole–thiomethyl side-chain at the C-3 position of the molecule. This substituent has been implicated in causing hypoprothrombinaemia in some patients treated with these compounds.

Penicillins

The original preparations of penicillin were found on analysis to be mixtures of four closely related compounds which were called penicillin F, G, K, and X. Benzylpenicillin (penicillin G), often simply called 'penicillin', was chosen for further development because it exhibited the most attractive properties and because a manufacturing process was developed in which *Penicillium chrysogenum* was persuaded to produce benzylpenicillin almost exclusively.

Benzylpenicillin revolutionized the treatment of many potentially lethal bacterial infections, particularly those caused by the pyogenic cocci, such as scarlet fever, puerperal sepsis, bacterial endocarditis, pneumococcal pneumonia, staphylococcal sepsis, meningococcal meningitis, and gonorrhoea. The overwhelming importance of benzylpenicillin as a major breakthrough in therapy may be gauged from the fact that it remains today the treatment of choice for all these diseases. However, resistance has eroded the value of benzylpenicillin. Nearly all staphylococci and many strains of gonococci are now resistant. Moreover, pneumococci exhibiting reduced susceptibility to benzylpenicillin are increasingly prevalent. Such strains are of two types: those for which the minimum inhibitory concentration (MIC) of benzylpenicillin is increased from the usual value of about 0.02 mg/l to between 0.1 and 1 mg/l, and those for which the MIC exceeds 1 mg/l. The former are sufficiently sensitive to enable the antibiotic to be successfully used in high dosage, except in pneumococcal meningitis. However, penicillin is not clinically reliable in infections with strains exhibiting the higher level of resistance.

Despite its attractive properties benzylpenicillin is not the perfect antimicrobial agent: it exhibits a restricted antibacterial spectrum; it causes hypersensitivity reactions in a small proportion of persons to whom it is given; it is broken down by gastric acidity when administered orally; it is eliminated from the body at a spectacular rate by the kidneys; and it is hydrolysed by β-lactamases produced by many bacteria including staphylococci. Subsequent developments in β-lactam agents have been aimed at overcoming these inherent disabilities whilst retaining the attractive properties of benzylpenicillin: high intrinsic activity and lack of toxicity.

Acid stability

The first major success in improving the pharmacological properties of penicillin was achieved with phenoxymethylpenicillin (penicillin V). This compound has properties very similar to those of benzylpenicillin, but is acid stable and thus achieves better and more reliable serum levels when given orally, at the expense of some intrinsic antibacterial activity.

Prolongation of serum levels

Four approaches have been tried in order to maintain effective levels of penicillin in the body. First, the blockbuster approach is simply to give enormous doses of this non-toxic drug. Second, the slow-release approach is to mix penicillin with oily or waxy excipients; these preparations are injected intramuscularly, where they act as depots from which penicillin is slowly liberated. The third approach is a variant of this in which insoluble derivatives of penicillin are prepared. Three such 'long-acting' penicillins are in use: procaine penicillin, benethamine penicillin, and benzathine penicillin. The last will maintain low levels of penicillin in the blood for many days. The fourth manoeuvre, the competitive approach, is to administer probenecid orally at the same time as the penicillin. Probenecid competes for sites of active tubular secretion in the kidney, slowing down the elimination of penicillin.

Extension of spectrum

The first success with extending the spectrum of benzylpenicillin to encompass Gram-negative bacilli was achieved by adding an amino group to the side-chain to form ampicillin. Ampicillin is slightly less active than benzylpenicillin against Gram-positive cocci and is equally susceptible to staphylococcal β-lactamase. However, it displays much improved activity against some enterobacteria, including *Escherichia coli*, *Salmonella* spp., and *Shigella* spp. as well as against *Haemophilus influenzae*. It is not particularly well absorbed when given orally, but absorption can be improved by esterifying the molecule to form so-called *pro-drugs* which are split by non-specific tissue esterases in the intestinal mucosa to release ampicillin during absorption.

Examples of esterified pro-drugs include pivampicillin, bacampicillin, and talampicillin. Improved absorption has also been achieved by minor modifications to the molecule to produce amoxycillin and the ampicillin condensates hetacillin and metampicillin.

A peculiar change of spectrum was brought about by altering the form of the linkage at the 6-position of the penicillanic acid nucleus to amidino (N–CH=N) instead of acyl (CO–NH). The only penicillin of this type to become available, mecillinam (known as amdinocillin in the United States), is extremely active against ampicillin-sensitive enterobacteria and further extends the ampicillin spectrum to embrace some of the more resistant Gram-negative rods. However, mecillinam displays no useful activity against Gram-positive cocci. Mecillinam is poorly absorbed when given orally, but a pro-drug form, pivmecillinam, can be given by mouth.

Temocillin, a penicillin in which the β-lactam ring carries a stabilizing methoxy group (as in cephamycins; see below), is not hydrolysed by most β-lactamases elaborated by Gram-negative bacilli, but has no useful activity against Gram-positive or anaerobic organisms.

Antipseudomonal penicillins

None of the agents so far mentioned has any activity against *Pseudomonas aeruginosa*, an important opportunist pathogen in burns, cystic fibrosis, and immunocompromised patients. However, carbenicillin, a simple carboxyl derivative of benzylpenicillin, exhibits limited antipseudomonal activity. This has since been improved upon by ticarcillin, the thienyl variant of carbenicillin, and by a group of *N*-acyl substituted ureido derivatives of ampicillin which include azlocillin, mezlocillin, piperacillin, and apalcillin. These antipseudomonal penicillins must be administered by injection, but two esterified pro-drugs of carbenicillin, carfecillin and carindacillin, are available in some countries.

Antistaphylococcal penicillins

By the end of the 1950s 80 per cent of staphylococci isolated in hospitals were resistant to benzylpenicillin because of their ability to produce penicillinase (β-lactamase). The rise to prominence of these resistant organisms, which often gave rise to serious cross-infection problems, stimulated research into derivatives which were insusceptible to β-lactamase hydrolysis. Success was achieved with nafcillin, methicillin, and the isoxazolylpenicillins: oxacillin, cloxacillin, dicloxacillin, and flucloxacillin. All except methicillin can be given orally. The isoxazolylpenicillins are highly bound to serum protein in the body (see Chapter 16), but this does not seem to affect their therapeutic efficacy; flucloxacillin achieves higher serum levels than the others and is probably to be preferred in therapy.

A form of resistance to penicillinase-stable penicillins may be encountered in staphylococci which is caused not by inactivating enzymes but by alterations in the penicillin target. Such strains may fully display the resistance phenotype only under abnormal laboratory conditions (at a reduced growth temperature or in the presence of high salt concentrations). Staphylococci of this type are usually detected in the laboratory in tests with methicillin, so they have become known as methicillin-resistant staphylococci. Such strains are, however, resistant to all β-lactam agents. Some are also resistant to gentamicin and many other antibiotics (multi-resistant staphylococci). Methicillin-resistant *Staphylococcus aureus* strains (MRSA) have become endemic in some units where they cause persistent problems; some strains have a propensity to spread to give rise to mini-epidemics (EMRSA).

The spectrum of activity of the most important penicillins in clinical use is shown in Table 1.1.

Cephalosporins

Cephalosporin C was originally detected as a minor component of a mixture of antibiotics produced by a *Cephalosporium* mould. Such a substance could easily have been dismissed, but it was pursued because it exhibited the attractive properites of activity against Gram-negative bacilli and stability to staphylococcal penicillinase. In the event cephalosporin C was never marketed, but has given rise to a large family of compounds which continues to expand.

The earliest cephalosporins, cephalothin and cephaloridine, are not absorbed when given orally. Moreover, it soon became clear that the Gram-negative organisms within their spectrum were capable of elaborating a wide variety of enzymes that exhibited potent cephalosporinase activity (see Chapter 12). Consequently, as with penicillins, developments within the cephalosporin family were aimed at devising compounds with more attractive properties, viz. oral absorption or other improved pharmacological properties, stability to inactivating enzymes, better intrinsic activity, or a combination of these features.

In medical jargon it is commonplace to hear cephalosporins described as first, second, third, or even fourth generation compounds. These loose terms, which are best avoided, refer to: early compounds like cephaloridine and cephalexin that were available before about 1975 (first generation); β-lactamase stable compounds such as cefuroxime and cefoxitin (second generation); compounds like cefotaxime that combine β-lactamase stability with improved intrinsic activity (third generation); and a group of newer compounds that the manufacturers would like to persuade us have special properties (fourth generation).

In fact, the cephalosporins display such diverse properties that they defy any rigid categorization, but it is helpful to distinguish between those cephalosporins (the majority) that have to be administered

Table 1.1. Summary of the antibacterial properties of penicillins

Penicillin	Compounds with similar antibacterial properties	Staphylococci Activity	Staphylococci Stability*	Streptococci	Neisseria	Haemophilus	Enterobacteria Activity	Enterobacteria Stability*	Pseudomonas*	Anaerobes
Benzyl-penicillin†	Procaine-† Benethamine- Benzathine- penicillins	Very good	Poor	Very good	Very good	Fair	—— No useful activity ——			Variable
Phenoxy-methyl-penicillin†	Azidocillin Phenethicillin Propicillin	Very good	Poor	Very good	Good	Poor	—— No useful activity ——			Variable
Ampicillin†	Amoxycillin† Ampicillin-esters† Ciclacillin	Good	Poor	Very good	Very good	Good	Good	Poor	No useful activity	Variable
Carbeni-cillin†	Ticarcillin† Azlocillin† Mezlocillin Piperacillin† Apalcillin	Fair	Poor	Fair	Good	Good	Variable	Variable	Good	Fair
Cloxa-cillin†	Flucloxacillin† Oxacillin Dicloxacillin Methicillin Nafcillin	Good	Good	Fair	Fair	Poor	—— No useful activity ——			Fair
Mecillinam	Pivmecillinam†	—— No useful activity ——			Fair	Poor	Good	Variable	Poor	No useful activity —
Temocillin†		—— No useful activity ——			Good	Good	Good	Very good	— No useful activity —	

* Stability to β-lactamases of these organisms.
† Compounds on the market in the UK (1995).

parenterally and those that can be given orally. Among injectable compounds, it is useful to consider separately those with improved β-lactamase stability and those notable for their antipseudomonal activity (Table 1.2).

Parenteral compounds hydrolysed by enterobacterial β-lactamases

Cephalosporins in this group are of limited clinical value and have been largely superseded by other derivatives. Only two are presently available in the UK: cephazolin, which has the interesting property of being excreted in fairly high concentration in bile, and cephamandole, which exhibits a modestly expanded spectrum (Table 1.3).

Some cephalosporins of this group, including cephacetrile and cefapirin, offer no discernible advantage over earlier congeners like cephaloridine and cephalothin. Among newer derivatives, ceforanide and cefonicid exhibit extended serum half-lives.

Parenteral compounds with improved β-lactamase stability

An important advance was achieved with the development of cephalosporins that exhibit almost complete stability to the common enterobacterial β-lactamases. The first of these were cefuroxime and cefoxitin, the latter being one of a group of cephalosporins, collectively called *cephamycins*, which bear a stabilizing methoxy grouping on the β-lactam ring. Other cephamycins available in some countries include cefotetan, cefbuperazone, cefmetazole, and cefminox. The cephamycins are the only cephalosporins with useful activity against anaerobes of the *Bacteroides fragilis* group.

These compounds have been somewhat overshadowed by the appearance of cephalosporins that combine almost complete stability to most β-lactamases with exceptional intrinsic activity. Cefotaxime was the forerunner of this group of compounds, but several others are available: ceftizoxime and cefmenoxime are similar to cefotaxime; ceftriaxone displays a very long plasma half-life; cefodizime also has an extended half-life and is said to possess immunomodulating properties.

Latamoxef (known as moxalactam in the USA), which is strictly an oxa-cephem (see below), also displays activity analogous to that of cefotaxime and its relatives, but differs in possessing useful activity against *B. fragilis* and related anaerobes. However, latamoxef has lost favour owing to toxicity problems and it is no longer available in the UK.

Compounds distinguished by antipseudomonal activity

The important opportunist pathogen, *Ps. aeruginosa*, is not susceptible to most cephalosporins and, as with penicillins, considerable efforts have been made to find derivatives that include this organism in their

Table 1.2. Categorization of cephalosporins in clinical use

Cephalosporins

Parenteral compounds			Oral compounds	
Cephalothin	Cephacetrile	Ceforanide	Cephalexin*	Cephaloglycin
Cephaloridine	Cefapirin	Cefonicid	Cephradine*	Cefatrizine
Cephazolin*	Cefazedone		Cefaclor*	Cefroxadine
Cephamandole*	Ceftezole		Cefadroxil*	Cefprozil

Compounds with improved β-lactamase stability

			Compounds with improved β-lactamase stability	
Cefuroxime*	Cefmetazole	Cefotiam	**Non-esterified**	**Esterified**
Cefoxitin*	Cefbuperazone			
Cefotetan	Cefminox		Cefixime*	Cefuroxime axetil*
			Ceftibuten*	Cefpodoxime proxetil*
				Cefetamet pivoxil
				Cefteram pivoxil

Compounds with improved intrinsic activity and β-lactamase stability

Cefotaxime*	Cefmenoxime
Ceftizoxime*	Cefodizime*
Ceftriaxone*	Latamoxef†

Compounds distinguished by activity against *Pseudomonas aeruginosa*

Broad spectrum	Medium spectrum	Narrow spectrum
Ceftazidime*	Cefoperazone	Cefsulodin*
Cefpirome	Cefpimazole	
Cefepime	Cefpiramide	

* Compounds on the market in the UK (1995).
† Strictly an oxa-cephem.

Table 1.3. Summary of the spectrum of antibacterial activity of cephalosporins available in the UK (1995)

Cephalosporin	Staphylococci	Streptococci*	Neisseria spp.	Haemophilus influenzae	Enterobacteria	Pseudomonas aeruginosa	Bacteroides spp.
Cephazolin	Good	Good	Fair	Poor	Variable	No useful activity	—
Cephamandole	Good	Good	Good	Good	Variable	No useful activity	—
Cefuroxime	Good	Very good	Good	Good	Good	No useful activity	Poor
Cefoxitin	Fair	Good	Good	Fair	Good	No useful activity	Good
Cefotaxime ⎫ Ceftizoxime ⎬ Ceftriaxone ⎭	Good	Very good	Very good	Very good	Very good	Poor	Poor
Cefodizime	Fair	Good	Very good	Very good	Very good	Poor	Poor
Ceftazidime	Fair	Good	Very good	Very good	Very good	Good	Poor
Cefsulodin	Poor	Poor	Poor	No useful activity	No useful activity	Good	No useful activity
Cephalexin ⎫ Cephradine ⎬ Cefadroxil ⎭	Good	Good	Poor	Poor	Variable	No useful activity	—
Cefaclor	Good	Good	Fair	Good	Variable	No useful activity	—
Cefixime	Poor	Very good	Very good	Very good	Very good	Poor	No useful activity
Cefpodoxime	Fair	Very good	Very good	Very good	Very good	Poor	Poor

* Enterococci are resistant to all cephalosporins.

spectrum. Some cephalosporins with antipseudomonal activity, like cefoperazone, cefpimazole, and cefpiramide, are not distinguished by any unusual activity against other organisms and cefsulodin is extraordinary in being virtually inactive against bacteria other than *Ps. aeruginosa*. Among other derivatives, ceftazidime, cefpirome, and cefepime exhibit broad-spectrum activity comparable to that of cefotaxime and its congeners. Ceftazidime has been available for some years and has established a useful role in the management of *Ps. aeruginosa* infections in seriously ill patients. However, the antistaphylococcal activity of this compound is suspect and cefpirome may have some advantage in this respect. Cefepime retains activity against some opportunist Gram-negative bacilli that may develop resistance to cefotaxime and its relatives.

Oral cephalosporins

Early development of the cephalosporins yielded cephalexin, a compound that is considerably less active than cephalothin or cephaloridine, particularly in terms of its bactericidal activity against Gram-negative bacilli, but which displays the attraction of being virtually completely absorbed when given orally. The property of oral absorption is unusual among cephalosporins and many oral derivatives are structurally minor variations on the cephalexin theme. Such compounds include: cephradine (the properties of which are indistinguishable from those of cephalexin); cefaclor (which is more active against the important respiratory pathogen *Haemophilus influenzae*); and cefadroxil (which exhibits a modestly extended plasma half-life). Cephaloglycin, cefroxadine, cefatrizine, and cefprozil are similar compounds available in certain countries.

Cefixime and ceftibuten are structurally unrelated to cephalexin. They display much improved activity against most Gram-negative bacilli, but at the expense of antistaphylococcal (and, in the case of ceftibuten, antipneumococcal) activity, which is very poor.

The principle of esterification to produce pro-drugs with improved oral absorption has also been applied to cephalosporins. Two such compounds, cefuroxime axetil and cefpodoxime proxetil, are available in the UK; cefteram pivoxil and cefetamet pivoxil are marketed elsewhere. These compounds are about 50 per cent absorbed by the oral route and deliver the parent drug into the bloodstream. Cefpodoxime and cefetamet are more active than is cefuroxime against most organisms within the spectrum, although cefetamet has poor activity against staphylococci.

Other β-lactam agents

In addition to penicillins and cephalosporins, various other compounds display a β-lactam ring in their structure (Fig. 1.4). The cephamycins and the oxa-cephem, latamoxef, both of which share the general properties of

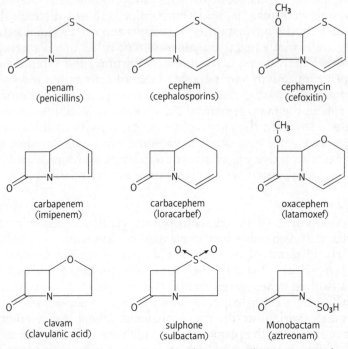

Fig. 1.4. Basic molecular structures of β-lactam antibiotics currently available (examples in parentheses).

cephalosporins (see above) are examples of such structural variants. Fundamentally different are clavulanic acid, a naturally occurring substance obtained from *Streptomyces clavuligerus*, and two penicillanic acid sulphones, sulbactam and tazobactam. These compounds have been developed as β-lactamase inhibitors for use in combination with β-lactamase-labile agents with a view to restoring their activity (see Chapter 9).

Among structurally novel compounds that exhibit antibacterial activity in their own right are: the carbapenems, imipenem (formerly called *N*-formimidoyl thienamycin), and meropenem; the carbacephem, loracarbef; and aztreonam, the first of a group of compounds collectively known as *monobactams*, which have a β-lactam ring but no associated fused-ring system. Imipenem exhibits the broadest spectrum of all β-lactam antibiotics, with high activity against nearly all Gram-positive and Gram-negative aerobes and anaerobes (but not intracellular bacteria such as chlamydia). Although it is extremely stable to most bacterial β-lactamases, it is readily hydrolysed by a dehydropeptidase located in the mammalian kidney and is administered together with a dehydropeptidase inhibitor, cilastatin. The activity of aztreonam, in contrast, is restricted to aerobic Gram-negative bacteria. These compounds thus typify two diametrically opposed approaches to the war on pathogenic microbes: blanket eradication and targeted therapy.

Meropenem is a carbapenem which shares the very broad spectrum of imipenem, but does not require administration with a dehydropeptidase inhibitor. Loracarbef also has carbon replacing sulphur in the fused-ring structure, but is otherwise structurally identical to cefaclor. Not surprisingly its properties resemble that of cefaclor: oral absorption, useful activity particularly against respiratory pathogens, and modest β-lactamase stability.

Mode of action of β-lactam agents

At one time it could be confidently stated that penicillins and cephalosporins act simply by interfering with the cross-linking reaction which gives the bacterial peptidoglycan its final rigidity. Bacterial death was thought to be secondary to this event in that continued growth led to osmotic rupture of cells no longer protected by an intact wall. It is now known that the situation is a good deal more complicated.

Penicillin-binding proteins

The chief complicating observation, so far as the mode of action was concerned, was that several distinct proteins were discovered in isolated cell membranes which efficiently bound penicillin (penicillin-binding proteins: PBPs). In *Esch. coli*, the best-studied species, there are seven of these proteins numbered 1a, 1b, 2, 3, 4, 5, and 6 according to the order in which they are separated by polyacrylamide gel electrophoresis. PBPs 4, 5, and 6 are thought to be unconnected with the antibacterial effect of β-lactam agents, since mutants lacking these proteins do not seem to be disabled in any way. Binding to the remainder has been correlated with the various morphological effects of β-lactam antibiotics. Thus, a number of β-lactam agents including cephalexin and its close congeners as well as aztreonam and temocillin bind almost exclusively to PBP 3 and inhibit the division process only, causing the bacteria to grow as long filaments. The amidinopenicillin, mecillinam, binds preferentially to PBP 2 and causes a generalized effect on the cell wall so that the bacteria gradually assume a spherical shape. Most other β-lactam antibiotics bind to PBPs 1–3 and induce the formation of osmotically fragile, wall-deficient forms (spheroplasts) which typically emerge through cell wall lesions situated at incipient division points. The morphological events are illustrated in Fig. 1.5.

Bactericidal action

The osmotic theory of the bactericidal effect of β-lactam agents has also undergone some modification in recent years, although it remains valid for Gram-negative bacilli, where cell death can be quantitatively

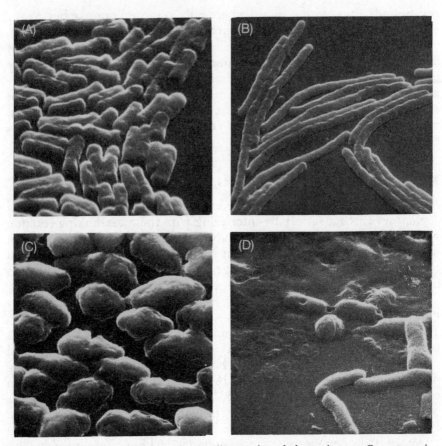

Fig. 1.5. Morphological effects of penicillins and cephalosporins on Gram-negative bacilli (scanning electron micrographs). (A) Normal *Esch. coli* cells. (B) *Esch. coli* exposed to cephalexin, 32 mg/l, for 1 h. (C)*Esch. coli* exposed to mecillinam, 10 mg/l, for 2 h. (D) *Esch. coli* exposed to ampicillin, 64 mg/l, for 1 h, showing lysed debris, central cell wall lesions, and a spheroplast; higher concentrations of most β-lactam agents cause this effect. [A–C from D. Greenwood and F.O'Grady (1973). *Journal of Infectious Diseases* **128**, 791–4. D from D. Greenwood and F.O'Grady (1969). *Journal of Medical Microbiology* **2**, 435–41.]

prevented by raising the osmolality of the growth medium. However, in the case of Gram-positive organisms one of the first events to occur following exposure to β-lactam antibiotics is a release of lipoteichoic acid from the cell wall, an event which appears to trigger a generalized autolytic dismantling of the peptidoglycan.

Optimal dosage effect
A further complication in Gram-positive organisms is that increasing the concentration of β-lactam antibiotics often results in a reduced

bactericidal effect. The mechanism of this effect (known as the *Eagle phenomenon* after its discoverer) is obscure, but may be related to the multiple sites of penicillin action, in that rapid bacteristasis achieved by blocking one cellular function may prevent the lethal events which normally follow inhibition of another by lower drug levels.

Persisters and penicillin tolerance

In both Gram-positive and Gram-negative bacteria, a proportion of the population survive exposure to concentrations of β-lactam antibiotics lethal to the rest of the culture. These *persisters* are apparently unaffected morphologically. They remain dormant so long as the antibiotic is present and resume growth when it is removed. In addition, some strains of staphylococci and streptococci display *tolerance* to β-lactam antibiotics in that they succumb much more slowly than usual to the lethal action of β-lactam agents. The therapeutic significance, if any, of persisters is unknown, but penicillin tolerance has been implicated in therapeutic failures in bacterial endocarditis where bactericidal activity is crucial to the success of treatment.

Post-antibiotic effect

Much has also been made of laboratory observations that the antimicrobial activity of β-lactam agents may persist for an hour or more after the drug is removed. This effect is not confined to β-lactam agents and is more consistently demonstrated with Gram-positive than with Gram-negative organisms. Theoretically, knowledge of post-antibiotic effects might influence the design of dosage regimens, but in practice they are too erratic to be used in this way, even if the *in vitro* observations could be convincingly shown to have clinical relevance, which is presently not the case.

2

Inhibitors of bacterial protein synthesis

D. Greenwood

The remarkable process by which proteins are manufactured on the ribosomal conveyor belt according to a blueprint provided by the cell nucleus is so fundamentally important and intrinsically fascinating that no one who has studied any aspect of modern biology can fail to have encountered it.

For the present purpose it is sufficient to outline the main features of the process. The first step is the formation of an initiation complex, consisting of messenger RNA (mRNA), transcribed from the appropriate area of a DNA strand, the two ribosomal subunits, and methionyl transfer RNA (tRNA) (*N*-formylated in bacteria) which occupies the 'peptidyl donor' site ('P' site) on the larger ribosomal subunit. Aminoacyl tRNA appropriate to the next codon to be read slots into place in the aminoacyl 'acceptor' site ('A' site), and an enzyme called peptidyl transferase attaches the methionine to the new amino acid with the formation of a peptide bond. The mRNA and the ribosome now move with respect to one another so that the dipeptide is translocated from the A to the P site and the next codon of the mRNA is aligned with the A site in readiness for the next aminoacyl tRNA. The process continues to build up amino acids in the nascent peptide chain according to the order dictated by mRNA until a 'nonsense' codon is encountered, which signals chain termination.

Although the general mechanism of protein synthesis is thought to be universal, the process as it occurs in bacterial cells is sufficiently different from mammalian protein synthesis to offer scope for the selective toxicity required of therapeutically useful antimicrobial agents. The chief difference that is exploited involves the actual structure of the ribosomal workshop in both protein and RNA components. These structural differences are reflected in the sedimentation characteristics of the two types of ribosome when they are subjected to ultracentrifugation analysis. Bacterial ribosomes exhibit a sedimentation coefficient of 70S and dissociate into 50S and 30S subunits; mammalian ribosomes, on the other hand, display an 80S sedimentation coefficient and are composed of 60S and 40S subunits.

The selective activity of therapeutically useful inhibitors of protein synthesis is far from absolute. Some, like tetracyclines and clindamycin, have sufficient activity against eukaryotic ribosomes to be of some value against certain protozoa. Moreover, the mitochondria of mammalian and other eukaryotic cells (which may have been derived from endosymbiotic bacteria during the course of evolution) carry out protein synthesis that is susceptible to some antibiotics used in therapy.

The selective action of this group of antibiotics is, therefore, a product not only of fundamental structural differences in the ribosomal targets, but also of access to, and affinity for, those targets.

Inhibitors of bacterial protein synthesis with sufficient selectivity to be useful in human therapy include aminoglycosides, chloramphenicol, tetracyclines, fusidic acid, macrolides, lincosamides, streptogramins, and mupirocin.

AMINOGLYCOSIDES

The discovery of the first aminoglycoside, streptomycin, in 1943 was a major landmark in the development of therapeutically useful antibiotics, particularly as it extended the sphere of influence of chemotherapy to embrace one of the major microbial scourges—tuberculosis. Later discoveries disclosed the fact that streptomycin was just one of a large

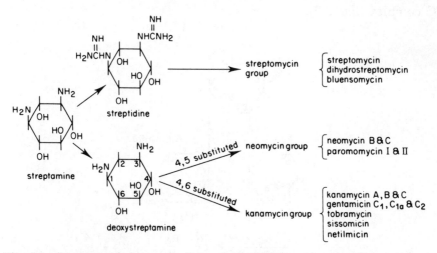

Fig. 2.1. Grouping of therapeutically useful aminoglycosides according to characteristics of the aminocyclitol ring. In most aminoglycosides the aminocyclitol moiety is either streptidine or deoxystreptamine, both derivatives of streptamine. The deoxystreptamine group can be subdivided into those in which sugar substituents are linked at the 4- and 5-hydroxyls, and those substituted at the 4- and 6-hydroxyl positions.

family of related antibiotics produced by various species of *Streptomyces* and *Micromonospora*. Those derived from the latter genus, such as gentamicin and sissomicin, are distinguished in their spelling by an 'i' rather than a 'y' in the 'mycin' suffix.

Structurally, most aminoglycosides consist of a linked ring system composed of aminosugars and an aminosubstituted cyclic polyalcohol (aminocyclitol). For this reason the group is sometimes given the cumbersome designation 'aminoglycosidic-aminocyclitol' group. One antibiotic usually included with the group, spectinomycin, contains no aminoglycoside substituent and is properly regarded as a pure aminocyclitol. Astromycin (fortimicin A), an aminoglycoside used in Japan, is also characterized by an unusual aminocyclitol group.

The aminocyclitol moiety of other aminoglycosides consists of one of two derivatives of streptamine: streptidine (present in streptomycin and its relatives) or deoxystreptamine (present in most other therapeutically useful aminoglycosides) (Fig. 2.1). Deoxystreptamine-containing aminoglycosides can, in their turn, be subdivided into two major groups: the *neomycin group* and the *kanamycin group*. The aminglycosides most commonly used in present-day medicine, including gentamicin and tobramycin, belong to the kanamycin group. The designation 'kanamycin', 'gentamicin', or 'neomycin' indicates a family of closely related compounds and commercial preparations usually contain a mixture of these. For example, gentamicin, as used therapeutically, is a mixture of three structural variants of the gentamicin C complex (Fig. 2.2).

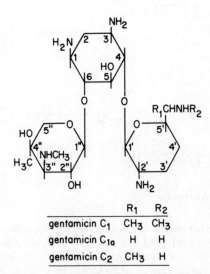

	R_1	R_2
gentamicin C_1	CH_3	CH_3
gentamicin C_{1a}	H	H
gentamicin C_2	CH_3	H

Fig. 2.2. Structure of the gentamicin C complex, showing the ring numbering system and variations in structure of the different gentamicins.

General properties of aminoglycosides

The aminoglycosides are potent, broad-spectrum bactericidal agents which must be injected for systemic use, since they are very poorly absorbed when administered orally. They lack useful activity against streptococci and anaerobes, but the activity against streptococci can often be improved by using them in conjunction with penicillins, with which they interact synergically (Chapter 9). They also penetrate poorly into mammalian cells and are of limited value in infections caused by intracellular bacteria. Some members of the group display important activity against *Mycobacterium tuberculosis* or *Pseudomonas aeruginosa* (Table 2.1).

As a group the aminoglycosides display considerable toxicity, affecting both the ear and the kidney, and their use may require careful laboratory monitoring (Chapter 8). In the laboratory the activity of aminoglycosides is markedly affected by pH and other variables (Chapter 7).

Mode of action

Most of the work on the mode of action of aminoglycosides has concentrated on streptomycin. This drug has been shown to bind to a particular protein in the 30S ribosomal subunit. Alteration of this protein results in streptomycin resistance but aminoglycosides of the kanamycin and neomcyin groups, which bind at a different site on the 30S subunit and also to the 50S subunit, are generally unaffected. Several effects of the binding of streptomycin and other aminoglycosides have been noted, including a tendency to cause misreading of certain codons of mRNA resulting in the production of defective proteins. It is unlikely that this effect is sufficient to account completely for the antibacterial activity of aminoglycosides, and other convincing lines of evidence suggest that the primary site of action (at least of streptomycin) lies in the formation of non-functioning initiation complexes. Other aminoglycosides may inhibit the translocation step in polypeptide synthesis. None of these hypotheses satisfactorily explains the potent bactericidal activity of aminoglycosides compared with other inhibitors of protein synthesis. Definitive solutions to these and other paradoxical aspects of aminoglycoside action are still the subject of dispute.

Aminoglycosides enter bacteria by an active transport process involving respiratory quinones. Since these are absent in streptococci and anaerobes this is thought to be the basis of the relative insusceptibility of those organisms.

Streptomycin

Once a drug of major chemotherapeutic importance, use of streptomycin has declined with the appearance of other aminoglycosides,

Table 2.1. Summary of the antibacterial spectrum and toxicity of aminoglycosides

Aminoglycoside	Staphylococci	Streptococci	Enterobacteria	Pseudomonas aeruginosa	Mycobacterium tuberculosis	Relative degrees of	
						ototoxicity	nephrotoxicity
Streptomycin	Good	Poor	Good	Poor	Good	+++	+
Kanamycin	Good	Poor	Good	Poor	Good	++	++
Gentamicin	Good	Fair	Good	Good	Poor	++	++
Tobramycin	Good	Poor	Good	Good	Poor	++	++
Sissomicin	Good	Poor	Good	Good	Poor	++	++
Netilmicin	Good	Poor	Good	Good	Poor	+	+
Amikacin	Good	Poor	Good	Good	Good	++	+
Neomycin	Good	Poor	Good	Poor	Fair	+++	+++

although it is still a common component of several antituberculosis regimens recommended by the WHO (see Chapter 26). It has also been traditionally recommended in the treatment of some rarer conditions, including plague, brucellosis, bartonellosis, and tularaemia, possibly for want of adequate evidence that more modern agents might be effective.

Neomycin group

Neomycin is among the most toxic of all aminoglycosides that have been developed for therapeutic use and it is now little used, except in topical preparations; even such usage is discouraged because of the risk of promoting the emergence of bacteria displaying non-specific aminoglycoside resistance. The poor oral absorption is exploited in the use of neomycin as a method of sterilizing the gut prior to abdominal surgery, but the inactivity of aminoglycosides against anaerobes ensures that the majority of the gut flora escapes, and the procedure is not without risk of systemic toxicity. Framycetin, a common component of topical preparations, is identical to neomycin B.

One aminoglycoside of the neomycin group, paromomycin, is unusual in exhibiting activity against the amoebae causing amoebic dysentery. However, the drug does not appear to offer any advantage over nitroimidazoles and other drugs in the treatment of this condition.

Kanamycin group

This group includes kanamycin itself, gentamicin, tobramycin, netilmicin, sissomicin, ribostamycin, and two semi-synthetic derivatives of kanamycin: amikacin and dibekacin.

Kanamycin, in the naturally occurring form obtained from the producer organism, is a mixture of three closely related compounds, kanamycin A, B, and C. Pharmaceutical preparations of kanamycin consist almost exclusively of kanamycin A, although kanamycin B (bekanamycin) is available in some countries. Kanamycin was the aminoglycoside which ousted streptomycin from its pedestal in the early 1960s. Its spectrum of activity is similar to that of streptomycin (and, like it, includes *M. tuberculosis*), but it retains activity against streptomycin-resistant strains and is less likely to cause vestibular damage.

In its turn kanamycin has been virtually superseded by gentamicin and tobramycin (deoxykanamycin B), which are more active against many enterobacteria and, more importantly, include *Ps. aeruginosa* in their spectrum. This has been a major factor in the popularity of these agents for the 'blind' therapy of serious infection before the results of laboratory tests are known.

The relative merits of gentamicin and tobramycin have been the subject of much debate. Tobramycin appears to be marginally less nephrotoxic and slightly more active against *Ps. aeruginosa*; against other susceptible bacteria, gentamicin probably has the edge.

Other agents of the kanamycin group, including sissomicin (sometimes spelt sisomicin) and dibekacin (dideoxykanamycin B), seem to offer little or no advantage over gentamicin or tobramycin. Netilmicin (*N*-acetyl sissomicin) is claimed to be less toxic than its predecessors and is more stable to some aminoglycoside-modifying enzymes (see Chapter 12).

Amikacin, a semi-synthetic derivative of kanamycin A in which an α-aminobutyric acid substituent has been added to an amino group on the deoxystreptamine ring, was specifically developed as a compound resistant to most aminoglycoside-modifying enzymes. Although it is somewhat less active than gentamicin or tobramycin, higher serum levels are achieved on conventional dosage and the drug has found some use in those units troubled by gentamicin resistance. Strains of bacteria that are resistant to gentamicin by non-enzymic mechanisms are, however, cross-resistant to amikacin and other aminoglycosides.

Spectinomycin

The aminocyclitol antibiotic, spectinomycin, exhibits properties that separate it from the true aminoglycosides. It displays inferior antibacterial activity against most species and generally achieves a bacteristatic rather than a bactericidal effect. Spectinomycin has found a niche for itself in the treatment of gonorrhoea in patients who are either hypersensitive to penicillin, or infected with gonococci that are resistant to penicillin.

CHLORAMPHENICOL

Chloramphenicol was one of the first therapeutically useful antibiotics to appear from systematic screening of *Streptomyces* strains in the wake of the discovery of streptomycin in the 1940s. Although it is a naturally occurring compound the molecular structure is relatively simple (Fig. 2.3) and can readily be synthesized. Attempts to modify the structure of chloramphenicol have generally resulted in a marked loss of activity, but thiamphenicol, a compound which possesses a sulphomethyl group in place of the nitro group of chloramphenicol, displays antibacterial activity comparable to that of chloramphenicol itself. Fluorinated derivatives

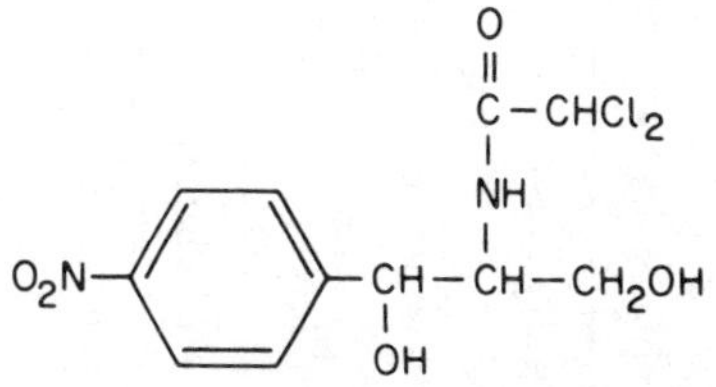

$$O_2N-\text{〈benzene ring〉}-\overset{\underset{|}{OH}}{CH}-\overset{\underset{|}{NH}}{CH}-CH_2OH$$

with NH connected to $\overset{O}{\overset{||}{C}}-CHCl_2$

Fig. 2.3. Structure of chloramphenicol.

of chloramphenicol and thiamphenicol that exhibit good antibacterial activity and retain activity against chloramphenicol-resistant strains have also been described, but have not been developed for therapeutic use.

Pure chloramphenicol is very insoluble in water and is extremely bitter to the taste. Both of these problems have been overcome by pro-drug forms of the antibiotic: chloramphenicol palmitate and stearate to improve palatability and chloramphenicol succinate to improve solubility for injection. These compounds have no antibacterial activity *per se*, but serve to release chloramphenicol in the body; they should not be used for laboratory tests of bacterial sensitivity.

Chloramphenicol acts by inhibiting the peptidyl transferase reaction—the step at which the peptide bond is formed—on 70 S ribosomes. The spectrum of activity embraces most Gram-positive and Gram-negative bacteria, and also extends to chlamydia and rickettsia, those strictly intracellular bacteria that cause a variety of infections, including trachoma, psittacosis, and typhus (Table 2.2). Resistance when it occurs is usually due to bacterial enzymes that acetylate the two hydroxyl groups.

The action of chloramphenical against enterobacteria is purely bacteristatic and this has led to its reputation as a generally bacteristatic drug. However, against some bacteria, including the Gram-positive cocci, chloramphenicol may display quite potent bactericidal activity. The drug also possesses the important properties of diffusing well into cerebrospinal fluid and of penetrating into cells—a very useful feature in the treatment of diseases such as typhoid, typhus, and other conditions where intracellular bacteria are involved. Resistance to chloramphenicol is generally uncommon, although resistant strains of *Salmonella typhi* have caused serious problems in areas of the world where typhoid is endemic. Strains of *Haemophilus influenzae* that are resistant to chloramphenicol are also being encountered with increasing frequency.

Given its attractive qualities it is a great pity that chloramphenicol displays one grave drawback: potentially fatal depression of the bone marrow. This side-effect, though extremely rare, has been sufficient to relegate chloramphenicol to the role of a reserve drug for special

Table 2.2. Summary of the antibacterial spectrum of inhibitors of bacterial protein synthesis

Antibiotic	Staphylococci	Streptococci	Neisseria spp.	Haemophilus influenzae	Enterobacteria	Pseudomonas aeruginosa	Anaerobes	Rickettsia and chlamydia	Mycoplasma
Aminoglycosides	Good	Poor	Fair	Fair	Good	Variable	—— No useful activity ——	—— No useful activity ——	Fair
Chloramphenicol	Good	Good	Good	Good	Good	Poor	Good	Good	Fair
Fusidic acid	Very good	Fair	Good	—— No useful activity ——	—— No useful activity ——	—— No useful activity ——	Fair	—— No useful activity ——	Variable
Lincosamides	Very good	Good	—— No useful activity ——	—— No useful activity ——	—— No useful activity ——	—— No useful activity ——	Good	(Fair)*	Good
Macrolides	Very good	Very good	Good	Good	—— No useful activity ——	—— No useful activity ——	Fair	Variable	Good
Mupirocin	Very good	Very good	Good	Good	—— No useful activity ——	—— No useful activity ——	—— No useful activity ——	—— No information ——	—— No information ——
Streptogramins	Very good	Very good	Good	Good	—— No useful activity ——	—— No useful activity ——	Fair	—— No information ——	Good
Tetracyclines	Good	Good	Good	Good	Good†	Poor	Fair	Good	Good

NB Individual strains of susceptible species may be resistant to any of these agents.
* Lincomycin, poor; clindamycin, fair.
† Poor activity against *Proteus* spp.

purposes. Use of thiamphenicol is also commonly associated with toxicity to the bone marrow, but the irreversible effects are said not to occur with this drug. Chloramphenicol is sometimes still used in typhoid fever and meningitis, including neonatal meningitis when, however, the other potentially fatal side-effect of the antibiotic ('grey baby' syndrome) may follow if the dosage is not properly adjusted.

TETRACYCLINES

The first tetracycline, chlortetracycline (Fig. 2.4), was described in 1948 as a product of *Streptomyces aureofaciens*. Oxytetracycline and tetracyline itself (so-called because it lacks both the chlorine of chlortetracycline and the hydroxyl of oxytetracycline) quickly followed. These, and other members of the group including clomocycline, demeclocycline, doxycycline, lymecycline, and minocycline, are closely related structural variants of the same tetracyclic molecule.

The tetracycline group is among the most broad-spectrum of all antimicrobial agents, displaying good activity against most Gram-positive and Gram-negative bacteria, rickettsiae, chlamydiae, mycoplasmas, and spirochaetes (Table 2.2). The different tetracyclines do not differ much in their antibacterial activity and are distinguished more by their pharmacokinetic behaviour. Doxycycline and minocycline are the most widely used; unlike the others they do not aggravate renal failure so that they can be used in patients suffering renal impairment; they also exhibit marginally better antibacterial activity, and they display sufficiently long serum half-lives to allow them to be given only twice daily.

Susceptible bacteria concentrate tetracyclines by an active transport process. In the cell they interact with the 30 S ribosomal subunit and thereby interfere with the binding of aminoacyl tRNA to the A site on the ribosome. Like chloramphenicol, the tetracyclines are predominantly bacteristatic, but some species are affected bactericidally. The therapeutic importance of the group as a whole has declined over the years with the upsurge of resistant strains, particularly among enterobacteria and streptococci. The mechanism of the most common

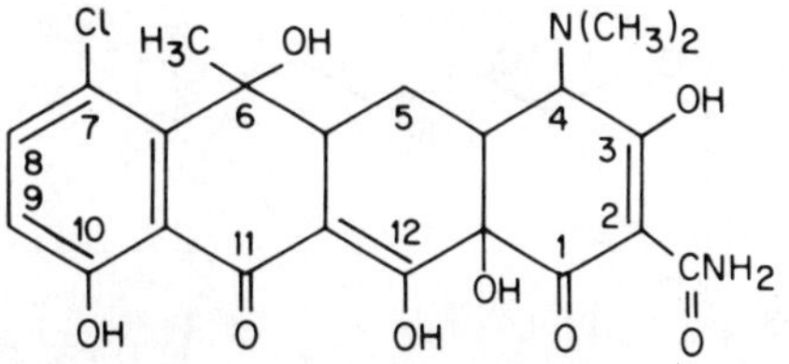

Fig. 2.4. Structure of chlortetracycline.

form of resistance is unusual in that a new protein is produced which appears to prevent uptake of the drug (Chapter 12). There is almost complete cross-resistance between tetracyclines, although minocycline may retain activity against some tetracycline-resistant strains.

Tetracyclines are still widely used for the treatment of respiratory infections, particularly chronic bronchitis and mycoplasma pneumonia. They are the drugs of choice for rickettsial and chlamydial infections of all types but their position may be eroded by the newer macrolides (see below). Their use should be avoided in young children, since they chelate calcium and are deposited in calcifying tissue so that their yellow pigment can permanently discolour growing teeth.

FUSIDIC ACID

Fusidic acid is the only therapeutically useful member of a group of naturally occurring antibiotics that display a steroid-like structure (Fig. 2.5). The antibiotic acts to prevent the translocation step in bacterial protein synthesis by inhibiting one of the substances (factor G) essential for this reaction.

Fusidic acid is active *in vitro* against Gram-positive and -negative cocci, *Mycobacterium tuberculosis, Nocardia asteroides*, and many anaerobes; the ribosomes of Gram-negative bacilli are susceptible to the action of the drug, but access is denied by the Gram-negative cell wall.

Staphylococcus aureus is particularly susceptible to fusidic acid and the compound is usually regarded simply as an antistaphylococcal agent. The antibiotic penetrates well into infected tissues, including bone, and it is favoured by some authorities for the treatment of staphylococcal osteomyelitis. A potential drawback to use of the drug is the presence

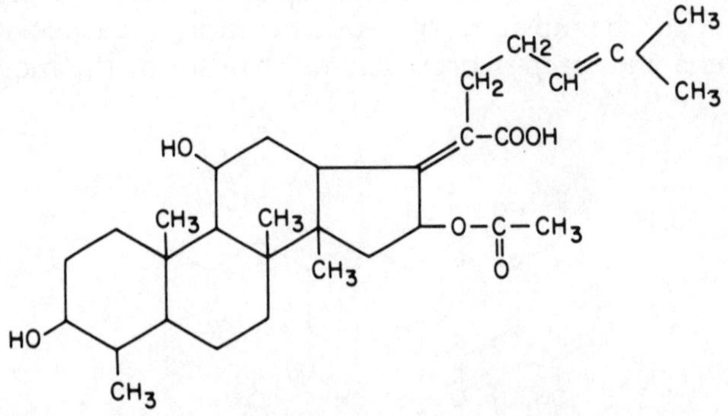

Fig. 2.5. Structure of fusidic acid.

in any large staphylococcal population of a small number of fusidic-acid-resistant variants which might proliferate during therapy. For this reason, fusidic acid is usually administered together with another antibiotic, often a penicillin. Fusidic acid is usually free from side-effects when given orally. Intravenous administration of the diethanolamine salt is sometimes accompanied by a reversible jaundice.

MACROLIDES

The earliest macrolide, erythromycin, was discovered in 1952 as a product of *Streptomyces erythreus*. This and related antibiotics share a similar molecular structure characterized by a 14- to 16-membered macrocyclic lactone ring substituted with some unusual sugars (Fig. 2.6). All members of the group are thought to act by causing the growing peptide chain to dissociate from the ribosome during the translocation step in bacterial protein synthesis.

Macrolides are most notable for their antistaphylococcal and antistreptococcal activity, though the spectrum may encompass other important pathogens, including chlamydiae, mycoplasmas, legionellae, and some mycobacteria (Table 2.2). Resistance is fairly common among staphylococci; it is less prevalent in streptococci, but erythromycin-resistant *Streptococcus pyogenes* strains have caused problems in some places.

The macrolide antibiotics have many attractive properties as well-tolerated oral compounds that display good tissue penetration. Their spectrum of activity makes them particularly suitable for the treatment

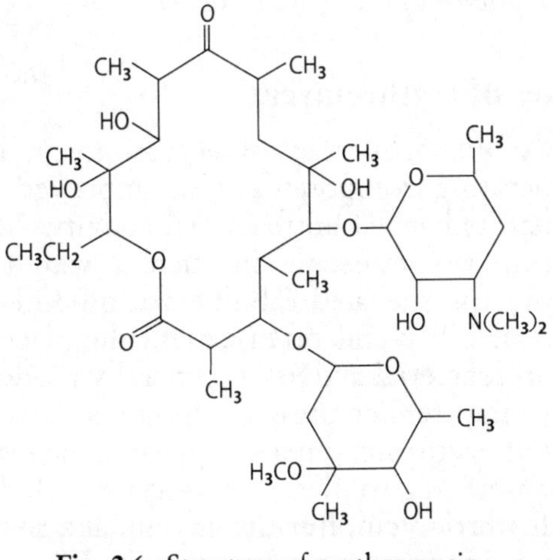

Fig. 2.6. Structure of erythromycin.

of respiratory and soft-tissue disease and for infections caused by susceptible intracellular bacteria.

Erythromycin

Erythromycin, the oldest and most widely used macrolide antibiotic, exists in four forms: erythromycin A, B, C, and D. Erythromycin A is the most active form and predominates in pharmaceutical preparations. The native form is broken down in the acid conditions of the stomach and is administered in the form of enteric-coated tablets which protect the antibiotic until it reaches the absorption site in the duodenum.

Alternatively, the stearate salt or esterified pro-drug forms are used for oral administration. Two ester formulations are in general use: the ethylsuccinate and the estolate. Erythromycin lactobionate and erythromycin gluceptate are available for intravenous use. The estolate has been generally regarded as the most toxic formulation because of its propensity to cause reversible cholestatic jaundice. However, this uncommon complication can arise with any of the preparations.

Erythromycin was originally discovered at a time when resistance of staphylococci to penicillin was first becoming a serious problem. In the fear that the usefulness of erythromycin might be similarly compromised, the drug was mainly used as a reserve antistaphylococcal agent, or as a second-line antistreptococcal agent for use in patients allergic to penicillin. Erythromycin is liable to cause nausea and abdominal cramps and this has also limited its popularity.

In common with most other macrolides, the antibiotic lacks useful activity against enterobacteria and *Ps. aeruginosa*, but is active against *Mycoplasma pneumoniae*. Erythromycin is also used in campylobacter enteritis when the severity of infection warrants antimicrobial treatment, and in *Legionella pneumophila* pneumonia.

Newer derivatives of erythromycin

Efforts to modify the properties of erythromycin have been more successful in generating compounds with improved pharmacological features rather than enhanced antibacterial activity. Much interest has centred on altering the molecule in such a way that the reactive groups responsible for the acid lability are modified. Such changes increase the bioavailability and often extend the plasma half-life. Any improvement in antibacterial activity is generally modest, but enhanced tissue penetration may render these compounds more effective. Acid-stable derivatives of erythromycin also appear to be less prone to cause gastrointestinal upset. Macrolides of this type include azithromycin, clarithromycin, dirithromycin, flurithromycin, and roxithromycin. The first two of these are presently marketed in the UK.

Azithromycin

In this semi-synthetic macrolide, a methyl-substituted nitrogen atom has been inserted into the lactone ring of erythromycin to produce a 15-membered ring structure that is described as an *azalide*. Azithromycin has a considerably improved bioavailability and a much extended plasma half-life of about 12 h, compared with about 2–4 h in the case of erythromycin.

The intrinsic antibacterial activity of azithromycin is roughly similar to that of erythromycin, although it is somewhat more active against some important respiratory pathogens such as *Haemophilus influenzae* and *Legionella pneumophila*; there is also some improvement in activity against enteric Gram-negative bacilli, but this is unlikely to be of great therapeutic benefit. Of particular interest are indications that azithromycin is effective in the single-dose treatment of chlamydial and gonococcal infections of the genital tract; if this early success is confirmed in long-term use it will represent a genuine therapeutic advance.

Clarithromycin

This compound is the 6-0-methyl derivative of erythromycin; it is metabolized in the body to yield the 14-hydroxy metabolite, which retains antibacterial activity, but has altered pharmacokinetic properties. The activities of clarithromycin and its hydroxy metabolite are similar to that of erythromycin, although concentrations required to inhibit legionellae and chlamydiae are generally lower; the compounds exhibit a slightly extended plasma half-life of about 3–7 h.

There have been claims of much enhanced penetration into pulmonary sites, beneficial interactions between the parent compound and the hydroxy metabolite, and other minor advantages, but whether these translate into significantly improved therapeutic efficacy compared with other macrolides is presently unclear.

Other macrolides

Other macrolides that have been used in various parts of the world include oleandomycin (or its better absorbed derivative triacetyloleandomycin) and a series of compounds with a 16-membered ring, including spiramycin, josamycin, midecamycin (and its diacetyl derivative, miocamycin), kitasamycin, and rokitamycin. None of them seems to offer much therapeutic advantage over erythromycin. Spiramycin is sometimes used as an alternative to pyrimethamine in infections caused by the protozoan parasite, *Toxoplasma gondii*. It has also been tentatively suggested, on the basis of little evidence, that it might be of value in cryptosporidiosis, a protozoal disease that is highly refractory to antimicrobial therapy.

LINCOSAMIDES

There are only two therapeutically important lincosamides—lincomycin, a naturally occurring product of *Streptomyces lincolnensis*, and clindamycin, a chemically modified derivative (7-chloro-7-deoxylincomycin; Fig. 2.7) which exhibits improved antibacterial activity and is thus generally preferred in therapy.

Lincosamides interfere with the process of peptide elongation in a way that has not been precisely defined. The ribosomal binding site is probably similar to that of erythromycin, since resistance to erythromycin caused by an inducible methylation of the ribosomal binding site affects lincosamides as well.

Lincomycin and clindamycin possess good antistaphylococcal and antistreptococcal activity and have also proved therapeutically useful in the treatment of infections due to *Bacteroides fragilis* and some other anaerobes. Enterobacteria and *Ps. aeruginosa* lie outside the spectrum of activity (Table 2.2). Clindamycin exhibits some activity against parasitic protozoa and has been used with modest success in toxoplasmosis, malaria, and babesiosis.

Clindamycin hydrochloride, like chloramphenicol, is extremely bitter. For oral administration the drug is formulated in capsules or as the biologically inactive palmitate, which liberates the parent compound *in vivo*. Clindamycin phosphate, which is used for intravenous administration, is similarly inactive in the test-tube but is transformed to the active form in the body.

Patients treated with clindamycin (or lincomycin) commonly experience diarrhoea, which may occasionally develop into a potentially fatal pseudomembranous colitis caused by a clostridial toxin (see Chapter 22). Other antibiotics, notably ampicillin and broad-spectrum

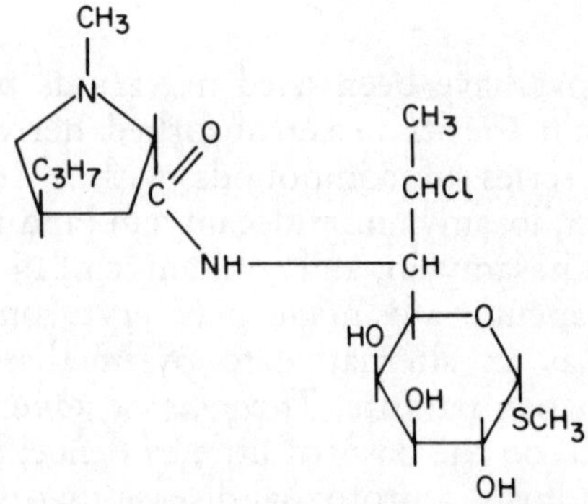

Fig. 2.7. Structure of clindamycin.

cephalosporins, may also cause this side-effect, but the incidence of toxin-associated colitis appears to be somewhat higher following clindamycin therapy than with other agents.

STREPTOGRAMINS

Each member of the streptogramin family is not one antibiotic, but two: they are produced as synergic mixtures by various species of *Streptomyces*. Two of these compounds, pristinamycin and virginiamycin, are used as antistaphylococcal agents in continental Europe; neither is available for human use in the UK, but virginiamycin is used as a growth promoter in animal husbandry.

The two components of streptogramin antibiotics are both macrolactones, but they are structurally different. Alone they exhibit feeble bacteristatic activity, but in combination the effect is bactericidal. Component A is a polyunsaturated peptolide that causes distortion of the aminoacyl-tRNA-binding site, hindering further growth of the peptide chain. The action of component B, a hexadepsipeptide, is less well understood, but it is proposed that it binds to an adjacent site and that the combined effect is to constrict the channel through which the nascent peptide is extruded from the ribosome. Protein synthesis is completely blocked and the consequences are lethal to the bacterial cell.

Pristinamycin and virginiamycin are best regarded solely as antistaphylococcal agents although the spectrum includes other organisms, notably streptococci. Their major claim to attention is that they retain activity against multiresistant staphylococci. However, plasma concentrations of the drugs after oral administration do not greatly exceed inhibitory levels. Solubility problems have militated against the production of parenteral formulations, but more soluble derivatives of pristinamycin are under development.

MUPIROCIN

Mupirocin (formerly known as pseudomonic acid) is a component of the antibiotic complex produced by the bacterium *Pseudomonas fluorescens*. The novel structure consists of monic acid with a short fatty acid side-chain (Fig. 2.8). The terminal portion of the molecule distal to the fatty acid resembles iso-leucine, and mupirocin inhibits protein synthesis by blocking incorporation of the amino acid into polypeptides.

The spectrum of activity embraces staphylococci and streptococci, but excludes most enteric Gram-negative bacilli (Table 2.2). Hopes

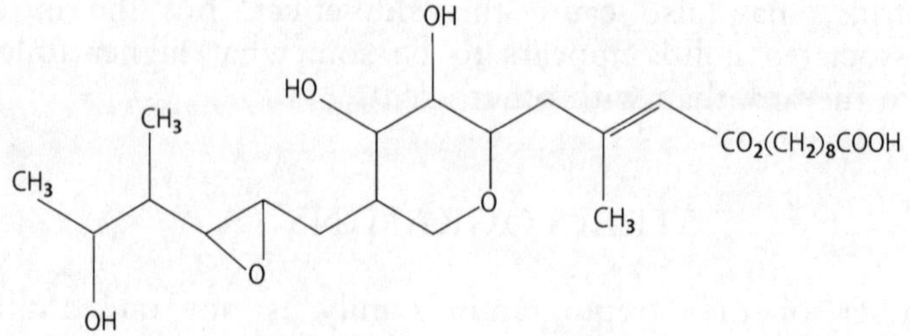

Fig. 2.8. Structure of mupirocin.

that mupirocin might be useful in systemic therapy were thwarted by the realization that the compound is inactivated in the body. Consequently, its use is restricted to topical preparations. Mupirocin has proved particularly useful in the eradication of staphylococci from nasal carriage sites (see Chapter 32).

3

Synthetic antibacterial agents and miscellaneous antibiotics

D. Greenwood

Various targets other than the cell wall and ribosome are open to attack by chemotherapeutic agents. These include the bacterial nucleic acid and cell membrane. There is also the possibility of interfering with essential metabolic processes within the cell, as sulphonamides and some antimycobacterial agents do. Hexamine (methenamine), a urinary antiseptic that is chiefly of historical interest, acts by liberating formaldehyde in the acidic conditions usually found in infected urine.

This chapter will consider the properties of inhibitors of bacterial nucleic acid synthesis, membrane-active compounds, and agents used solely for the treatment of mycobacterial disease. Many, but not all, of these compounds are synthetic chemicals rather than antibiotics in the strict sense.

INHIBITORS OF NUCLEIC ACID SYNTHESIS

Given the universality of nucleic acid as the basis of life, it is surprising that so many antimicrobial agents have been discovered that selectively interfere with the functions of DNA and RNA. Some, like the sulphonamides and diaminopyrimidines, achieve their effect indirectly by interrupting metabolic pathways that lead to the manufacture of nucleic acids; others, of which the quinolones and nitroimidazoles are prime examples, exert a more direct action.

Sulphonamides

The discovery of prontosil in the 1930s was a major breakthrough in the chemotherapy of bacterial infections (see Historical Introduction). Prontosil was found to be inactive *in vitro*, but it was quickly realized that its activity in the body was due to the liberation of sulphanilamide, an analogue of *para*-aminobenzoic acid (PABA; Fig. 3.1), which is essential for bacterial folate synthesis. Most bacteria synthesize folic acid and cannot take it up preformed from the environment. Mammalian cells, in contrast, use preformed folate and cannot make their own.

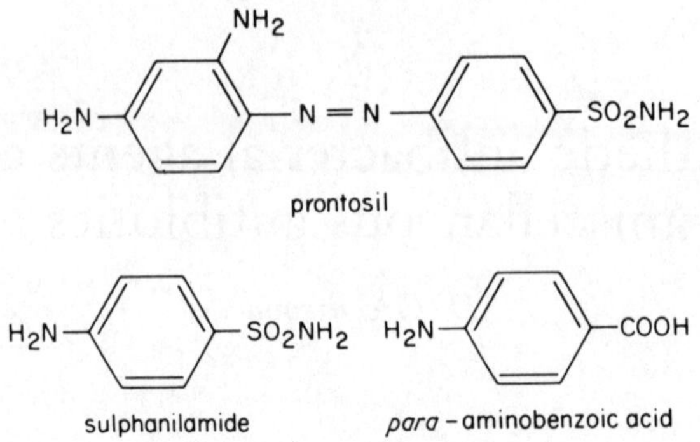

Fig. 3.1. Structures of prontosil, sulphanilamide, and *para*-aminobenzoic acid.

Sulphonamides block an early stage in folate synthesis: the condensation of PABA with dihydropteridine to form dihydropteroic acid. Depletion of folate leads to a number of effects, including a failure to synthesize purine nucleotides and thymidine.

Chemical modification of the sulphanilamide molecule has resulted in the production of hundreds of different sulphonamides which differ chiefly in their pharmacological properties. Few are now in regular clinical use.

Sulphonamides are broad spectrum (Table 3.1), predominantly bacteristatic, and relatively slow to act: several generations of bacterial growth are needed to deplete the folate pool before inhibition of growth occurs. Resistance emerges readily, and bacteria resistant to one sulphonamide are cross-resistant to the others. Sensitivity tests present problems in the laboratory since results depend critically on the composition of the culture medium and the inoculum size (see Chapter 7).

The emergence of resistant strains and the appearance of more potent antimicrobial agents has relegated the sulphonamide group to a minor therapeutic role, chiefly as agents for use in uncomplicated urinary infection. Sulphonamides (usually sulphadiazine) also remain useful for the protection of close contacts of cases of meningococcal meningitis, providing the strain of *Neisseria meningitidis* involved is sulphonamide sensitive.

Some sulphonamides are applied topically. Silver sulphadiazine is used in burns, but the activity probably owes as much to the silver as to the sulphonamide. Sulphacetamide, a component of some eye drops and vaginal creams, has little value.

In curious extension of the good fortune that attended the discovery of the sulphonamides, sulphasalazine, an agent used in ulcerative colitis and rheumatoid arthritis, probably owes its efficacy to a breakdown product, 5-aminosalicylic acid.

Table 3.1. Summary of the antibacterial spectrum of inhibitors of nucleic acid synthesis

Antibacterial compound	Staphylococci	Streptococci	Enterococcus faecalis	Escherichia coli	Proteus spp.	Other coliforms	Pseudomonas aeruginosa	Anaerobes
Fluoroquinolones	Good	Fair	Fair	Very good	Very good	Very good	Good	Poor
Nalidixic acid*	Poor	Poor	Poor	Good	Good	Good	Poor	Poor
Nitrofurantoin	Fair	Fair	Poor	Good	Poor	Good	Poor	Fair
5-Nitroimidazoles	——————————————— No useful activity ———————————————							Very good
Novobiocin	Good	Good	Fair	——————— No useful activity ———————				
Rifampicin	Very good	Very good	Good	Fair	Fair	Poor	Poor	Fair
Sulphonamides	(Good)	(Good)	Poor	(Good)	(Good)	(Good)	Poor	Poor
Trimethoprim	Good	Good	Good	Good	Good	(Good)	Poor	Fair

Brackets indicate that resistant strains are common.

* And congeners of nalidixic acid (see text).

Most sulphonamides are well absorbed when given orally and are chiefly excreted in the urine, partly in an antibacterially inactive acetylated form. The compounds diffuse relatively well into cerebrospinal fluid (CSF) and were successfully used for treating meningitis before resistance became common. Sulphonamides that are poorly absorbed when given orally (including sulphaloxate and derivatives of sulphathiazole) have been used for intestinal infections, but are not recommended.

Less soluble sulphonamides (e.g. sulphathiazole and sulphadiazine) are prone to cause renal damage due to the deposition of crystals in the urinary collecting system. Sulphafurazole (known as sulfisoxazole in the USA), sulphadimidine (sulfamethazine), sulphasomidine (sulfisomidine), and sulphamethizole lack this side-effect and are preferred in the treatment of urinary infection.

Some other sulphonamides in clinical use are distinguished by long plasma half-lives $(T_{1/2})$ and are known as *long-acting sulphonamides*. The most important are sulphamethoxypyridazine $(T_{1/2} = 35h)$, sulphadimethoxine $(T_{1/2} = 40h)$, sulfametopyrazine $(T_{1/2} = 60h)$, and sulfadoxine $(T_{1/2} = 120h)$. The latter two are excreted so slowly that they need be given only weekly.

Diaminopyrimidines

Diaminopyrimidines inhibit dihydrofolate reductase, the enzyme which generates tetrahydrofolate (the active form of the vitamin) from metabolically inactive dihydrofolate. Trimethoprim (Fig. 3.2), the most important antibacterial agent of this type, exhibits far greater affinity for the dihydrofolate of bacteria than for the corresponding mammalian enzyme; this is the basis of the selective toxicity of the compound.

Since sulphonamides and trimethoprim act at different points in the same metabolic pathway they interact synergically: bacteria are inhibited by much lower concentrations of the combination than by either agent alone. For this reason trimethoprim and sulphonamides

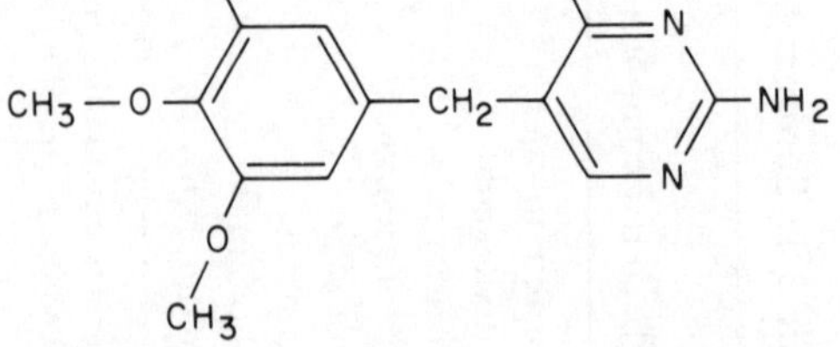

Fig. 3.2. Structure of trimethoprim.

are often combined in therapeutic formulations, although trimethoprim alone is probably as effective and less toxic. The most commonly used combination is trimethoprim and sulphamethoxazole (co-trimoxazole), but combinations of trimethoprim with sulphadiazine (co-trimazine) and sulphamoxole (co-trifamole) are also available in some countries.

Trimethoprim is active in low concentration against most common pathogenic bacteria, although *Pseudomonas aeruginosa* is a notable exception (Table 3.1). Resistance is on the increase; up to 30 per cent of urinary isolates have been reported to be resistant in some series, but this is not a universal experience. The drug is rapidly absorbed from the gut and excreted almost exclusively by the kidneys with a plasma half-life of about 10 h. Toxic side-effects are uncommon, but residual effects on folate metabolism may cause haematological changes in folate-depleted patients.

The chief use for trimethoprim is in urinary tract infection. The combination with sulphamethoxazole has also been extensively used in many other clinical situations, including respiratory tract infections, typhoid fever, and brucellosis.

Other diaminopyrimidines include: tetroxoprim, which is less active than trimethoprim, but is marketed in combination with sulphadiazine as co-tetroxazine in some countries; brodimoprim and metioprim, which are very similar to trimethoprim; the antimalarial agents pyrimethamine and proguanil (Chapter 5); the antipneumocystis agent, trimetrexate; and the antineoplastic agent, methotrexate.

Quinolones

Nalidixic acid and its early congeners
Nalidixic acid (Fig. 3.3a) was the first representative to appear of a family of compounds which share close similarities of structure. Early members of the group, developed in the 1960s and 1970s and available in various countries throughout the world, include nalidixic acid, cinoxacin, oxolinic acid, pipemidic acid, piromidic acid, flumequine,

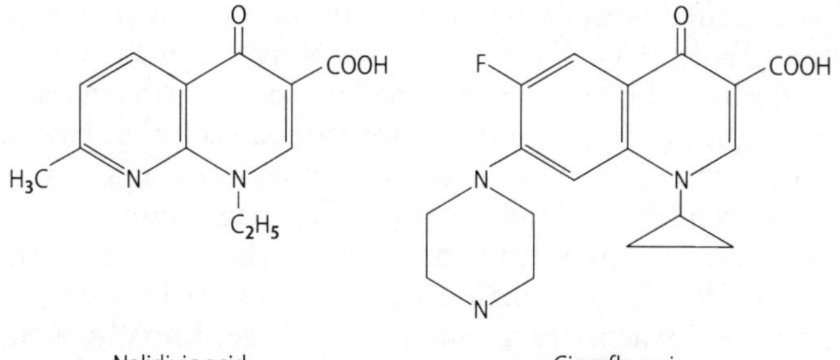

Nalidixic acid   Ciprofloxacin

Fig. 3.3. Structures of nalidixic acid and ciprofloxacin.

and acrosoxacin. These agents are generically known as quinolones, although they embrace a variety of structural variants, depending on the arrangement of nitrogen atoms within the heterocyclic structure.

The site of action of these compounds has been pinpointed with unusual precision to a subunit of that remarkable enzyme, DNA gyrase, which unwinds the supercoiled DNA helix prior to replication and transcription.

Nalidixic acid and its congeners are all well absorbed when taken by mouth and are more or less extensively metabolized in the body before being excreted into the urine. Nalidixic acid itself is largely converted to hydroxynalidixic acid (which retains antibacterial activity) and glucuronide conjugates (which do not).

Most Gram-negative bacteria, with the exception of *Ps. aeruginosa*, are susceptible to nalidixic acid and its early congeners, but Gram-positive organisms are usually resistant (Table 3.1). Susceptible bacteria can readily be converted to resistance in the laboratory and the emergence of resistance sometimes causes treatment failure. However, 'wild' strains resistant to nalidixic acid are uncommon, perhaps because resistance, when it occurs, is not spread by plasmids (see Chapter 13). These drugs are normally used only in urinary infection. Acrosoxacin exhibits good activity against *Neisseria* and is sometimes used for the treatment of gonorrhoea.

Fluoroquinolones

Among the earlier quinolones are two that display modestly improved antibacterial activity: flumequine (which bears a fluorine atom at the C-6 position) and pipemidic acid (with a piperazine substituent at C-7). During the 1980s a new series of quinolones appeared in which the 6-fluoro, 7-piperazinyl features were combined; in some subsequent derivatives, piperazine has been replaced by aminopyrrolidine or other substituents, and this group of compounds are now generally referred to as fluoroquinolones.

These agents have generated much interest because they exhibit greatly enhanced activity against enterobacteria and expand the spectrum of the earlier quinolones to include Gram-positive cocci and *Ps. aeruginosa* (Table 3.1). They are also active against some problem organisms such as chlamydiae, legionellae, and mycobacteria, but hopes that they might display useful antiprotozoal activity have not been realized. Antibacterial activity is somewhat reduced in acidic conditions and in the presence of divalent cations like magnesium.

Fluoroquinolones presently on the market in the UK include ciprofloxacin (Fig. 3.3b), norfloxacin, and ofloxacin; enoxacin, lomefloxacin, and pefloxacin are available elsewhere. Enrofloxacin, a ciprofloxacin-like compound, is used in veterinary practice. Other derivatives are waiting in the wings; some of these display further improved activity, especially against Gram-positive cocci (clinafloxacin, tosufloxacin), extended plasma half-lives (fleroxacin, rufloxacin), or both (sparfloxacin). Numerous other compounds are under development.

Fluoroquinolones are usually administered by the oral route, although some, including ciprofloxacin and ofloxacin, can also be given intravenously. Therapeutic dosages achieve relatively low concentrations in plasma, but the compounds are well distributed in tissues and are concentrated within mammalian cells. The major route of excretion is renal, in the form of native compound and various metabolites, some of which retain antibacterial activity. In general, they are less extensively metabolized than is nalidixic acid.

The broad spectrum of activity of ciprofloxacin and its congeners, and their ease of administration by the oral route, make them attractive candidates for 'blind' therapy in hospital and domiciliary practice. However, while these compounds have undoubted value in many infective conditions, they are not universal panaceas and should not be used indiscriminately. They cannot be recommended unreservedly for respiratory tract infection since the antipneumococcal activity is unreliable.

Ciprofloxacin is the most active of the fluoroquinolones in current use, although the pharmacological properties of ofloxacin and pefloxacin may compensate for their somewhat inferior antibacterial potency. Norfloxacin, enoxacin, and lomefloxacin are not reliably effective in systemic infection; these drugs are almost exclusively used in urinary tract infection but they may also be of value in other situations, notably gonorrhoea and certain enteric infections.

Resistance is presently not a major problem, although alterations in the permeability characteristics of bacteria, or to the DNA gyrase target, may reduce the susceptibility sufficiently to render the drugs therapeutically ineffective. This is a particular worry with organisms like staphylococci, streptococci, and *Ps. aeruginosa*, for which the margin of safety between therapeutically achievable concentrations and inhibitory activity is not large. Indeed, failures of therapy due to small increments in resistance in these organisms are well documented.

Fluoroquinolones are generally well tolerated, but rashes and gastrointestinal disturbances may occur; photophobia and various non-specific neurological complaints are also sometimes encountered. These compounds also affect the deposition of cartilage in experimental animals, and licensing authorities have cautioned against their use in children and pregnant women.

Novobiocin

Novobiocin is a coumarin-like antibiotic first described in 1955. The heterocyclic structure is unrelated to those of other antibiotics and cross-resistance is not a problem. The target site of the drug is the same DNA gyrase enzyme that is inhibited by nalidixic acid and other quinolones, but novobiocin binds to a different subunit. Curiously, this leads to a spectrum of activity that is the mirror image of that of nalidixic acid: good activity against Gram-positive organisms, but no useful activity against enteric Gram-negative rods (Table 3.1).

Since side-effects are common in patients treated with novobiocin, and bacterial resistance develops readily, the drug is seldom used. It is no longer available in the UK.

Nitroimidazoles

As a group, the imidazoles are synthetic antimicrobials which are remarkable in that derivatives are known which between them cover bacteria, fungi, viruses, protozoa, and helminths—in fact, the whole antimicrobial spectrum. Outside the antimicrobial field certain imidazoles have been shown to exhibit radio-sensitizing properties and have attracted attention as adjuncts to radiation therapy for some tumours.

The members of this family of compounds used as antibacterial agents are 5-nitroimidazoles, of which metronidazole (Fig. 3.4) is best known. Related 5-nitroimidazoles include tinidazole, ornidazole, secnidazole, and nimorazole; they share the properties of metronidazole but have somewhat extended plasma half-lives.

Metronidazole was originally used for the treatment of protozoal infections, first for trichomoniasis, then later for amoebiasis and giardiasis. The antibacterial activity of the compound was only recognized when a patient suffering from acute ulcerative gingivitis responded spontaneously while receiving metronidazole for a *Trichomonas vaginalis* infection. Anaerobic bacteria are commonly incriminated in gingivitis, and it was subsequently shown that metronidazole possesses potent antibacterial activity that was at first thought to be confined to strict anaerobes (the protozoa against which the drug is effective are also anaerobes) since even oxygen-tolerant species like *Actinomyces* and *Propionibacterium* are resistant. However, it is now known that some micro-aerophilic bacteria, including *Gardnerella vaginalis* and *Helicobacter pylori*, are

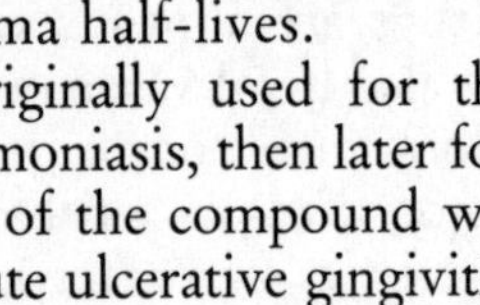

Fig. 3.4. Structure of metronidazole.

commonly susceptible to nitroimidazoles, and metronidazole features in drug regimens for the treatment of infections with these organisms.

Metronidazole is so effective against anaerobic bacteria and resistance is so uncommon that it is now widely considered the drug of choice for the treatment of anaerobic infections. It is also commonly used as a prophylactic drug in some surgical procedures in which post-operative anaerobic infection is a frequent complication and as an alternative to vancomycin in the treatment of antibiotic-associated colitis.

The basis of the selective activity against anaerobes resides in the fact that the antibacterially active form of the drug is a reduced derivative produced intracellularly at the low redox values attainable by anaerobes, but not by aerobes. The reduced form of metronidazole is thought to act by inducing strand breakage in DNA by a mechanism that has not been precisely determined.

Nitrofurans

A number of nitrofuran derivatives have attracted attention over the years, but only one, nitrofurantoin (Fig. 3.5), has found widespread use, and this is restricted to the treatment of urinary infection. The reason for this is that after oral absorption it is rapidly excreted into urine and the small amount that finds its way into tissues is inactivated there. Nausea is fairly common after administration of nitrofurantoin, but gastrointestinal intolerance is improved with the macrocrystalline formulation.

Nitrofurantoin is active against most urinary tract pathogens, but *Proteus* spp. and *Ps. aeruginosa* are usually resistant (Table 3.1). The occurrence of resistant strains among susceptible species is uncommon. The activity of nitrofurantoin is affected by pH—acid conditions favouring the activity.

The mode of action of nitrofurantoin has not been precisely elucidated. It appears likely that, as with metronidazole, a reduced form of the drug is produced intracellularly and this interacts with DNA in some way.

Nitrofurans related to nitrofurantoin that are available outside the UK include nitrofurazone (marketed for topical use and bladder irrigation), nifuratel (used in some countries for *T. vaginalis* infection),

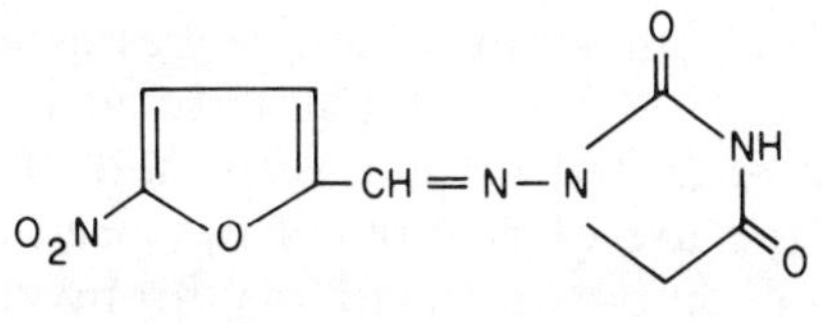

Fig. 3.5. Structure of nitrofurantoin.

furazolidone, an orally non-absorbed compound sometimes used for intestinal infections), and nifurtimox (used in Chagas' disease; see Chapter 5).

Rifamycins

The clinically useful rifamycins, of which rifampicin (known in the USA as rifampin) is the most important, are semi-synthetic derivatives of rifamycin B, one of a group of structurally complex antibiotics produced by *Streptomyces mediterranei*. These compounds interfere with mRNA formation by binding to the β-subunit of DNA-dependent RNA polymerase. Mutations in the subunit readily occur and render the bacteria resistant.

Rifampicin

Rifampicin has established a special place for itself in antimicrobial therapy as one of the most effective weapons against the major mycobacterial scourges of mankind: tuberculosis and leprosy. It also exhibits potent bactericidal activity against a range of other bacteria (Table 3.1), notably staphylococci and legionellae; the compound even displays some antiviral activity, but this is not of any clinical value.

Rifampicin is well absorbed by the oral route, although it may also be given by intravenous infusion. Serious side-effects are relatively uncommon, but can be more troublesome when the drug is used intermittently, as it may be in antituberculosis regimens. Hepatotoxicity is well recognized and the antibiotic induces hepatic enzymes, leading to self-potentiation of excretion and antagonism of some other drugs handled by the liver, including oral contraceptives. A potentially alarming side-effect arising from the fact that rifampicin is strongly pigmented is the production of red urine and other bodily secretions; contact lenses may become discoloured. Patients should be warned of these potential problems.

The chief drawback to the use of rifampicin is the frequency with which resistant mutants develop. For this reason, the drug is normally used in combination with other agents.

Rifampicin has established itself as such a useful antimycobacterial drug that there has been a move to confine its use to tuberculosis and leprosy on the grounds that more widespread use might inadvertently encourage the emergence of resistant strains of mycobacteria. Critics of this view claim that an agent which possesses exceptionally good antistaphylococcal activity and useful activity against other bacteria is being unnecessarily restricted on unproven and unlikely grounds. In fact, restriction of the use of rifampicin has been steadily eroded; it is now often used in combination with erythromycin in Legionnaires' disease and is also used to eliminate meningococci from the throats of carriers as well as the protection of close contacts of meningococcal and *Haemophilus influenzae* type b disease.

Other rifamycins

Two other rifamycin derivatives are of some interest: rifapentine exhibits an extended plasma half-life, but is otherwise similar to rifampicin; rifabutin (ansamycin) also has a prolonged half-life and retains activity against some rifampicin-resistant bacteria. Much interest has focused on the possibility that these agents may be useful in infections caused by organisms of the *Mycobacterium avium* complex, which often cause disseminated disease in patients with cancer or acquired immune deficiency syndrome (AIDS). Although these mycobacteria are commonly resistant to standard antituberculosis drugs, rifabutin and rifapentine display good activity *in vitro*. Clinical success has been modest, but rifabutin has proved of sufficient value to warrant its inclusion in some multidrug regimens. Rifabutin also inhibits replication of human immunodeficiency virus (HIV) *in vitro*, but it seems unlikely that this translates into clinical benefit.

AGENTS AFFECTING MEMBRANE FUNCTION

Polymyxins

The polymyxins are a family of five compounds (polymyxins A, B, C, D, and E) produced by *Bacillus polymyxa* and related bacteria. Only polymyxins B and E are used therapeutically. Polymyxin E is usually known by its alternative name, colistin.

Structurally, the polymyxins are polypeptides with a long hydrophobic tail. Most of the peptide portion is arranged in a cyclic fashion, reminiscent of bacitracin and the cyclic peptides. The polymyxins act like cationic detergents by binding to the cell membrane and causing the leakage of essential cytoplasmic contents. The effect is not entirely selective, and both polymyxin B and colistin exhibit considerable toxicity.

Derivatives of the polymyxins in which up to five diaminobutyric acid residues are substituted with sulphomethyl groups are better tolerated and more quickly excreted than are the parent compounds. These sulphomethylpolymyxins exhibit diminished antibacterial activity, but the precise loss in activity is difficult to estimate because the substituted compounds spontaneously break down to the more active parent.

The antibacterial spectrum of the polymyxins encompasses most Gram-negative bacteria except *Proteus* spp., but the importance of these antibiotics has hinged on their activity against *Ps. aeruginosa*. With the appearance of antipseudomonal β-lactam agents, aminoglycosides, and fluoroquinolones, the polymyxins have virtually fallen into disuse for systemic therapy, although they are still used in some topical preparations. They are also included in selective decontamination regimens aimed at preventing endogenous infection in profoundly neutropenic patients (Chapter 19).

Other membrane-active agents

Antibiotics of the tyrothricin complex (gramicidin and tyrocidine), which are used in some topical preparations, are cyclic decapeptides which bind to the cell membrane to form channels that allow leakage of potassium ions. Monensin, a polyether used in animal husbandry as a growth promoter and coccidiostat, acts in a similar manner. These agents possess good activity against Gram-positive organisms, but they also bind to mammalian cell membranes and are far too toxic to be used systemically.

Toxicity also precludes the systemic use of the many disinfectants, including phenols, quaternary ammonium compounds, biguanides, and others, that achieve their antibacterial effect wholly or in part by interfering with the integrity of the cell membrane.

ANTIMYCOBACTERIAL AGENTS

Compared with the number of agents at the disposal of the prescriber for the therapy of most bacterial infections, the resources available to treat mycobacterial disease are precariously meagre. Part of the reason for this may be that mycobacteria are unusual organisms with a relatively impermeable waxy coat, but the fact that they are very slow growing and are able to survive and multiply within macrophages and necrotic tissue also makes them difficult targets.

In general, the development of drugs for the treatment of tuberculosis and leprosy has tended to evolve along specialized lines, but some important antimycobacterial agents, such as rifampicin and certain aminoglycosides, have wider uses (see above and Chapter 2). Agents specifically used for the treatment of tuberculosis include isoniazid (isonicotinic acid hydrazide; INH), pyrazinamide, ethambutol, and thiacetazone (thioacetazone); *p*-aminosalicylic acid (PAS), which was formerly much used in antituberculosis regimens, is no longer recommended, but this and other compounds with activity against *Mycobacterium tuberculosis*, such as capreomycin, cycloserine, and viomycin, may be considered if first-line treatment fails. In leprosy, the most important agents (apart from rifampicin) are dapsone (or its prodrug, acedapsone) and clofazimine. The thioamides, ethionamide, and prothionamide (protionamide) are sometimes used, but are hepatotoxic.

The fluoroquinolones and macrolides display quite good activity against mycobacteria, including *M. leprae* and organisms of the *M. avium* complex, and there are hopes that these agents might widen the options for treating mycobacterial disease at a time when resistance is emerging as a serious problem.

Because of the difficulties in studying mycobacteria in the laboratory, less is known about the mode of action of antimycobacterial drugs than about other antibacterial agents. Isoniazid is a nicotinic acid derivative that arose from early studies with thiosemicarbazones (of which thiacetazone is an example). It has been suggested that isoniazid is incorporated into nicotinamide coenzymes, but this would not explain its selective action against mycobacteria, and other evidence suggests that the drug inhibits the formation of the mycolic acids that are peculiar to the cell walls of acid-fast bacilli. Other derivatives of nicotinic acid, including pyrazinamide, ethionamide, and prothionamide, presumably act in the same way, and such evidence as is available suggests that the diamine, ethambutol, also interferes with mycolic acid synthesis. Dapsone (diaminodiphenyl sulphone) and *p*-aminosalicylic acid, like the sulphonamides to which they are related, are analogues of *p*-aminobenzoic acid. Their idiosyncratic spectrum of activity may be due to differential uptake, or to subtle differences in the way folic acid is synthesized in *M. tuberculosis* and *M. leprae*.

Further information on antimycobacterial agents is given in the context of their use in Chapter 26.

4

Antifungal agents

D. Greenwood

Fungi may cause benign, but unsightly infection of the skin, nail, or hair (dermatophytosis), relatively trivial infection of mucous membranes (thrush), or systemic infection causing progressive, often fatal disease.

It is common practice to classify medically important fungi into four morphological groups:

(1) true yeasts (e.g. *Cryptococcus neoformans*);

(2) yeast-like fungi that produce a pseudomycelium (e.g. *Candida albicans*);

(3) filamentous fungi that produce a true mycelium (e.g. *Aspergillus fumigatus*);

(4) dimorphic fungi that grow as yeasts or filamentous fungi, depending on the cultural conditions (e.g. *Histoplasma capsulatum*).

There is now some evidence that *Pneumocystis carinii*, an organism of uncertain affiliation that is an important opportunist pathogen of patients with AIDS, may be a fungus; if so, it is unclear to which group it belongs. This organism has morphological features resembling some protozoa and it is insusceptible to antifungal agents. Consideration of antimicrobial compounds active against *P. carinii* will be deferred to the next chapter.

Fungi are eukaryotic organisms and antibacterial agents have no effect on them. Specialized antifungal agents must therefore be used, and some are quite toxic. In order to minimize problems of toxicity, superficial lesions are usually treated by topical application, but deep mycoses, which are serious life-threatening infections, need vigorous systemic therapy. Unfortunately, therapeutic resources are slender: the polyene, amphotericin B, is the mainstay of systemic treatment; otherwise choice is limited to flucytosine, a handful of azole derivatives, and, possibly, the new allylamine, terbinafine.

The differential activity of the chief antifungal agents in common use is summarized in Table 4.1. Precise assessment of the activity of antifungal agents *in vitro* is beset with methodological difficulties and susceptibility tests are not generally available.

Table 4.1. Summary of the differential activity of antifungal agents against the more common pathogenic fungi

Fungus	Principal diseases caused	Polyenes	Flucytosine	Griseofulvin	Azoles	Allylamines
Yeast						
Cryptococcus neoformans	Meningitis	+	+	−	+	−
Yeast-like fungus						
Candida albicans	Thrush; Systemic candidiasis	+	+	−	+	±
Filamentous fungi						
Trichophyton spp.	Infection of skin,	−	−	+	+	+
Microsporum spp.	nail or hair	−	−	+	+	+
Epidermophyton floccosum	('ringworm')	−	−	+	+	+
Aspergillus fumigatus	Pulmonary aspergillosis	+	−	−	(+)*	+†
Dimorphic fungi						
Histoplasma capsulatum	Histoplasmosis	+	−	−	+	+†
Coccidioides immitis	Coccidioidomycosis	+	−	−	+	+†
Blastomyces dermatitidis	Blastomycosis	+	−	−	+	+†

+ = Useful activity; − = no useful activity.

* = limited activity, itraconazole may be useful.

† = clinical efficacy not yet established.

POLYENES

The polyenes are naturally occurring compounds exhibiting a macrocyclic lactone structure with an extensive conjugated system of double bonds. The most commonly used members of the group are nystatin and amphotericin B (Fig. 4.1). Related polyenes include candicidin, natamycin (also known as pimaricin), trichomycin (also known as hachimycin), and pentamycin, none of which is marketed in the UK. All of these compounds act by binding to sterols in the fungal cell membrane, thereby interfering with membrane integrity and causing leakage of essential metabolites.

The activity of the polyenes embraces a variety of pathogenic fungi, and yeasts are particularly susceptible. Nystatin has been extensively used for treating candida infections of the mucous membranes. Natamycin, trichomycin, and pentamycin display some activity against the protozoon *Trichomonas vaginalis*, and have been used for treating vaginitis in which either *Candida* or *T. vaginalis* may be involved.

Most polyenes are restricted to topical use, but amphotericin B remains the most important weapon in the antifungal armamentarium for the treatment of systemic fungal infections, including disseminated candidiasis, cryptococcosis, aspergillosis, and deep mycoses caused by dimorphic fungi.

Toxicity is a major problem in systemic therapy with amphotericin B and it needs to be used with care. The drug is highly insoluble and for parenteral use it is normally formulated in a surfactant vehicle from which it readily precipitates; for this reason, other drugs should not be added to intravenous infusions of amphotericin B.

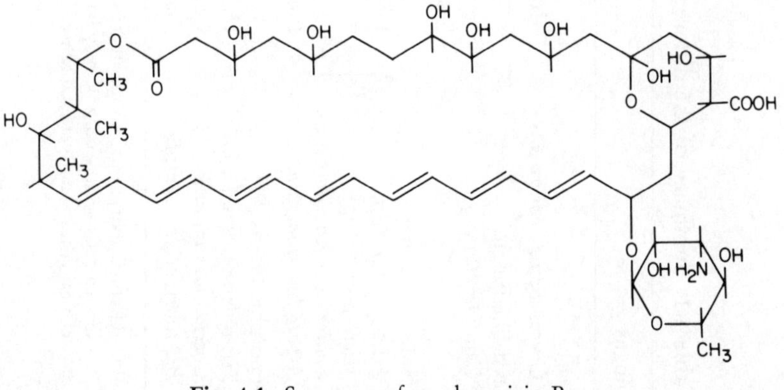

Fig. 4.1. Structure of amphotericin B.

Various ways have been tried to minimize toxicity problems. Amphotericin B methyl ester was developed as a water-soluble form with reduced nephrotoxicity, but, disappointingly, it proved to be neurotoxic. Lipid-complexed colloidal formulations appear to exhibit improved safety. The most successful manoeuvre so far has been the use of phospholipid vesicles (liposomes) as carriers of the drug; packaged in this way, the drug is delivered to the site of infection. Such evidence as is presently available suggests that this is an effective mode of drug delivery which may allow the use of higher doses without compromising safety. An alternative approach, at least in systemic candidiasis, is to administer amphotericin B in reduced dosage in combination with flucytosine (see below).

AZOLES

Many imidazole and triazole derivatives display antifungal activity and, in fact, these compounds offer the nearest approximation we have to broad-spectrum antifungal agents. They act selectively against fungi (and some protozoa) by interfering with the demethylation of lanosterol during the synthesis of ergosterol, which is the principal sterol in the fungal cell membrane. The structure of clotrimazole, the first imidazole to be introduced into clinical medicine, is shown in Fig. 4.2.

Antifungal imidazoles are most widely used for topical application in superficial fungal infections and as pessaries for use in vaginal candidiasis. Indeed, these are virtually the only useful roles for clotrimazole, miconazole, econazole, isoconazole, and sulconazole (and several others available outside the UK), all of which have very similar properties and indications. Miconazole is also available as an intravenous preparation for use in deep-seated *Candida* infections, but toxicity has restricted its value.

One antifungal imidazole, tioconazole, is available in a formulation

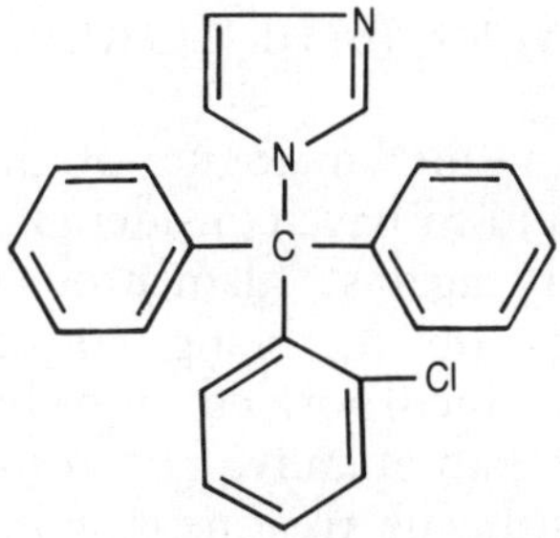

Fig. 4.2. Structure of clotrimazole.

which is painted on infected nails. It is unlikely to be effective alone in severe nail infections, but may be useful as an adjunct to oral therapy with griseofulvin (see below).

A significant advance in the oral therapy of systemic fungal infections was achieved with the introduction of ketoconazole. This imidazole derivative is well absorbed when given orally and achieves therapeutic concentrations for several hours. However, early enthusiasm for ketoconazole waned when it was realized that the drug was occasionally implicated in fatal hepatotoxic reactions. Nevertheless, ketoconazole remains a useful drug in the treatment of some systemic mycoses, when the benefits outweigh the risks. It should not be used for trivial dermatophyte infections.

The decline in popularity of ketoconazole is likely to be further accelerated by the appearance of fluconazole and itraconazole, both of which are associated with fewer side-effects. These compounds are triazoles rather than imidazoles. Both are well absorbed after oral administration and have long plasma half-lives (20–30 h), properties that make them suitable for once-daily administration. However, fluconazole appears to have several advantages over itraconazole: it achieves higher plasma concentrations, it is less extensively metabolized and protein bound, and it penetrates into cerebrospinal fluid in therapeutically useful concentrations. Itraconazole is also more liable to give rise to hepatic injury. On the credit side, itraconazole exhibits better activity against *Aspergillus* spp.

Fluconazole and itraconazole can be used to treat superficial infections with *Candida* if oral therapy is thought to be necessary or more acceptable than, for example, vaginal pessaries. More importantly, they appear effective in many forms of systemic mycosis, including in the case of fluconazole, cryptococcosis and, in the case of itraconazole, aspergillosis. One area in which the azoles are becoming more widely used is in chemoprophylactic regimens for profoundly neutropenic patients. Resistance is presently uncommon, but extensive use of these compounds could compromise their value in the long term.

FLUCYTOSINE (5-FLUOROCYTOSINE)

Flucytosine is a pyrimidine analogue originally developed as an anticancer drug, but found to have considerable activity against yeasts; it has no useful activity against filamentous fungi. The activity of the compound depends on its being converted intracellularly to 5-fluorouracil, which is incorporated into fungal RNA. The drug can be given orally or parenterally, but resistance develops readily and sometimes emerges during treatment. For this reason flucytosine is administered together with amphotericin B, an arrangement that has the additional advantage of allowing a lower dose of amphotericin B to be used. It has also been suggested that amphotericin B, by interfering with the permeability of the fungal membrane, may facilitate entry of flucytosine into the fungal cell.

Flucytosine is usually well tolerated, but marrow toxicity may occur, particularly if the drug is allowed to accumulate in patients with impaired renal function. Adjustment of dosage according to the results of drug assays is therefore indicated.

GRISEOFULVIN

Griseofulvin was the first antifungal antibiotic to be described. Use of the drug is confined to the treatment of dermatophyte infections of the skin, nail, or hair, and griseofulvin is peculiarly suited to this purpose since it is deposited in newly formed keratin. Treatment is prolonged to allow time for the infected nail to grow out, but even so only about one-third of toenail infections respond completely. The compound is well absorbed when administered orally, particularly if a fine-particle formulation is used, and serious side-effects are uncommon.

The mode of action of griseofulvin has not been definitively established, but its activity appears to be directed against the process of mitosis, perhaps by interfering with the microtubules of the mitotic spindle.

ALLYLAMINES

With so few agents available for the systemic treatment of fungal disease, the appearance of an active compound with a novel structure is particularly welcome. Such a compound is terbinafine (Fig. 4.3), an allylamine derivative that exhibits broad-spectrum antifungal activity. An earlier allylamine, naftifine, is insufficiently active to be useful systemically, but is marketed in some countries for topical use. These compounds, like the antifungal azoles, interfere with ergosterol synthesis, but act

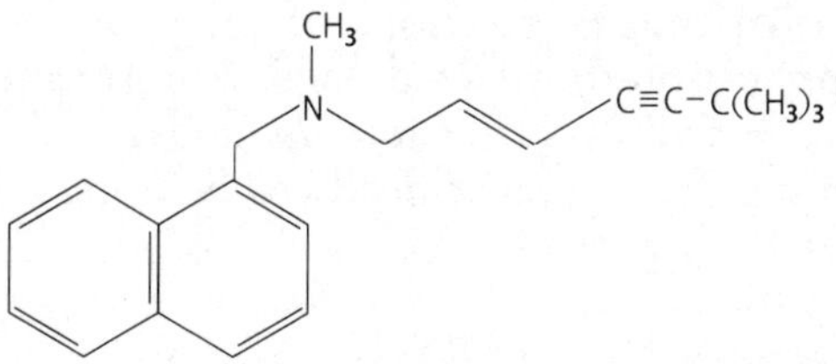

Fig. 4.3. Structure of terbinafine.

at an earlier stage by inhibiting the formation of squalene epoxide, a precursor of lanosterol.

Terbinafine is almost completely absorbed when given orally. Despite being almost entirely protein bound and extensively metabolized in the body, it accumulates in keratin, where it persists after treatment is stopped. This is particularly important in dermatophyte infections of the toenails, which are notoriously refractory even to prolonged therapy with griseofulvin or azole derivatives, whereas early experience with terbinafine suggests that relatively short courses of treatment may be curative.

The broad spectrum of activity of terbinafine includes *Apergillus* spp. and dimorphic fungi as well as dermatophytes, but at the time of writing it is too soon to assess whether the drug will offer a useful alternative to older antifungal agents in these conditions. *Candida albicans* seems to be more susceptible in the mycelial phase than in the yeast form and, whereas the drug is generally fungicidal, the action against *Candida* is fungistatic.

Terbinafine is likely to become the drug of choice for dermatophyte infections that require systemic therapy, but any wider role remains to be defined.

TOPICAL ANTIFUNGAL AGENTS

Apart from the wide selection of azole and polyene derivatives that are available for topical use, a range of other agents is available in some countries for the treatment of ringworm and pityriasis versicolor, a mild but chronic infection of skin. These include tolnaftate, haloprogin, and ciclopirox olamine. None of these agents exhibits useful activity against *Candida*. A variety of ointments containing benzoic acid (e.g. Whitfield's ointment: benzoic acid and salicylic acid in an emulsifying base) have been used traditionally for treating dermatophyte infections of the skin. Though old-fashioned and a little messy, they are cheap and effective, and still have a place in treatment. Undecanoic acids are also widely used in proprietary preparations for conditions such as 'athlete's foot'.

One additional novel compound, amorolfine, is marketed for the topical treatment of fungal infections of the skin and, in the form of a lacquer, for application to infected nails. Amorolfine is a morpholine derivative that is active against *Candida* and the dermatophytes. Its action is said to persist so that it needs to be applied to infected nails only once or twice a week.

5

Antiprotozoal and anthelminthic agents

D. Greenwood

Pathogenic protozoa and helminths are among the most important causes of morbidity and mortality in the world. An estimated 700 million people suffer from malaria, filariasis, and schistosomiasis alone, and two-thirds of the world's population lives in conditions in which parasitic diseases are unavoidable.

Some parasitic diseases were among the first to be treated by specific remedies; indeed, cures for malaria, amoebic dysentery, and tapeworm infection have been known for centuries. Nevertheless, the therapeutic armamentarium for parasitic infection remains severely restricted. Many of the antiparasitic drugs that are available leave much to be desired in terms of efficacy and safety, and a few parasitic infections remain for which there is no effective remedy at all.

PROTOZOA

Protozoa are all unicellular organisms. Those of medical importance are conveniently classified into four groups: amoebae, flagellates, sporozoa, and 'others' (Table 5.1).

Amoebae

Parasitic amoebae
Several species of parasitic amoebae may be found in humans. Only one, *Entamoeba histolytica*, the causative parasite of amoebic dysentery and amoebic liver abscess, is commonly incriminated in disease. Invasive disease is caused by the motile trophozoite form, but the disease is transmitted by non-motile cysts which represent a more resistant resting phase.

An effective treatment for amoebiasis has been available for many years in the form of emetine, an alkaloid of ipecacuanha. Emetine, whether as the hydrochloride, as the dehydroemetine derivative, or as the bismuth iodide complex, all of which are used therapeutically, acts by inhibiting protein synthesis in amoebae.

Emetine has largely been replaced by metronidazole (or one of

Table 5.1. Principal pathogenic protozoa infecting humans, and the drugs used in treatment

Species	Diseases caused	Useful drugs
Amoebae		
Entamoeba histolytica	Amoebic dysentery	Metronidazole,
	Invasive amoebiasis	etc.
Naegleria fowleri	Meningoencephalitis	Amphotericin B
Acanthamoeba spp.	Amoebic keratitis	Propamidine (topical)
Flagellates		
Trypanosoma brucei rhodesiense	Sleeping sickness	Melarsoprol; suramin;
Trypanosoma brucei gambiense		pentamidine; eflornithine*
Trypanosoma cruzi	Chagas' disease	Nifurtimox
Leishmania tropica	Oriental sore	
Leishmania major	Oriental sore	
Leishmania donovani	Kala-azar	Sodium stibogluconate;
Leishmania braziliensis	Espundia	liposomal amphotericin B
Leishmania mexicana	Chiclero's ulcer	
Trichomonas vaginalis	Vaginitis	Metronidazole
Giardia lamblia	Diarrhoea	Metronidazole
	Steatorrhoea	
Sporozoa		
Plasmodium falciparum	Malignant tertian malaria	
Plasmodium vivax	Benign tertian malaria	Chloroquine, etc.
Plasmodium ovale	Benign tertian malaria	(see Chapter 31)
Plasmodium malariae	Quartan malaria	
Toxoplasma gondii	Congenital malformation	Pyrimethamine +
	Ocular toxoplasmosis	sulphonamide;
	Encephalitis (AIDS)	spiramycin
Cryptosporidium parvum	Diarrhoea	None
Others		
Balantidium coli	Diarrhoea	Tetracycline
Babesia spp.	Babesiosis	Quinine + clindamycin
Pneumocystis carinii†	Pneumonia	Co-trimoxazole; pentamidine; atovaquone

* Eflornithine is not active against *T. brucei rhodesiense*.
† Taxonomy uncertain; may be a fungus.

the other 5-nitroimidazoles), which has proved a very effective and non-toxic substitute in acute amoebiasis and amoebic liver abscess. Other drugs sometimes used in amoebiasis include chloroquine and diloxanide furoate, which have the virtue of being cheap. Diloxanide furoate is particularly useful for the elimination of cysts from symptomless excreters. Di-iodohydroxyquinoline (diodoquin; iodoquinol) is no longer recommended because of its toxicity.

Two antibiotics, tetracycline and the aminoglycoside paromomycin, also have some activity against amoebae. Problems in treating the various manifestations of *E. histolytica* infection are discussed in more detail in Chapter 31.

Free-living amoebae

Although *E. histolytica* is, to all intents and purposes, the only parasitic amoeba pathogenic to humans, certain species of free-living amoebae (especially *Naegleria* spp.) occasionally cause primary amoebic meningo-encephalitis. The condition is almost invariably fatal and only amphotericin B, an antifungal agent, has shown any useful activity in *in vitro* tests. Free-living amoebae of the *Acanthamoeba* group may occasionally be involved in serious eye infections (amoebic keratitis). Suitable antimicrobial chemotherapy for this condition remains to be defined, but local application of propamidine together with topical neomycin or polymyxin may be useful.

Flagellates

Trypanosomes

Trypanosomes have a complex life cycle involving developmental stages in an insect, and their distribution is restricted to those areas where the insect vector is found. In tropical Africa, tsetse flies transmit *Trypanosoma brucei*, of which two subspecies (*T. brucei gambiense* and *T. brucei rhodesiense*) cause 'sleeping sickness' in humans, an ultimately fatal infection. *T. brucei gambiense* infection responds to eflornithine, which may be effective even in the late stages of the disease—a property that has caused it to be dubbed the 'resurrection' drug in Africa. Unfortunately, *T. brucei rhodesiense* is resistant to eflornithine. Other drugs used include organic arsenicals such as melarsoprol (mel B). If treatment can be started before the trypanosomes invade the central nervous system, pentamidine or suramin may be curative.

South American trypanosomiasis, Chagas' disease, is a different disease caused by *T. cruzi* and transmitted by reduviid bugs, nicknamed 'kissing bugs' because of their predilection for feeding round the mouths of sleeping persons. There is presently no drug of proven efficacy in Chagas' disease, although some modest success has been obtained with the nitrofuran derivative, nifurtimox, and the imidazole, benznidazole. Unfortunately, production of nifurtimox has now been stopped, although at the time of writing stocks are still available in South America.

Leishmania

Leishmania, which are related to the trypanosomes, also cause a variety of clinical conditions and are also transmitted by biting insects, in this case sandflies. Cutaneous leishmaniasis (oriental sore) caused by *Leishmania tropica* or *L. major* is usually self limiting, but visceral leishmaniasis (kala-azar) in which the reticuloendothelial system is infected by *L. donovani*, is potentially fatal. Leishmaniasis occurs in the Middle East, India, parts of Africa, and countries on the south European coast of the Mediterranean. Various species of *Leishmania* have also been incriminated in disease in Central and South America, including *L. braziliensis* (mucocutaneous leishmaniasis, or espundia) and *L. mexicana* (Chiclero's ulcer, a form of cutaneous leishmaniasis).

The drugs traditionally used for the treatment of leishmaniasis are the pentavalent antimonials, of which sodium stibogluconate and meglumine antimonate are in universal use, and pentamidine. The purine analogue, allopurinol, halts protein synthesis in leishmania and appears to potentiate the activity of antimonials. Evidence is accumulating that the antifungal polyene, amphotericin B, may be effective, especially when administered in a liposomal formulation that carries the drug into macrophages. The antifungal azoles also exhibit some activity against leishmania and may offer an alternative in recalcitrant cases.

Other flagellates

Two other flagellates cause disease in humans: *Giardia lamblia* (also known as *G. intestinalis*)—a common cause of diarrhoea, abdominal pain, and steatorrhoea, and *Trichomonas vaginalis*—a common cause of vaginitis or, more rarely, urethritis. *G. lamblia* is transmitted in the cyst form, often in infected water; *T. vaginalis* is transmitted venereally. Both of these parasites are susceptible to nitroimidazoles such as metronidazole. Mepacrine (known in the United States as quinacrine) is also efficacious in giardiasis, and there is growing realization that the anthelminthic benzimidazoles, such as albendazole, have antigiardial activity.

Sporozoa

The sporozoa are all parasitic; they have a complex life cycle involving alternate sexual and asexual phases. Two kinds of sporozoa infect humans: the malaria parasites and the coccidia.

Malaria parasites

Malaria is, without doubt, the most important of all parasitic diseases. Despite sustained efforts to eradicate the disease it remains the commonest cause of fever in the world and is a major cause of morbidity and mortality in areas of high endemicity throughout the tropical belt. Four species infect humans: *Plasmodium falciparum* is the most dangerous, since primary infections are often rapidly fatal if left untreated; *P. vivax* and *P. ovale*, which cause benign tertian malaria, and *P. malariae*, which causes quartan malaria, rarely kill but give rise to debilitating infections. The most common species world-wide is *P. falciparum*, which accounts for over 90 per cent of infections in tropical Africa; in some parts of the world, however, notably the Indian sub-continent, *P. vivax* is the dominant species.

The malaria parasite is transmitted by the bite of infected female *Anopheles* mosquitoes. The parasites first infect liver cells; then after 1–2 weeks the liver parasites mature and infect circulating red blood cells to commence the cycle of erythrocytic schizogony which is responsible for the overt signs of disease. *P. vivax* and *P. ovale* can also set up a cryptic infection in the liver, which may cause the relapse of symptoms for up to 2 years after the infection is acquired.

A proportion of erythrocytic parasites differentiate into male and female gametocytes, which do not develop further in the mammalian host but complete the sexual phase of development in the anopheline vector when ingested during a blood meal.

The traditional mainstay of the treatment of malaria is quinine, originally derived from the bark of the cinchona tree in Peru, but during the course of the present century various other effective antimalarials have been developed. These include the 4-aminoquinolines, chloroquine and amodiaquine, and the acridine dye, mepacrine. Amodiaquine and mepacrine are no longer widely used, the former because of bone marrow toxicity and the latter because of the pigmentation that it imparts to the skin.

Pyrimethamine, a dihydrofolate reductase inhibitor related to trimethoprim, exhibits a selectively high affinity for the plasmodial enzyme. It has been used alone, but is usually formulated in combination with sulfadoxine, a long-acting sulphonamide, or with dapsone, a sulphone also used for treating leprosy. The combination of pyrimethamine with sulfadoxine has been associated with some fatal reactions and is no longer recommended for routine prophylaxis. Proguanil, a substance that is metabolized in the body to a compound closely related structurally to pyrimethamine and having an identical mode of action, is used alone as a prophylactic agent.

Since the 1960s resistance to chloroquine and other antimalarials has become common in *P. falciparum* in many parts of the world. For the present, most of these strains are susceptible to the newer agents, mefloquine (a quinolinemethanol) and halofantrine (a phenanthrenemethanol), but resistance to these is also beginning to appear. Promising results have been obtained with artemisinin, the active principle of an ancient Chinese herbal remedy, qinghaosu. Derivatives of this drug, including artemether and sodium artesunate are in use in parts of South East Asia and are under trial elsewhere.

Some antibiotics, notably tetracyclines and clindamycin, have some antimalarial activity and have been used as adjuncts to quinine therapy in chloroquine-resistant falciparum malaria. A hydroxynaphthoquinone, atovaquone, is under trial. Results have been disappointing when the drug was used alone, but the combination with proguanil seems to produce a useful synergic interaction.

All the above drugs act solely, or predominantly, on erythrocytic parasites; to eradicate parasites undergoing exoerythrocytic replication in the liver it is necessary to use the 8-aminoquinoline, primaquine, which is selectively active against the liver forms.

The factors governing the choice of antimalarial for treatment and prophylaxis are discussed in Chapter 31.

Coccidia

Phylogenetically related to the malaria parasites are the coccidia, which share many features of the complex life cycle, but are not transmitted by insect vectors. Several species of coccidia may infect humans. *Isospora belli* and *Cryptosporidium parvum* cause diarrhoea which is usually self limiting. However, in immunocompromised patients, especially those suffering from AIDS, cryptosporidia (and to a lesser extent *Isospora*) may cause a profuse, intractable diarrhoea for which no suitable antimicrobial therapy has yet been devised. Spiramycin, paromomycin, and eflornithine have been used experimentally, but success has been, at best, modest.

The most important human coccidian parasite is *Toxoplasma gondii*. Intrauterine infections with this organism are an important cause of congenital malformations and still birth throughout the world. AIDS sufferers may develop toxoplasma encephalitis, apparently by reactivation of latent infection. Cats often harbour the parasite and liberate the infectious oocysts in their faeces; this probably represents a major reservoir of infection. Pyrimethamine, in combination with a sulphonamide (usually sulphadiazine) is the treatment of choice in toxoplasmosis. Clindamycin and the macrolide antibiotic spiramycin have also been used with some success, especially in combination with pyrimethamine. Spiramycin has been recommended during pregnancy, when antifolates are considered by some to be best avoided.

Other protozoa

Balantidium coli

This ciliate is a rare cause of severe diarrhoea; it is cosmopolitan in distribution. Treatment of balantidiasis has never been properly defined, but tetracyclines and metronidazole appear to be effective.

Babesia

Although *Babesia* spp., like malaria parasites, infect red blood cells, they are unrelated. They are predominantly animal parasites, but are occasionally transmitted to humans by the bite of ixodid ticks. Recorded European cases have mostly been in splenectomized patients and have usually been caused by *B. divergens*, but infection in previously healthy persons caused by *B. microti* has been reported from North America. Most cases of babesiosis have been treated with chloroquine, following a mistaken diagnosis of malaria. However, chloroquine treatment often fails and this is clearly not the drug of choice. There is evidence that the combination of quinine and clindamycin might be effective.

Pneumocystis carinii

This organism is of uncertain taxonomic status and it may be a fungus. It used to be found only as a rare cause of interstitial pneumonia in infants, but has lately come into prominence as a respiratory pathogen of immunocompromised individuals, notably those with AIDS, in whom it commonly causes a life-threatening pneumonia. Co-trimoxazole and pentamidine are active against the organism, but both carry problems of toxicity, which seem to be increased in patients suffering from AIDS. The isethionate salt is the preferred formulation of pentamidine.

The hydroxynaphthoquinone derivative, atovaquone, is licensed in some countries for the treatment of *P. carinii* pneumonia. The drug is administered orally and appears to be a safe alternative to co-trimoxazole and pentamidine. However, bioavailability problems of the oral formulation have not yet been entirely overcome. Atovaquone is also under trial in toxoplasmosis.

Microsporidia

Encephalitozoon cuniculi and some other microsporidia occasionally cause infection, usually in immunocompromised patients. Although these protozoa have ribosomes of the prokaryotic type, inhibitors of bacterial protein synthesis do not seem to work. There is anecdotal evidence that albendazole may be useful.

Blastocystis hominis

The pathogenicity of this organism is disputed, but it has been incriminated in some cases of diarrhoea. Metronidazole appears to eliminate the parasite.

HELMINTHS

Helminths are parasitic worms. They often have a complex life cycle involving a period of development outside the definitive host either in soil or in some intermediate host. Helminths of medical importance fall into three major groups: nematodes (roundworms), trematodes (flukes), and cestodes (tapeworms) (Table 5.2).

Nematodes

Filarial worms

The most important group of nematodes are the filarial worms, which are transmitted by biting insects. Filariae infecting humans include *Wuchereria bancrofti*, which causes elephantiasis throughout the tropics, *Onchocerca volvulus*, the cause of 'river blindness' in West Africa, and *Loa loa*, the African 'eye worm'. The antitrypanosomal drug, suramin, has some effect in filariasis and may effect a radical cure by killing the adult worms. However, it is too toxic for routine use and diethylcarbamazine (DEC), a derivative of piperazine, has been most widely used, although it may cause unpleasant side-effects as well as evoking severe reaction to dead filarial larvae (Mazzotti reaction). The mode of action of DEC is something of a mystery since it appears to have no effect on the viability of microfilariae (the larval forms found in blood or skin) *in vitro*. One possibility is that the drug has a relatively trivial effect on the surface integument of the worms, which then succumb to immune clearance mechanisms. This explanation is perfectly feasible since it is known that the worms provoke an immune response, but in the absence of drug they are able to avoid its consequences.

DEC has, in its turn, been replaced by ivermectin as the drug of choice for the treatment of onchocerciasis, and possibly other filarial infections. The latter compound is a derivative of avermectin B_1, one of a family of macrocyclic lactone antibiotics produced by *Streptomyces avermitilis*. It has been extensively used in animals, in which it exhibits the astonishing property of dealing with not only helminths, but also many of the arthropod ectoparasites that cause problems in animal husbandry. In human disease, ivermectin has so far been most widely used in infection with *O. volvulus*, but evidence is accumulating of its

Table 5.2. Principal helminth parasites of humans and the drugs used in treatment

Species	Intermediate host	Geographical distribution	Useful drugs
Nematodes			
Wuchereria bancrofti	Mosquitoes	Tropical belt	Diethylcarbamazine, ivermectin
Loa loa	*Chrysops* spp.	Tropical Africa	
Brugia malayi	Mosquitoes	SE Asia	
Onchocerca volvulus	*Simulium* spp.	Tropical Africa, Central America	Ivermectin
Dracunculus medinensis	Cyclops (water flea)	Africa, Arabia, India, Pakistan	Niridazole, thiabendazole
Trichinella spiralis	Pig, etc.	World-wide	Mebendazole
Ancyclostoma duodenale	None	Tropics and subtropics	Mebendazole, etc. (see Table 31.1, Chapter 31)
Necator americanus	None	Tropics and subtropics	
Ascaris lumbricoides	None	World-wide	
Trichuris trichura	None	World-wide	
Strongyloides stercoralis	None	Tropics and subtropics	
Enterobius vermicularis	None	World-wide	
Trematodes			
Schistosoma mansoni	Snail	Africa, W. Indies, S. America	Praziquantel, etc. (see Table 31.2, Chapter 31)
Schistosoma haematobium	Snail	Africa	
Schistosoma japonicum	Snail	Far East	
Fasciola hepatica	Snail/vegetation	World-wide	Triclabendazole, bithionol
Clonorchis sinensis	Snail/fresh-water fish	Far East	Praziquantel
Paragonimus westermani	Snail/crabs, crayfish	Far East	
Fasciolopsis buski	Snail/water chestnut	Far East	
Cestodes			
Echinococcus granulosus	Human, sheep	World-wide	Albendazole
Taenia saginata	Cattle	World-wide	Niclosamide, praziquantel
Taenia solium	Pig	World-wide	
Hymenolepis nana	None	World-wide	
Diphyllobothrium latum	Cyclops/fish	Chiefly Finland	

value in other filarial infections. Use of ivermectin does not seem to be accompanied by the severe side-effects sometimes associated with the administration of DEC. A bonus is the concomitant expulsion of some intestinal worms.

Intestinal nematodes

Less important than filariae as causes of clinical disease, but extremely common world-wide, are the intestinal nematodes, which include the hookworms *Ancylostoma duodenale* and *Necator americanus*, the common roundworm *Ascaris lumbricoides*, the threadworm *Enterobius vermicularis*, and the whipworm *Trichuris trichiura*. These are not restricted in distribution to the tropics, but are, with the possible exception of *E. vermicularis*, more common in countries with poor standards of hygiene. Treatment of infection with these and related intestinal worms has traditionally relied on a variety of compounds of variable efficacy, including tetrachloroethylene, piperazine, bephenium, levamisole, and pyrantel pamoate (see Table 31.1). More reliable, but also more expensive, are benzimidazoles, a group of broad-spectrum anthelminthics active against most intestinal roundworms. The benzimidazoles currently available—thiabendazole, mebendazole, and albendazole—have become the drugs of choice for the elimination of intestinal roundworms.

Roundworms other than filariae that invade tissues include *Trichinella spiralis*, now an uncommon cause of human infection, and the Guinea worm, *Dracunculus medinensis*, which is the target of a World Health Organization eradication campaign. Anthelminthic therapy is probably unnecessary in either of these infections, but benzimidazoles have some activity against both parasites and the antischistosomal drug niridazole (see below) has been used against Guinea worm.

Larvae of the dog ascarid, *Toxocara canis*, sometimes infect children who come into contact with dogs. Thiabendazole and DEC have been traditionally used in treatment, but there is some evidence that albendazole or ivermectin may be preferable.

Trematodes

Trematodes (flukes) generally have a complex life cycle involving a stage of development in a snail and a secondary intermediate host, as well as in the definitive host where the mature adult forms develop.

Schistosomes (blood flukes)

The most important trematodes are the schistosomes, which cause human infection in many parts of Africa as well as the Far East, the West Indies, and South America. Schistosomes are unusual among flukes in having no secondary intermediate host; infection is acquired when cercaria (the infective form) penetrate the skin following exposure to water inhabited by infected snails. Mature adults develop in the portal vessels from where they migrate to the small veins of the rectum (*Schistosoma mansoni* and *S. japonicum*) or the bladder (*S. haematobium*). Eggs are then passed through the rectal or bladder mucosa into the faeces or urine.

For many years, treatment relied on trivalent antimonials of which sodium (or potassium) antimony tartrate (tartar emetic) was the mainstay. Now at least half a dozen compounds are available that offer advantages over antimonials. These include: the nitrothiazole derivative niridazole; the thioxanthones, lucanthone and hycanthone; metriphonate, (originally developed as an organophosphate insecticide); and the hydroxyquinoline derivatives oxamniquine and praziquantel (see Chapter 31). The last named is the only one that is highly active against all three species of *Schistosoma* that commonly infect humans.

Other flukes

Other important trematodes include *Fasciola hepatica* (liver fluke), *Clonorchis sinensis* (Chinese liver fluke), and *Paragonimus westermani* (lung fluke). *F. hepatica* is predominantly a parasite of sheep, and human infection usually follows eating wild watercress gathered near pastures. *C. sinensis* is acquired from eating uncooked freshwater fish and is extremely common in parts of the Far East where raw fish is widely eaten. Similarly, *P. westermani* infection is acquired from eating raw or undercooked crabs and crayfish.

No entirely satisfactory treatment of these fluke infections exists, but evidence is accumulating that praziquantel is effective. There have been reports of failures of praziquantel therapy in fascioliasis, and the benzimidazole derivative, triclabendazole or the halogenated phenol, bithionol, probably offer the best chance of cure.

Cestodes

Tapeworms usually have a simpler life cycle than do flukes, but transmission generally involves an intermediate host.

Hydatid worms

By far the most important tapeworms are *Echinococcus granulosus* and the closely related *E. multilocularis* (the hydatid worms). These parasites are unusual in that man is an intermediate host, harbouring the larval form in hydatid cysts which arise, usually in the liver, following ingestion of eggs from an infected dog. The internal wall of the hydatid cyst consists of a germinal layer from which 'brood capsules' containing protoscolices develop. Each protoscolex is capable of forming the head of a mature worm when ingested by the definitive host (usually the dog), or to initiate a fresh hydatid cyst within the intermediate host if the mother cyst is ruptured.

Hydatid disease occurs in many countries, including parts of the UK, where sheep and sheepdogs maintain the cycle of infection.

There is no effective chemotherapy for hydatid disease, although claims have been made for success with benzimidazoles, including mebendazole and albendazole. Praziquantel may also be of benefit, but chemotherapy remains an adjunct to surgical removal, which is not without risk from the spillage of viable protoscolices into the peritoneal cavity.

Other tapeworms

Other tapeworms infecting humans include: *Taenia saginata* the beef tapeworm, *T. solium* the pork tapeworm (now rare), *Hymenolepis nana* the dwarf tapeworm, and *Diphyllobothrium latum* the fish tapeworm. Despite their reputation, none of these well-adapted parasites causes much mischief under normal circumstances, although autoinfection with the larval form of *T. solium* can cause an epileptiform condition known as cerebral cysticercosis.

The ancient, and effective treatment for tapeworm infection is extract of male fern (*Dryopteris filix-mas*); the acridine dye, mepacrine, is also effective. These old drugs have now been replaced by niclosamide, which is at least 90 per cent effective in all forms of intestinal tapeworm infection. However, niclosamide treatment causes disruption of the worm and in *T. solium* infection there is a small risk of cysticercosis caused by autoinfection with liberated eggs. Praziquantel exhibits good activity against intestinal tapeworms and offers a useful alternative to niclosamide. Cerebral cysticercosis may respond to treatment with praziquantel given together with steroids. Albendazole is also effective and, since it penetrates better into the cerebrospinal fluid, it may be preferable.

6

Antiviral agents

W. L. Irving

Viruses are almost as versatile as bacteria in the range of diseases they can cause. Vertebrates, insects, plants, and even bacteria are all open to attack. Some viruses of vertebrates (arboviruses) develop in and are transmitted by mosquitoes or other arthropods; others—rabies is a good example—can infect a wide range of mammalian hosts. In general, however, viruses are highly specific in their host range.

All viruses are *obligate intracellular parasites*; that is, they replicate only within living cells and cannot usually survive for long outside the host cell. Selectivity usually extends not only to the host, but also to the type of cell within the host, as viruses infect only cells that express appropriate receptors on their surface. The preference of a virus for certain types of cell is known as the *tropism* of the virus, and this often accounts for the characteristic clinical manifestations of particular viral infections. Thus, some viruses preferentially infect liver cells, giving rise to hepatitis.

Intact skin is impermeable to viruses and access to sites within the body can occur only through mucous membranes, damaged skin, insect bites, or direct inoculation. Most viruses that infect humans gain entry to the body by adsorption to superficial cells of the mucous membranes of the respiratory, intestinal, and genital tracts, or of the conjunctivae.

The principal types of virus causing human disease are listed in Table 6.1.

PROPERTIES OF VIRUSES

Viruses are deceptively simple. Their sizes range from about 20 nm (parvovirus) to 300 nm (poxvirus); consequently, even the biggest viruses fall barely within the limits of resolution of conventional light microscopy, and the electron microscope must be used to visualize them.

Complete virus particles (*virions*) consist of a nucleic acid core (the genome of the virus), surrounded by a few proteins, and possibly a lipid envelope. The nucleic acid may be DNA or RNA (never both), single or double stranded, circular or linear, and continuous or segmented. This provides all the information needed for viral replication once it is released within the host cell. The proteins serve a number of functions. The *capsid*, or protein coat surrounding the nucleic acid,

Table 6.1. Principal types of virus causing human disease

Family	Examples	Diseases	Mode of transmission
RNA viruses			
Orthomyxoviruses	Influenza A and B viruses	Influenza	
Paramyxoviruses	Mumps virus	Mumps	Respiratory
	Measles virus	Measles	
	Respiratory syncytial virus	Lower respiratory tract infection esp. babies	
	Parainfluenza virus		
Rhabdoviruses	Rabies virus	Rabies	Bite of rabid animals
Arenaviruses	Lassa virus	Lassa fever	?Respiratory/contact rodent reservoir
Togaviruses	Rubella virus	German measles	Respiratory/congenital
Flaviviruses	Many arboviruses	Yellow fever	Arthropod vectors
	Hepatitis C virus	Hepatitis	Inoculation
Picornaviruses	Enteroviruses:		
	polio	Meningitis/paralysis	Faecal–oral
	echo		
	coxsackie A & B	Meningitis	
	hepatitis A	Infectious hepatitis	
	Rhinoviruses	Colds	Respiratory
Retroviruses	Human immunodeficiency virus (HIV)	AIDS	Inoculation/sexual/vertical
	Human T cell lymphotropic viruses (HTLV)	T cell leukaemia/lymphoma	
Reoviruses	Rotavirus	Infantile diarrhoea	Faecal–oral

Table 6.1. cont.

Family	Examples	Diseases	Mode of transmission
DNA viruses			
Poxviruses	Variola	Smallpox (now eradicated)	Mainly respiratory
	Vaccinia	Smallpox vaccine	Vaccination
	Molluscum contagiosum	Skin disease	Contact
	Orf		Contact with sheep
Herpesviruses	Herpes simplex	Cold sores/genital herpes	Saliva/contact/sexual
	Varicella-zoster	Chickenpox	Respiratory
	Cytomegalovirus	Non-specific illness	Close contact/congenital
	Epstein–Barr virus	Glandular fever	Saliva, e.g. kissing
	Human herpesvirus type 6	Roseola infantum (sixth disease)	Saliva
Adenoviruses	Many serotypes	Conjunctivitis/pharyngitis	Respiratory
Papovaviruses	Papillomavirus	Warts	Contact
Hepadnaviruses	Hepatitis B virus	Serum hepatitis	Inoculation/sexual/vertical
Parvoviruses	Parvovirus B19	Erythema infectiosum (fifth disease)	Respiratory

consists of repeating structural units made up of 1–3 different protein molecules that are generally arranged in helical or cubic symmetry. The nucleic acid surrounded by its capsid is referred to as the *nucleocapsid* of the virus. Many viral proteins have enzymatic properties. These include polymerases and proteases that are necessary for replication and assembly of viral particles. Proteins protruding from the surface coat of the virus act as ligands which will bind to cellular receptors during the first stage of infection of a cell. The lipid envelope possessed by some viruses is derived from membranes of the host cell.

TARGETS FOR ANTIVIRAL DRUGS

Virus infection of and replication within cells proceed via a number of distinct steps, each of which, theoretically, provides a possible target for attack (Fig. 6.1). Although the exact details of these steps vary between different viruses, they can be broadly summarized as follows:

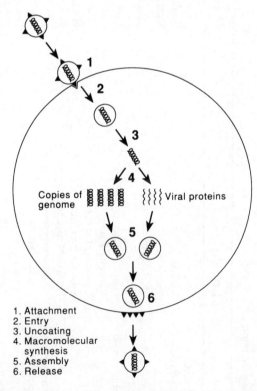

1. Attachment
2. Entry
3. Uncoating
4. Macromolecular synthesis
5. Assembly
6. Release

Copies of genome   Viral proteins

Fig. 6.1. Schematic representation of the virus replication cycle within the host cell showing the stages that are theoretically open to inhibition by antiviral agents.

1. *Adsorption to the cell surface*: this involves a specific interaction between proteins (ligands) on the surface of the virus and receptors on the surface of the cell. The nature of the viral ligands and cellular receptors is known in great detail for some viruses (e.g. the gp120 of human immunodeficiency virus and the CD4 molecule on T lymphocytes), but not at all for others.

2. *Uptake into the host cell*: some viruses are able to enter cells by fusion of their own outer lipid membrane with the plasma membrane of the cell, resulting in release of viral nucleocapsid into the cell cytoplasm. For other viruses, the process of translocation of the viral particle from the outside of the cell to the inside is very poorly understood.

3. *Uncoating of the viral genome*: the viral nucleic acid must be released from its capsid before replication. This process may be mediated by cellular lysosomal enzymes.

4. *Macromolecular synthesis*: within the cell, multiple copies of the viral genome are made, and mRNA derived from the virus is translated into multiple copies of the proteins encoded by the viral genome. Many viruses use enzymes present within the host cell to perform these activities, but some viruses carry their own enzymes for certain synthetic processes which are not present within the host cell. A good example is HIV, which copies its RNA genome into a DNA intermediate. Since host cells are not able to convert RNA into DNA, the necessary *reverse transcriptase* must be encoded by the HIV genome itself.

5. *Assembly*: before final assembly into new viral particles, viral proteins may be modified by host cell processes such as glycosylation and phosphorylation.

6. *Release*: the infected cell has by now become little more than a viral factory and complete viral particles may be released by destruction of the cell, or by continuous export through the cell membrane.

Virus–cell interactions

The viral replication cycle described above is representative of an *acute* viral infection: the virus enters the cell, replicates, disrupts normal cellular function, and is released, often resulting in cell death. However, viruses may interact with cells in other ways. Some viruses are able to undergo *latency* within cells; that is, the viral genome is present within the cell, and may even become incorporated into the host cell chromosomes, but no replication of the genome occurs, and no viral proteins are synthesized. The latent virus may cause the cell no harm, but it does have the propensity, under certain conditions, to become reactivated, with consequent viral replication and damage to the cell.

Another form of virus–cell interaction is the *chronic* or *persistent* infection. In this, there is a steady but low-level production and release of virus, but the host cell is able to survive. However, host cell function may be impaired, and the expression of viral antigens on the cell surface can lead to a chronic inflammatory state, as in chronic infection of hepatocytes with hepatitis B virus leading to chronic active hepatitis.

The final potential consequence of virus–cell interaction to be considered is *transformation*. This is the process whereby viral infection of a cell leads to uncontrolled cell division, resulting in an immortal cell line. For example, infection of B lymphocytes by Epstein–Barr virus (EBV) *in vitro* results in the stimulation of cell division and establishment of a continuous lymphoblastoid cell line. The molecular mechanisms underlying this process, and possible means of interfering with them, are obviously of great interest, especially as several viruses, including EBV, have now been implicated in initiating malignant change *in vivo*.

Limitations of antiviral therapy

Although all stages of the cycle of virus replication are potential targets for antiviral drugs, the intimate relationship between the virus and its host cell has meant that the design or discovery of compounds that are selectively toxic for the virus has been beset with considerable problems.

Moreover, antiviral therapy may be at a disadvantage for quite a different reason: in many viral diseases the initial infection and spread are commonly asymptomatic and the onset of illness, often at the peak of viral multiplication, occurs when the host defences have been fully mobilized. Unless the patient is immunodeficient in some way these defences are usually quite able to deal with the infection unassisted. Consequently, initiation of antiviral therapy at the onset of symptoms may have little influence on the course of the disease.

Viruses which undergo latency pose a further problem. Unless the latently infected cells can be killed or removed, the virus cannot be eliminated from the patient. Achieving such elimination by therapeutic intervention is a daunting task, as there are no virus-specific metabolic processes occurring in those cells, and there is no expression of viral antigens on the cell surface against which an immune response could be mounted.

Despite these discouraging considerations, a certain amount of success has been achieved in the development of antiviral compounds, and a handful of antiviral agents are now in regular use (Table 6.2). Most presently available agents are nucleoside analogues, which interfere with

Table 6.2. Antiviral agents available in the UK (1995)

Compound	Indication	Mode of action	Route of administration
Acyclovir	Herpes simplex	Nucleoside analogue	Oral; Topical; IV
Amantadine	Influenza A	Uncoating/assembly of virus particles	Oral
Didanosine	Human immuno-deficiency virus	Nucleoside analogue	Oral
Famciclovir	Herpes zoster	Nucleoside analogue	Oral
Foscarnet	Cytomegalovirus	DNA polymerase inhibitor	IV
Ganciclovir	Cytomegalovirus	Nucleoside analogue	IV
Idoxuridine	Herpes simplex	Nucleoside analogue	Topical
Interferons	Chronic hepatitis	Immunomodulation	IM
Tribavirin	Respiratory syncytial virus	Nucleoside analogue	Nebulizer
Vidarabine	Herpesviruses	Nucleoside analogue	IV
Zidovudine	Human immuno-deficiency virus	Nucleoside analogue	Oral
Zalcitabine	Human immuno-deficiency virus	Nucleoside analogue	Oral

IV = intravenous; IM = intramuscular.

viral replication; most clinical progress has been achieved with agents active against viruses of the herpes group.

PROPERTIES OF ANTIVIRAL AGENTS

Acyclovir

Acyclovir (now often spelt aciclovir) inhibits the replication of certain viruses and exhibits virtually no toxic side-effects on host cells. Structurally, it is acycloguanosine (Fig. 6.2)—that is, it is an analogue of the purine nucleoside, guanosine, in which the ribose moiety has lost its cyclic configuration. Acyclovir itself is inactive; in order to achieve its antiviral effect it must first be phosphorylated to the triphosphate form within the infected cell. Although the second and third phosphate groups are added by cellular enzymes, the first phosphorylation step is accomplished by a *viral* thymidine kinase enzyme, specified by certain herpesviruses; the cellular form of this enzyme is much less efficient in producing acyclovir monophosphate. This unique feature is the basis for the selective toxicity of acyclovir, for two reasons. Firstly, it means that the active form of the drug is produced only in cells infected with those viruses (herpes simplex

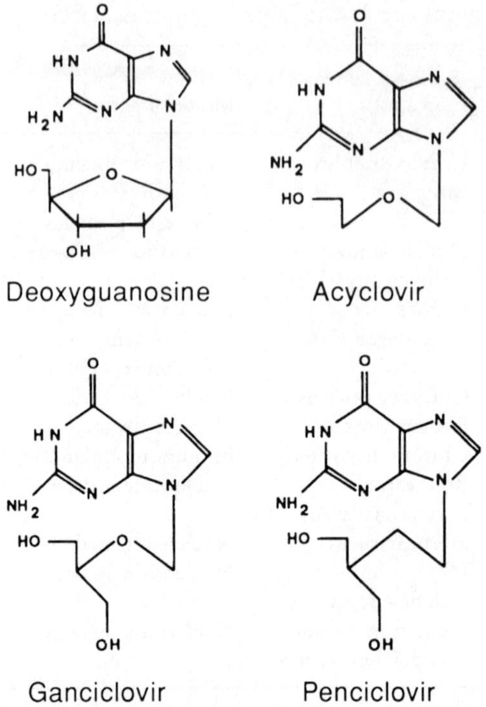

Fig. 6.2. Structures of deoxyguanosine and three antiviral agents that act as analogues of the nucleoside: acyclovir, ganciclovir, and penciclovir.

and varicella-zoster viruses; HSV and VZV) that possess the thymidine kinase. Secondly, by the law of mass action, once the equilibrium

$$\text{acyclovir} \rightleftharpoons \text{acyclovir monophosphate}$$

is shifted to the right within an infected cell, more free acyclovir will enter the cell from the extracellular space, thus resulting in concentration of the drug precisely where it is needed: in the infected cell.

Mode of action
Acyclovir triphosphate is able to inhibit viral DNA replication by two mechanisms. First, as an analogue of guanosine triphosphate it is incorporated into the growing DNA chain and causes chain termination, since acyclovir triphosphate lacks the 3'-hydroxyl group necessary to form the 5'–3' phosphodiester linkage with the next base. Acyclovir triphosphate is also a direct inhibitor of viral DNA polymerase.

Resistance
It is theoretically possible for a virus to become resistant to acyclovir by a number of mechanisms:

1. Strains of virus which lack the thymidine kinase enzyme, known as TK⁻ mutants, are inherently resistant to the drug, as they cannot generate the active form.

2. Mutations in the TK gene may alter the thymidine kinase molecule so that this enzyme becomes unable to perform the first phosphorylation step.

3. Alterations in viral DNA polymerase may reduce the ability of the enzyme to bind acyclovir triphosphate, thereby escaping the inhibitory properties of the drug.

All these mechanisms have been shown to occur in the laboratory and in nature. However, TK⁻ strains and those with altered thymidine kinases appear to exhibit reduced virulence, and DNA polymerase mutants are the ones that cause most clinical difficulties. These emerge particularly in immunocompromised patients including those with HIV infection, in whom recurrent HSV infections cause frequent and extensive disease necessitating prolonged treatment with acyclovir.

Acyclovir represents a prime example of what a good antiviral drug should be. It has potent antiviral activity, but is virtually free of toxic side-effects. It can be life saving in certain infections, and in others can significantly decrease morbidity (see Chapter 28). However, it is poorly absorbed when given orally, and in life-threatening infection it must be given intravenously.

Analogues of acyclovir

Following the success of acyclovir, a number of structural analogues have been developed. *Valaciclovir*, the L-valyl ester of acyclovir, is an oral pro-drug that is well absorbed when given by mouth to release acyclovir into the bloodstream. A similar relationship exists between *famciclovir* and *penciclovir*; the former is metabolized into the latter after oral administration. Penciclovir (Fig. 6.2) exhibits antiviral activity very similar to that of acyclovir, but the half-life of penciclovir triphosphate within cells is considerably longer than that of acyclovir triphosphate, so fewer doses of drug are necessary to achieve an antiviral effect.

Ganciclovir

Ganciclovir (dihydroxypropoxymethylguanine, DHPG, Fig. 6.2) is a derivative of acyclovir that exhibits useful activity against cytomegalovirus (CMV). Acyclovir has no activity against CMV, as this member of the herpesvirus family does not possess a thymidine kinase enzyme. As with acyclovir, ganciclovir must be activated by phosphorylation. The nature of the viral enzyme which phosphorylates the drug is unknown, but it is not thymidine kinase, as CMV can perform this step. Subsequent phosphorylation to the triphosphate generates a compound which acts as a chain terminator and viral DNA polymerase inhibitor.

Unfortunately, cellular enzymes can phosphorylate ganciclovir, so that active drug is also generated in uninfected cells. This mechanism presumably underlies the toxicity of ganciclovir, which is considerably greater than that of acyclovir. Thus ganciclovir impairs the function of the bone marrow, particularly affecting the production of neutrophils; it is also nephrotoxic. It is poorly absorbed when given orally, and has to be administered intravenously. Despite these drawbacks, the anti-CMV activity of ganciclovir can be sight or life saving in immunosuppressed patients with severe CMV infections (see Chapter 28).

Tribavirin (ribavirin)

Tribavirin (Fig. 6.3) is the British Approved Name for the substance known elsewhere as ribavirin. It is a triazole compound structurally related to guanosine. Like other nucleoside analogues it has to be activated intracellularly by phosphorylation. In the triphosphate form it inhibits viral protein synthesis, apparently by interfering with 'cap' formation at the 5′ end of mRNA.

Tribavirin has an unusually broad spectrum of activity against both RNA and DNA viruses, at least *in vitro*. Its main use is in the treatment of severe lower respiratory tract infection in young children caused by respiratory syncytial virus infection. The compound is administered by inhalation of an aerosolized solution.

In addition, oral tribavirin has been used successfully in the treatment of Lassa fever. Trials of this drug in the treatment of HIV-infected patients have been contradictory, with the weight of evidence now suggesting that it is of little use in this condition.

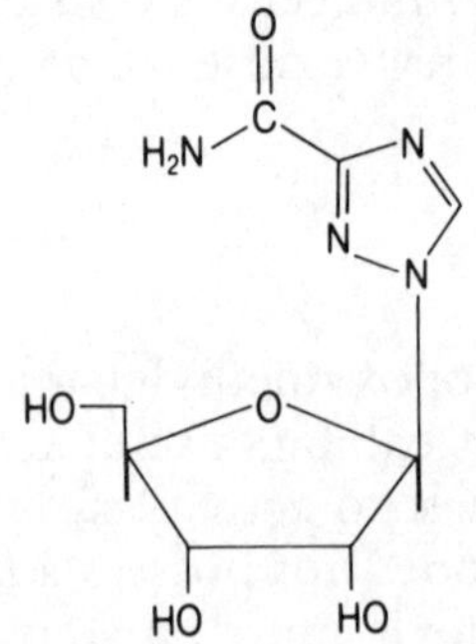

Fig. 6.3. Structure of tribavirin (ribavirin).

Tribavirin is relatively free of serious side-effects. It causes an increase in red cell volume (macrocytosis), and also a rise in serum bilirubin levels.

Zidovudine

Zidovudine (azidothymidine; often simply called AZT) is a dideoxy-nucleoside in which the 3′ hydroxyl group of thymidine has been replaced by an azido (N_3) group (Fig. 6.4). Like other nucleoside analogues, it is activated by phosphorylation to the triphosphate form, these steps being carried out by cellular enzymes. As with acyclovir triphosphate, incorporation of zidovudine triphosphate into a growing DNA chain will result in chain termination, as there will be no 3′ hydroxyl group available for formation of the next 5′–3′ phosphodiester linkage.

Zidovudine was originally investigated for use as an anticancer agent. However, when the HIV epidemic arose in the 1980s it was tested along with many other drugs sitting on the shelves of pharmaceutical companies for activity against the virus. It was found to inhibit the reverse transcriptase activity of retroviruses at concentrations considerably lower than those needed to interfere with synthesis of host cell DNA. This property of the drug has led to its use in the treatment of patients infected with HIV.

Non-specific side-effects such as headache, anorexia, and nausea are common with zidovudine therapy, but these effects often abate after 2–3 weeks. More serious toxicity to bone marrow cells is dose related, and hence much effort has been directed at defining the minimum dose of the drug which exhibits effective antiviral action. Temporary cessation of therapy usually results in restoration of marrow function, but some patients on zidovudine become transfusion dependent. Combination therapy with ganciclovir, whilst desirable as many HIV-infected patients

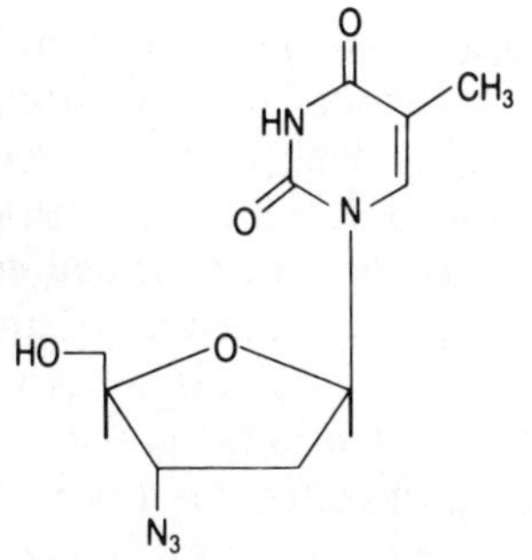

Fig. 6.4. Structure of zidovudine (AZT).

suffer serious CMV infection, is complicated by an additive effect on the bone marrow.

Isolates of HIV derived from patients who have been taking zidovudine for at least 6 months are invariably less sensitive to the drug *in vitro* than isolates taken from the same patient at the initiation of therapy. This arises from mutations in the gene coding for reverse transcriptase, leading to reduced binding of zidovudine triphosphate. The clinical significance of this relative resistance may be of considerable importance: the benefits of treating asymptomatic patients have to be weighed against the possibility that early treatment may lead to correspondingly early emergence of drug-resistant mutants.

Didanosine, zalcitabine, and stavudine

Three other deoxynucleosides have been approved in the USA and some other countries for the treatment of HIV infection: *didanosine* (dideoxyinosine), and *zalcitabine* (dideoxycytidine) and *stavudine* (didehydrodeoxythymidine). They act in the same way as zidovudine but their toxicity profiles differ considerably. Painful peripheral neuropathy is the principal dose-limiting side-effect of didanosine; pancreatitis, which may be life threatening, may also develop in patients taking didanosine or zalcitabine. Resistance may arise, but cross-resistance between zidovudine and didanosine appears to be the exception rather than the rule. The different properties of these drugs have led to the design of strategies of therapy involving alternating courses of the drugs, the idea being that as resistance to, say, zidovudine develops or its side-effects become intolerable the patient is switched to didanosine, or vice versa. Encouraging results have been reported with this approach, but much evaluation remains to be done to determine optimum doses and switchover times.

Foscarnet

Unlike the drugs discussed so far, foscarnet (Fig. 6.5) is not a nucleoside analogue; it is trisodium phosphonoformate, a derivative of phosphonoacetic acid. This drug does not require phosphorylation. It acts directly as a DNA and RNA polymerase inhibitor, with some selective toxicity for viral rather than host cell enzymes. It has activity against all the herpesviruses, and is used as an alternative to ganciclovir in the treatment of serious CMV infection, as well as in the treatment of acyclovir-resistant HSV infection. It also has some antiretroviral activity, but the clinical significance of this in the treatment of HIV infection is unclear. Like ganciclovir, oral bioavailability is poor, and it has to be administered by intravenous injection. It is nephrotoxic, and

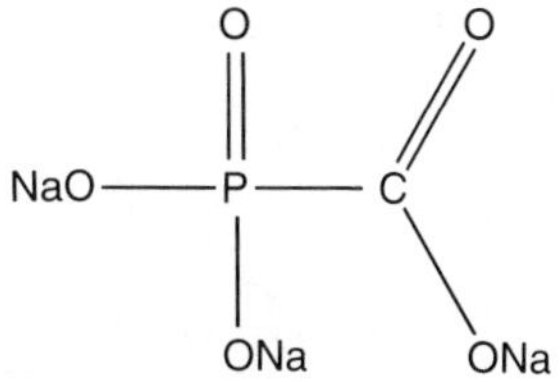

Fig. 6.5. Structure of foscarnet.

can cause acute renal failure. Other side-effects include symptomatic hypocalcaemia and penile ulceration.

Amantadine and rimantadine

Amantadine (Fig. 6.6) is a tricyclic amine derivative of adamantane, a compound that originally aroused interest because of its symmetrical three-dimensional structure which is composed entirely of carbon atoms and is thus related to the crystalline array of natural diamonds. The antiviral activity of amantadine was first described in 1964. Rimantadine is a closely related substance which has been widely used in the former USSR.

The activity of both amantadine and rimantadine is restricted to influenza A virus; other influenza viruses are virtually unaffected at therapeutically achievable concentrations. These compounds interfere with uncoating of the viral nucleic acid within the infected cell. Resistance may arise by mutation in a viral matrix protein, which is then unable to bind the drugs.

Amantadine binds to *N*-methyl-D-aspartate receptors in the brain, and therefore has dopaminergic effects. These effects can be therapeutically useful (amantadine is also licensed in the UK as an anti-Parkinsonian drug), but also account for the side-effects of the drug: restlessness, insomnia, agitation, and confusion. Unfortunately, amantadine is poorly tolerated, especially by the elderly, one of the groups who stand to

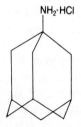

Fig. 6.6. Structure of amantadine.

benefit most from an effective anti-influenza drug. Rimantadine is said to give rise to fewer side-effects, but experience with this derivative is limited.

Amantadine is also licensed in the UK for use in shingles, but this has few advocates.

Interferon

Interferon was described in 1957 as an antiviral compound in chick embryo cells. It turns out that the activity is associated with a family of species-specific glycosylated proteins produced *in vivo* in response to viral or antigenic challenge. There are three types of human interferon: interferon-alpha (IFN-α) produced by many cell types, interferon-beta (IFN-β) produced by fibroblasts, and interferon-gamma (IFN-γ, sometimes referred to as immune interferon) produced by T lymphocytes. IFN-α and -β share 30 per cent structural homology, but they are quite distinct from IFN-γ, which shares only about 10 per cent homology in its amino acid sequence. Moreover, there are over fifteen different forms of IFN-α, each differing by a few amino acids, and, possibly, two forms of IFN-β. Interferons have a wide range of biological effects. They activate several different biochemical pathways within a cell, with the result that the cell is rendered resistant to virus infection. The relative importance of each of these pathways differs between different interferons, and indeed between different cells stimulated by the same interferon. One pathway results in the activation of a ribonuclease which digests viral RNA. Another results in phosphorylation of a protein known as initiation factor; phosphorylation of this factor, the normal function of which is to assist in the initiation of transcription of mRNA into protein, effectively prevents production of viral proteins.

Interferons also have a number of effects on cells of the immune system. As with their antiviral properties, these immunomodulatory effects vary in detail between different interferons, but they include stimulation of natural killer (NK) cells, induction or suppression of antibody production, stimulation of T cell activity, and stimulation of expression of human leucocyte antigen (HLA) class I and II molecules on the surface of cells. Finally, interferons also affect cell proliferation, which has led to their successful use in the management of certain malignant tumours.

When interferons were discovered, they were hailed as the antiviral equivalent of penicillin. As these substances were produced naturally, it seemed reasonable to imagine that their toxic effects on host cells would be minimal. Early studies were hampered by difficulties in obtaining sufficient quantities of interferons to conduct clinical trials. This problem has been solved by recombinant DNA technology, which has allowed cloning and expression of the relevant genes, and also by the use of Sendai virus to induce interferon production by a lymphoblastoid cell line (so-called *lymphoblastoid interferon*). Unexpectedly, clinical trials revealed that patients receiving interferon experienced 'flu-like side-effects: fever, headache, and myalgia. This led to the realization that individuals suffering from influenza complain of 'flu-like symptoms precisely because of the induction of interferons by the virus. Most patients become tolerant to these effects after the first few doses.

Clinical experience with interferons has, however, been disappointing. Interferon-α is successfully used in the management of patients with chronic viral hepatitis, but even here the therapeutic effect may be due to its immunomodulatory rather than antiviral properties.

PREVENTION OF VIRUS INFECTIONS

Despite the progress that has been made in antiviral therapy, the major impact on virus infections is currently achieved by prevention rather than by treatment. The successful eradication of smallpox by appropriate use of vaccinia vaccine is ample testament to this statement, and has lent credence to the notion that other viral infections may be similarly eradicated. The WHO campaign to eliminate polio by the year 2000 is currently on target, and in many countries measles, mumps, and rubella are becoming rare.

Immunization against infectious disease may be passive or active.

Passive immunization

The transfer of preformed antibodies from one individual to another can be achieved with normal human gammaglobulin derived from blood donors, provided that the antibody in question is present in a sufficiently large number of randomly selected donors, as in the case of anti-hepatitis A virus. If not, then hyperimmune globulin can be prepared specifically from individuals known to have high antibody titres. Examples of preparations in current use include hyperimmune hepatitis B immunoglobulin (HBIg), varicella-zoster immune globulin (VZIg), and human rabies immunoglobulin (HRIg).

Active immunization

Stimulating the host to produce a protective immune response is achieved by vaccinating the host with some form of the infectious agent that does not cause disease. Vaccines can be alive or dead.

Live vaccines consist of attenuated forms of the infectious agent. Examples include measles, mumps, rubella, and live poliovirus (Sabin) vaccines. Difficulties arise in ensuring that the attenuated variant is unable to revert to virulence: the few cases of paralytic polio that still occur in Europe and North America are nearly all caused by vaccine strains that have reverted to virulence.

Dead vaccines may consist of the whole agent, grown in the laboratory and subsequently killed by some means, or of a subunit of the agent, usually prepared by recombinant DNA technology. Dead vaccines have the advantage that there is no risk of reversion to virulence, although there is at least one infamous example of an inadequately killed poliovirus vaccine which led to an outbreak of paralytic polio. However, they are less immunogenic than live vaccines, and therefore more doses need to be given to achieve a satisfactory response. Examples of such vaccines include poliovirus (Salk), rabies virus, and hepatitis A and hepatitis B virus vaccines; the latter is a subunit vaccine, consisting only of the surface protein (HBsAg) prepared by cloning and expressing the appropriate gene into yeast cells.

Part II

Laboratory aspects of antimicrobial therapy

7

Antibiotic sensitivity testing

D. Greenwood

PURPOSE OF SENSITIVITY TESTING

Since therapy of infection normally begins, quite properly, before laboratory results are available, antibiotic sensitivity testing primarily plays a supplementary role in confirming that the organism is susceptible to the agent that is being used. Sometimes it may enable the clinician to change from a toxic to a less toxic agent, or from an expensive to a cheaper one.

Usually the laboratory report will influence treatment only if the patient is failing to respond. By this time, the laboratory should have succeeded in establishing the sensitivity pattern of the offending organism (if it is bacterial) sufficiently for the clinician to be able to make an informed decision as to how treatment might be modified. Sensitivity testing of non-bacterial pathogens is not usually possible, although limited antifungal testing is carried out in some centres.

The laboratory also has an important function in recording and storing data on the sensitivity patterns of common pathogens in the hospital and in the community, in order that reliable predictions of their probable sensitivity may be made. Patterns of bacterial sensitivity and resistance vary considerably from place to place and hospitals, or even wards, often have their own particular resistance problems. It is, therefore, important that each hospital keeps its own record of resistance trends.

Finally, sensitivity testing is used to establish the degree and spectrum of *in vitro* activity of new antibacterial agents, first of all in the laboratories of the pharmaceutical houses from whence most new developments emanate, but also in diagnostic laboratories where the new agent can be tested against the various types of organism encountered locally.

METHODS OF TESTING

The antibiotic sensitivity of bacteria can be assessed in a variety of ways according to individual preference, the constraints of cost, the nature of

the bacterium, the number of strains requiring investigation, and the
degree of accuracy required. Most methods fall into one of three main
categories.

1. *Agar diffusion tests*, in which the antibiotic is allowed to diffuse
    from a point source, commonly in the form of an impregnated
    filter paper disc, into an agar medium that has been seeded with
    the test organism.

2. *Broth dilution tests*, in which serial (usually twofold) dilutions
    of antibiotic in a suitable fluid medium are inoculated with the
    test organism. The highest dilution of the antibiotic to inhibit
    growth after overnight incubation is the *minimum inhibitory
    concentration* (MIC).

3. *Agar incorporation tests*, which are essentially similar to broth
    dilution tests except that the antibiotic dilutions are incorporated
    in an agar medium in a series of Petri dishes. These are spot-
    inoculated with a number of test organisms, usually by means
    of a semi-automatic inoculating device.

Agar diffusion tests

Most diagnostic microbiology laboratories test antibiotic sensitivity of
bacteria by some form of agar diffusion test in which the organism under
investigation is exposed to a diffusion gradient of antibiotic provided
by an impregnated disc of filter paper. When the bacterial population
reaches a certain critical concentration, no further inhibition of growth
can be achieved and the edge of an inhibition zone is formed. Up to
six antibiotics can be tested on one culture plate and several firms
manufacture disc dispensers or multiple discs to facilitate this.

Several versions of the disc diffusion test are in use in different countries, but none has achieved universal approval. A highly standardized
version of the method with a single high-content disc, the Bauer–Kirby
test, is officially sanctioned by the Food and Drug Administration in
the USA. This test, if properly performed, enables a highly reproducible
determination of sensitivity to be made.

The formation of inhibition zones represents the dynamic interaction
between antibiotic diffusion and bacterial growth. Within certain limits
the size of the inhibition zone is a measure of the MIC of the antibiotic
for the test organism, but for individual strains the relationship between
two may be far from perfect. By examining numerous strains of known
MIC, regression analysis can be applied and the relationship quantified
for each bacterial species and antibiotic (Fig. 7.1).

A specialized version of the agar diffusion test that has been introduced commercially is the 'E-test'. Antibiotic in a linearly decreasing
concentration is immobilized along the length of a carrier strip, which

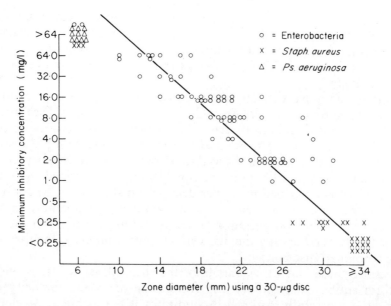

Fig. 7.1. Hypothetical example of correlation of disc diffusion zone sizes and minimum inhibitory concentration (MIC) values. Note that MIC values are plotted on a logarithmic scale and appear in discrete $\log_2$ steps, whereas disc zone sizes are measured on a continuous arithmetic scale. A zone size of 6 mm indicates no zone of inhibition, since this is the diameter of the antibiotic-containing disc. The example shown indicates that most *Staph. aureus* strains are fully susceptible to the antibiotic, but a few strains are fully resistant; all *Ps. aeruginosa* strains are resistant. A very wide spread of susceptibility values is observed with enterobacteria, and correlation is less than perfect. It is this group that presents interpretative difficulties.

is applied to the surface of an inoculated agar plate. An elliptical zone of inhibition is formed after incubation, and the point at which this intersects with the strip corresponds to the MIC of the antibiotic, which can then be read off from graduations on the strip. The test is said to be suitable for many types of organisms and provides a simple, if expensive, means of assessing the MIC if this is required.

Factors affecting disc tests

Many of the factors determining the outcome of disc tests are the same as those encountered in other methods of sensitivity testing (see below: factors affecting sensitivity tests), but some are peculiar to this method.

The size of the inhibition zone may be profoundly influenced by the physico-chemical characteristics of the antibacterial agent such as solubility, ionic charge, and molecular size. Large cyclic peptides, such as the polymyxins, diffuse poorly and produce small zones of inhibition even when sensitive organisms are tested against high drug concentrations.

The growth rate of the bacterial cell will also affect zone sizes, slow-growing organisms giving rise to large zones. A corollary of this is that if cultures are allowed to stand at room temperature before incubation at 37 °C an overestimate of bacterial susceptibility may be made.

One of the most difficult factors to control adequately is the initial amount of antibiotic in the disc. Commercially available discs usually contain the stated amount of drug with a tolerance of 67–150 per cent; i.e. a disc rated at 30 μg may contain between 20 and 45 μg of drug. If discs are incorrectly stored, allowed to become moist or used beyond the expiry date, the lower limit may be considerably overstepped. Note that disc content is described in μg per disc, which should not be confused with μg per ml, often used to specify antibacterial potency. In fact, in disc testing the concentration of antibiotic in μg per ml in the area immediately surrounding the disc can be a much higher value than that of the nominal disc content.

Despite these and other variables, the disc diffusion test is widely used for antibiotic sensitivity tests for reasons of speed, simplicity, and cost. Under carefully controlled conditions it is capable of producing satisfactory results with the more common rapidly growing pathogens such as *Staphylococcus aureus, Pseudomonas aeruginosa* and various enterobacteria; it is less suitable for fastidious or slow-growing bacteria such as anaerobes, streptococci, *Haemophilus* spp. and *Neisseria* spp., for which alternative procedures are preferable.

Control of disc diffusion tests

Since zone sizes are affected by many variable factors it is essential that all tests include adequate controls. A common method of control is to include a series of plates inoculated with a standardized inoculum of organisms of known sensitivity along with each batch of tests and to measure the size of the inhibition zones produced. This adequately controls culture medium composition (providing the same batch of medium is used for all tests) and incubation conditions, but makes no allowance for variations in disc content.

Disc content is more satisfactorily controlled by Stokes' 'comparative method', in which both test and control organisms are inoculated on the same culture plate so that a direct comparison of zone size and inoculum density can be made (Fig. 7.2). With this method it is preferable for control and test strains to be of the same species and it is essential that both strains should have similar growth characteristics on the medium used. Critics of the method point to the difficulty of reliably achieving these conditions in routine practice.

Stokes' method is particularly valuable in circumstances in which disc

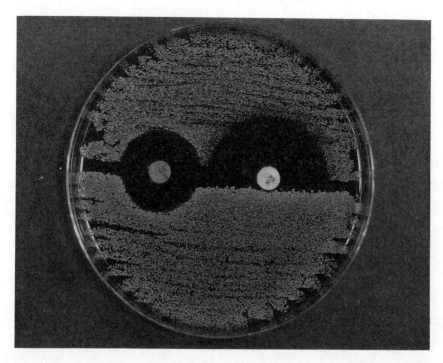

Fig. 7.2. Disc sensitivity testing by the Stokes' method, in which inhibition of the test organism by antibiotics is directly compared with that of a similar control organism of known sensitivity. In the example shown, the test organism (*Staph. aureus*) is resistant to penicillin (right-hand disc), but fully sensitive to erythromycin (left-hand disc). [Photograph courtesy of George Sharp and Richard Edwards.]

potency is uncertain—e.g. in countries in which supply is unreliable, refrigeration inadequate, and the climate humid.

Broth dilution tests

Conventional test

Conventional broth dilution tests are expensive in both time and materials and tend to be used when only a few strains of bacteria need to be tested or when an accurate MIC estimation is required. A series of twofold dilutions of the antibiotic under study is prepared in a suitable broth medium and a standard inoculum of the test strain (commonly 10^5 bacteria) is introduced into each tube. The test is incubated at 37°C overnight and the end-point is read as that concentration of antibiotic in which no turbidity can be seen. Uninoculated tubes containing broth plus antibiotic and broth alone act as sterility controls; an antibiotic-free tube inoculated with the test organism serves to indicate that the organism is alive and well in

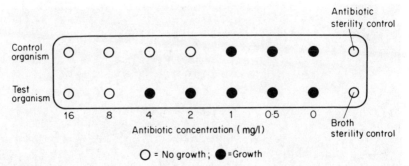

Fig. 7.3. Broth dilution test of antibiotic susceptibility. Twofold dilutions of antibiotic are inoculated with a known number of organisms and incubated at 37 °C overnight. The potency of the antibiotic is checked by titrating it against a control organism of known susceptibility. The minimum inhibitory concentration (MIC) is the highest dilution in which no turbidity develops (2 mg/l for the control organism and 8 mg/l for the test organism in the example shown).

case the end-point is missed. The whole test is controlled by a parallel titration of the antibiotic against an organism of known sensitivity (Fig. 7.3).

Micro-method
One-millilitre volumes are traditionally used for broth dilution MIC tests, but a micro-method with much smaller volumes in microtitration trays is also used. A further convenience is provided by using preprepared trays containing freeze-dried antibiotic. The antibiotic dilutions are reconstituted with preseeded culture medium and incubated as before.

Determination of MBC
A major advantage claimed for broth dilution procedures is that the *minimum bactericidal concentration* (MBC) of antibiotic for the test strain may additionally be determined if so desired. This is done by subculturing onto solid medium a standard volume of broth from those antibiotic dilutions showing no visible growth after overnight incubation. The number of colonies developing after a further overnight period of incubation is compared with the number originally inoculated. The MBC is arbitrarily defined as the lowest concentration which kills 99.9 per cent of the original inoculum, i.e. the concentration at which there is a thousand-fold reduction in bacterial numbers. Clearly if 10^5 bacteria were inoculated into 1 ml of broth, a 0.1 ml volume subcultured onto solid medium should yield less than 10 colonies if the antibacterial agent is bactericidal.

Killing curves

The MBC is a very crude estimate of bactericidal potency which reveals nothing about the kinetics of bacterial response. It is more satisfactory, but much more laborious, to construct killing curves in which sequential viable counts are carried out at regular intervals after exposure to various concentrations of the drug. This indicates the rate of bacterial killing and may detect recovery during the overnight incubation period which would be masked in the overnight end-point. It should be noted that viable counting methods detect colony-forming units, not absolute numbers of bacteria since chains and clumps give rise to single colonies. An antibiotic such as cephalexin, which affects the division process of Gram-negative bacteria, but does not stop them from growing during during the first few hours' exposure, will cause the viable count to stop rising even though growth continues.

Agar incorporation tests

In this method the antibiotic dilutions are made in solid agar medium by adding antibiotics to molten agar (at 45 °C) and pouring into Petri dishes. The test strains are inoculated onto the surface of the medium. This is the preferred method when large numbers of strains are to be examined since 20–36 strains can be accommodated on a single 9 cm plate. The inoculum is applied with a suitably designed multipoint inoculator which transfers a small drop of broth culture to each of the desired number of antibiotic-containing plates. A suitable inoculum yields a barely confluent spot of culture after overnight incubation on an antibiotic-free control plate. A series of control strains of known sensitivity are included on each plate.

Break-point tests

By using an appropriate series of antibiotic concentrations, MICs can be estimated by the agar incorporation method. The results are commonly found to be one or two twofold dilutions lower than those obtained by broth dilution. Since accurate MICs are seldom required for routine sensitivity tests the range of dilutions can be considerably reduced by using only one or two preselected 'break-point' concentrations related to agreed cut-off points of sensitivity or resistance (Table 7.1). Like the content of antibiotic discs these break-points are somewhat arbitrary, but are related to levels achievable in serum, tissue, or urine during therapy. Inaccuracies introduced in preparing appropriate antibiotic concentrations for the break-point method may be minimized by using commercially prepared antibiotic tablets of guaranteed potency which are simply dissolved in the correct volume of molten agar and poured into Petri dishes.

Mycobacteria

Most mycobacteria are slow growing and need special media for cultivation. Traditionally, sensitivity testing has been carried out by the 'resistance ratio' method, a variety of the agar incorporation test in which growth of the organisms on medium containing antimycobacterial agents is compared with that of a control. The method is cumbersome and an alternative technique, in which inhibition of growth is detected by failure to release radioactive CO_2 from a labelled substrate, is gaining popularity. This method can be automated and produces reliable results within 7 days. Molecular techniques aimed at the rapid detection of resistance genes are under development.

M. leprae can be grown only in certain experimental animals and sensitivity tests are not routinely available.

FACTORS AFFECTING SENSITIVITY TESTS

Inoculum size

The most important single factor affecting the result of sensitivity tests is the number of bacteria present in the original inoculum; this must be carefully standardized if reliable and reproducible results are to be obtained. Unfortunately, the therapeutically 'correct' inoculum has never been precisely defined and the inocula usually used are based on tradition rather than firm evidence. With some antibacterial agents, notably the sulphonamides, antibacterial activity is abolished *in vitro* if dense inocula are used and this clearly does not accord with clinical experience. However, the sulphonamides represent a special

Table 7.1. Example of antibiotic susceptibility testing by the 'break-point' method

| Test organism | Ampicillin concentration | | | Result |
	Plate 1 (nil)	Plate 2 (8 mg/l)	Plate 3 (64 mg/l)	
1	Growth	No growth	No growth	Fully sensitive
2	Growth	Growth	No growth	Reduced sensitivity*
3	Growth	Growth	Growth	Fully resistant
4	No growth	No growth	No growth	Void test†

* Susceptible to levels achievable in urine.
† Control failed to grow.

case because they achieve their effect only after bacterial growth has continued normally for 2 or 3 h, and it is unwise to assume that dense bacterial populations (such as are frequently present in infection) are generally inappropriate in sensitivity tests.

Composition of culture medium

Culture media used for sensitivity testing must be free of antibiotic antagonists and readily support growth of the bacteria under test. Several formulations of medium suitable for sensitivity testing of a wide range of bacterial pathogens are commercially available. Mueller–Hinton medium has become established for the purpose in the USA, but it is unclear that this has any special properties which single it out as being particularly suitable and other specially formulated sensitivity test media are usually preferred elsewhere. Media which contain thymidine are unsuitable for testing trimethoprim or sulphonamides, but the addition of lysed horse blood to the medium renders it suitable because horse blood contains the enzyme thymidine phosphorylase.

As well as being able to support growth of the major pathogens well, sensitivity test media should be standardized for carbohydrate content, pH, osmolality, and cation content. Excess fermentable carbohydrate will cause a change in pH of the medium during growth, which may alter the rate of growth of the bacteria and the activity of the antibiotic. The aminoglycosides and erythromycin, for example, are much less active in an acid than in an alkaline medium, whilst nitrofurantoin is more active at an acid pH. Aminoglycosides may be affected by a number of different constituents of culture media including divalent cations (Ca^{2+} and Mg^{2+}), NaCl, and phosphates. These factors may differentially affect the activity against different species of bacteria so that, for example, the activity of aminoglycosides against *Ps. aeruginosa* is particularly affected by alterations in divalent cations.

Osmolality of culture medium

The bactericidal activity of β-lactam antibiotics, which in general rely on osmotic rupture of the bacterial cell to achieve their lethal effect, is markedly influenced by the osmolality of the growth medium. Species of bacteria which have a naturally low internal osmolality, such as *Proteus mirabilis* and *Haemophilus influenzae*, are predominantly affected bacteristatically by β-lactam agents unless the osmolality of broth media is artificially reduced to below physiological levels.

Antibiotic formulation

An obvious factor which is sometimes overlooked in sensitivity testing is that the formulation of the antibiotic used must be appropriate. Although the esters of ampicillin, carbenicillin, mecillinam, cefuroxime, and erythromycin are used clinically these are antibacterially inactive pro-drugs which release the active parent compound in the body. Similarly, chloramphenicol succinate and clindamycin phosphate are inactive *in vitro* and the parent compounds should be used in laboratory tests. Sulphomethyl derivatives of polymyxins are much less active *in vitro* than are the non-sulphomethylated varieties, although they do spontaneously break down to the more active parent form on incubation.

NEWER METHODS OF SENSITIVITY TESTING

Alternative methods of assessing bacterial susceptibility to antibiotics are gradually coming into use in an effort to obtain results more quickly than by traditional procedures. Most rapid of all are the tests which detect resistance to β-lactam antibiotics by the demonstration of β-lactamase activity in the bacteria. Several methods are available which will accomplish this in a few minutes once a bacterial culture is available. However, since β-lactam agents display differential susceptibility to the various β-lactamases the tests are of limited value. They have been successfully used to detect β-lactamase-mediated resistance to penicillin and ampicillin in *Neisseria gonorrhoeae* and *H. influenzae*, which is due to one particular variety of β-lactamase (TEM-1, see Chapter 12).

Of wider applicability are those techniques which employ turbidimetry to detect antibacterial activity by comparing the growth of bacteria exposed to antibiotic with a drug-free control over a time span which for fast-growing organisms can be as little as 2 or 3 h. Several machines have been described which do this with various degrees of sophistication. Turbidimetric results show discrepancies with more traditional methods for certain bacterium/drug combinations and there is controversy about the correct interpretation of these.

Any method which measures bacterial growth or metabolism can theoretically be used to assess the influence of antibacterial agents on the normal course of events. Various techniques based on impedance measurements, bioluminescence, chemiluminescence, and microcalorimetry have been described, but none has achieved the status of a routine test.

An alternative approach that is gaining in popularity is the use of gene probes that are able to detect DNA sequences associated with resistance traits. These provide a specific and reliable means of detecting antibiotic resistance. However, because of the large array of resistance mechanisms that may be encountered, as well as other technical problems, it is likely to be some time before gene probes can be economically introduced into routine laboratory practice for sensitivity testing. They may have a particular value with problem organisms or for the detection of specific resistance mechanisms.

8
Antibiotic assay

R. C. B. Slack

In the context of antimicrobial chemotherapy, antibiotic assay means the estimation of antibiotic concentrations in serum, urine, or other body fluids at appropriate times after giving the drug. The indications to assay antimicrobial drugs in biological material in routine practice are few. However, in the development of a new drug, determination of the pharmacokinetic profile in health and disease forms an important part of the evaluation of the agent, and frequent assays in various body fluids are part of this process.

In the management of individual treatment, determination of antibiotic concentration is usually only necessary on two counts: first, with drugs of known toxicity where the adverse effect is dose related; second, to monitor efficacy when there is a narrow therapeutic range between adequate and toxic levels (Fig. 8.1). Occasionally, it may be useful to check antibiotic levels when there is reason to doubt that treatment is achieving adequate levels, for example in CSF, but this is seldom done.

In the management of some infections, of which tuberculosis is the most important, it may be necessary to check for compliance. In such cases, an indication of whether the patient is taking the medication is all that is required and the assay needs to detect only the presence of the drug rather than an accurate concentration. It is good practice to check for compliance during the months of therapy with antituberculosis drugs; rifampicin can be easily detected in urine by colorimetric methods and several qualitative tests are available for the detection of isoniazid or its metabolites.

Some workers advocate a special form of assay in the treatment of certain infections such as bacterial endocarditis, in which it is important to achieve bactericidal levels of drug. In this case a sample of the patient's serum, obtained at a period of time after administration of the antibiotic at which a peak concentration is anticipated, is titrated against the organism responsible for the infection (so-called *back-titration*). Since the object is to establish that a sufficiently high bactericidal titre is maintained it is necessary to measure the bactericidal, not just the bacteristatic end-point.

ASSAY OF AMINOGLYCOSIDES

In practice, aminoglycosides, and gentamicin in particular, are the most commonly assayed antibiotics in hospital laboratories. These drugs are excreted into urine by glomerular filtration. With degrees of renal impairment the usual interval of 8 hours between doses must be lengthened or accumulation will occur, with subsequent manifestation of the unpleasant nephrotoxic and ototoxic side-effects associated with this group of drugs (see Chapter 18). Serum for assay should be taken at a fixed time, usually 1 h after the dose is given (*peak*) and just before the next injection (*trough*). If the drug is given intravenously there will be rapid equilibration in the vascular compartment and the 1 h concentration is not a true peak, but if blood is taken at a standard time there will be comparability between assays.

The therapeutic range of gentamicin concentrations in serum is approximately 2–10 mg/l. This depends on the MIC of the infecting organism as well as the toxic concentration. As far as the latter is concerned, it is far from certain that high peak concentrations correlate simply with adverse effects. What may be of more importance is the

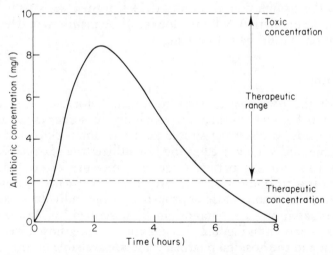

Fig. 8.1. The concept of 'therapeutic range'. An antibiotic administered to a patient at time 0 reaches a peak concentration in plasma and is subsequently eliminated. The therapeutic concentration needed to achieve an antibacterial effect (usually taken as the MIC for the infecting organism) is shown by the lower dashed line; the concentration above which toxic side-effects are known to be commonly encountered is shown by the upper dashed line. The difference between these values is the *therapeutic range*. The *therapeutic index* is the ratio of the toxic concentration to the therapeutic concentration.

area under the curve, i.e. the total concentration of drug related to time. Thus, relatively minor increases in trough levels, such as occur with minimal renal impairment, may be of more importance than high peaks.

With regular dosing a trough concentration above 2 mg/l is an indication to reduce the dose or to prolong the interval between doses. In most patients with normal renal function the gentamicin trough level is below 1 mg/l and may be undetectable by some assay methods; with a peak concentration above 5 mg/l this can be considered satisfactory. If the peak turns out to be very high, but the trough is below 2 mg/l, there is no cause to alter the dose immediately, but a further assay should be done to check the levels. If the peak is below 5 mg/l and the trough level undetectable, the dose must be increased and the assays repeated.

In patients with stable renal function it is usually necessary to perform only one set of assays (peak and trough) during therapy. Where there are fluctuations in serum creatinine (the indicator of glomerular function that is usually used) it will be necessary to monitor aminoglycoside therapy more closely.

Single daily dosing of aminoglycosides is becoming more commonly used for all patients, except the acutely ill. Peak concentrations are likely to exceed 10 mg/l soon after the large doses used in these regimens and there is little justification for assays of peak levels in these circumstances. However, the trough concentration at 24 h post-dose is vital because changes in accumulation will take longer to be manifested. The trough concentration should be below 1 mg/l.

Nomograms

Because of the necessity to start treatment before assay results are available and because of their unavailability in some areas, attempts have been made to construct simple guides to aminoglycoside dosage. A typical method widely used in the UK utilizes the sex-related serum creatinine level for the patient's age as a measure of renal function and relates this to body weight to provide a first (*loading*) dose and a subsequent *maintenance* dose appropriate to the individual patient. A nomogram based on such data, originally described by Mawer and his colleagues, is shown in Fig. 8.2. The instructions are those given by our department and the hospital pharmacy and are available on the wards in Nottingham hospitals so that junior doctors may reliably dose patients before assay results are known. The Mawer nomogram was originally devised for gentamicin and can also be used for tobramycin, but not for amikacin or netilmicin which are given in higher doses.

It should be noted that this nomogram does not apply to children or to those undergoing renal dialysis. In both these situations regular monitoring by assay is important. Children may be dosed on a weight

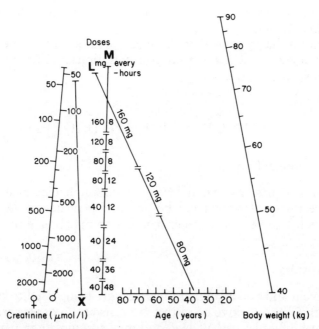

Fig. 8.2. Nomogram for determining a suitable dose regimen for gentamicin. *Instructions*—for patients not receiving dialysis treatment: 1. Join with a straight line the serum creatinine concentration appropriate to the sex on the left-hand scale, and the age on the lower scale. Mark the point at which the straight line cuts line X. 2. Join with a straight line the mark on line X and the body weight on the right-hand scale. Mark the points at which this cuts the dosage lines L and M. 3. The loading dose in milligrams is written against the mark on line L and the maintenance dose against the mark on line M.

The nomogram is designed to give serum concentrations of gentamicin within the range 5–10 mg/l 1 h after each dose. In patients with renal insufficiency it is essential to perform assays before and after the second or third maintenance dose, as this nomogram is only a guide to treatment. It is desirable in all seriously ill patients to perform at least one early assay to check that the nomogram has given an appropriate schedule for that individual patient.

NB. Patients with any degree of renal impairment are liable to ototoxicity after exposure to gentamicin, especially *if it is given with or after certain other drugs*. Patients who have had an earlier course of gentamicin, or who have had or are having any other aminoglycoside antibiotic, cephalosporin, frusemide, or other potentially nephrotoxic or ototoxic drug, should be treated with particular care—and alternative antibiotics wherever possible. [Adapted from G. E. Mawer *et al.* (1974). *British Journal of Clinical Pharmacology* 1, 45–50.]

basis; although great variations will be found when assaying their serum levels, this method is a useful guide.

Experience has shown that the manufacturers' recommended regimens often give inadequate serum concentrations, as they are calculated simply on a mg/kg basis.

ASSAY OF OTHER ANTIBIOTICS

Chloramphenicol

Monitoring of plasma and CSF levels of chloramphenicol may be needed in the treatment of neonates, who are at risk of developing the 'grey baby' syndrome because of their inability to metabolize the drug.

Glycopeptides

Vancomycin and teicoplanin are increasingly being used to treat infections with Gram-positive cocci that are resistant to other agents. These drugs have long plasma half-lives and may accumulate in patients with renal impairment. For this reason, and because of the reputation of vancomycin for toxicity, assay is often carried out. However, modern commercial preparations of vancomycin, which are of a much higher purity than earlier ones (which originally earned the nickname 'Mississippi mud'), appear to be less toxic and the necessity of monitoring plasma levels has been questioned.

ANTIBIOTIC ASSAY METHODS

Numerous methods have been described to assay various antimicrobial substances. Some compounds, such as β-lactam antibiotics and sulphonamides, lend themselves to chemical assay methods, but these are often insufficiently sensitive to measure the small amounts which may be present in body fluids and in some cases do not discriminate between active compound and inactivate metabolites. More attractive to microbiologists are bacteriological methods which directly quantify antibacterial activity.

Microbiological assay

The simplest method is to titrate the antibiotic-containing fluid against a known sensitive organism and to compare the result with a parallel titration of a standard solution of the drug in question. The standard solution should be initially prepared in a similar fluid to that of the test (serum, urine, etc.). Although the method has the virtue of simplicity it is not very accurate because test and standard are being compared in a discontinuous series of concentrations and because antibiotic titrations are inherently irreproducible within twofold limits.

More satisfactory from this point of view, and therefore more widely used, is the agar diffusion method of assay. In this test a sterile punch is used to cut a series of wells in a prearranged pattern in agar contained in a flat-bottomed plate. The agar may be seeded with the test organism prior to its distribution in dishes, so that the bacteria are in the agar, or the surface may be flooded with an appropriately diluted suspension of bacteria and allowed to dry before the wells are cut. The wells are filled with the test fluid (which may be diluted if high levels are anticipated) and a series of standard antibiotic concentrations prepared in the same body fluid as the test.

After overnight incubation at 37 °C the diameter of each inhibition zone is carefully measured (Fig. 8.3). A graph of the square of the zone diameter is plotted against the logarithm of the antibiotic concentration for the antibiotic standards. A linear relationship should be obtained if the test is working satisfactorily. The levels of antibiotic in the test fluid can then be determined by reference to the graph (Fig. 8.4).

The organism used in the assay should obviously be chosen for its sensitivity to the antibiotic in question, but should not be so sensitive that huge inhibition zones are produced by therapeutic concentrations. *Bacillus subtilis*, *Sarcinia lutea*, or the Oxford strain of *Staphylococcus aureus* are widely used. For gentamicin assay done by the microbiological method it is commonplace to use a fast-growing organism such as *Klebsiella aerogenes* so that results can be obtained within 4 or 5 hours if required. If a strain of *Klebsiella* is chosen which has a restricted susceptibility pattern, interference with the assay by other antibacterial agents can be minimized. Since the method merely detects antimicrobial activity, antibiotics other than the one being assayed may interfere with the result unless steps are taken to inactivate the other compound, or to use an organism that is resistant to it. It is essential that assay requests made to the laboratory should reveal *all* antimicrobial therapy that the patient is currently receiving.

Non-microbiological assay methods

Apart from chemical assays specifically designed for individual antimicrobial compounds and high-pressure liquid chromatography (see

Antimicrobial chemotherapy

below) most non-microbiological assays have been developed to cope with the demand for the rapid estimation of aminoglycoside levels in serum.

Enzymatic assays

Enzymatic methods utilize the susceptibility of aminoglycosides to specific adenylyl or acetyl transferase enzymes. In the presence of one or other of these enzymes, radio-labelled adenyl or acetyl groups can be transferred from ATP or acetyl coenzyme A to any gentamicin present in the sample. After removing unreacted ATP or acetyl CoA, the radio activity is measured in a scintillation counter. The method is specific, rapid, and accurate, but expensive.

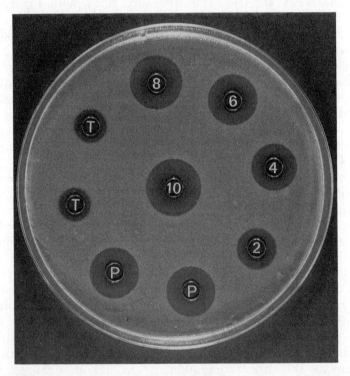

Fig. 8.3. Microbiological assay of antibiotic levels in patient's serum. Wells cut in agar (previously seeded with an indicator organism) are filled with patient's serum, or standard dilutions of antibiotic of known potency. After overnight incubation the zones of inhibition are measured, a graph is drawn from results obtained with the standards (see Fig. 8.4) and the concentration in the patient's serum is read off from the graph. In the example shown, the figures represent the concentrations of the antibiotic standards used; patient's serum was obtained 1 h after receiving a dose of antibiotic (peak level, P) and immediately before administration of the next dose (trough level, T). [Photograph courtesy of George Sharp and Richard Edwards.]

Immunoassay

Various kinds of immunoassay have been described. In all of them antibody against gentamicin, prepared in rabbits, is allowed to react with the patient's serum where it combines with any gentamicin that is present. A known amount of radio-, fluorescein-, or enzyme-labelled gentamicin is then added to the mixture and reacts with any remaining antibody. The radioactivity, fluorescence or enzyme activity is measured and the loss, compared to a control value, is proportional to the amount of gentamicin in the serum. The reagents for this test must be highly standardized and a scintillation counter, fluorimeter or spectrophotometer is required to read the result. As with transferase methods, immunoassay is rapid and precise, but expensive on reagents and equipment. These methods are available as diagnostic kits.

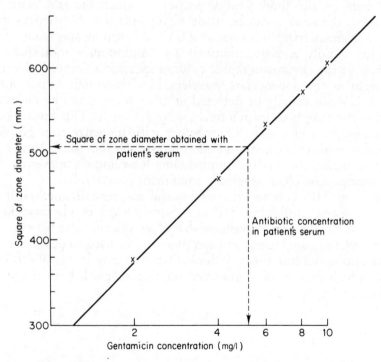

Fig. 8.4. Calibration graph used for estimating concentrations of an antibiotic in patient's serum. Values obtained with standard concentrations of the antibiotic in a test such as that depicted in Fig. 8.3 are plotted as shown. The concentration of antibiotic in the appropriate test sample can then be read off by reference to the graph. In the example shown, the patient's serum produced an inhibition zone measuring 22.5 mm in diameter (zone squared = 506 mm) indicating an antibiotic concentration of 5.1 mg/l. [Graph, based on an assay of gentamicin in serum, kindly provided by Anthony Cowlishaw.]

A commercially available polarization fluoro immunoassay system has now virtually replaced old-fashioned microbiological methods for the assay of aminoglycosides in most laboratories in the UK and other parts of the world where the cost of the machine and reagents is not prohibitive. In addition to those available for the assay of gentamicin, tobramycin, and amikacin, kits have also been developed for the assay of vancomycin and chloramphenicol.

High-pressure liquid chromatography (HPLC)

This is a development of traditional chromatographic procedures which have been used in biochemistry laboratories for many years. Compounds are separated according to their differential retention times as they are passed under pressure through a special column containing particles which delay the test substance to a greater or lesser degree depending on small variations in surface charge. By manipulating the conditions of the fluid (*mobile phase*) in which the test material is dissolved, the system can be made highly selective. Substances which have a characteristic ultra violet (UV) absorption spectrum can be detected rapidly and quantitatively by continuously monitoring the outflow of the chromatographic column spectrophotometrically, using UV light at the appropriate wavelength. Compounds which do not absorb UV can usually be detected in other ways, often by chemically treating the sample to form a fluorescent derivative. This must be done for aminoglycosides and this, together with the extraction procedure needed to remove proteins and other interfering substances from serum samples, makes the method cumbersome for routine use even in those laboratories where the necessary equipment is available.

However, HPLC is an extremely useful and versatile method for the assay of many antibiotics and it is widely used in pharmacokinetic studies. It has the great advantage that it can discriminate between very closely related compounds and can therefore be used to detect not only native antibiotic, but also any derivatives that may be produced in the body, which may display modified pharmacological, toxicological, or antibacterial properties.

9

Antibiotic interactions

D. Greenwood

When the antimicrobial activity of combinations of antibiotics is studied, several results are possible.

1. The combined effect may be greater than that which either agent alone could achieve—a small increase is generally due to simple additive effects; larger increases may indicate true *synergy*.
2. The overall effect may be reduced, in which case the combination is *antagonistic*.
3. Each compound may ignore the presence of the other and the more active compound prevails. In this case the compounds are said to show *indifference*.

SYNERGY

Antimicrobial synergy, implying the beneficial interaction between two drugs exceeding simple additive effects, may take several forms (Table 9.1). One compound may potentiate the activity of the other at a biochemical level, one may assist the other to penetrate into the bacterial cell, one may protect the other from destruction, or the two compounds may act on separate sections of the bacterial population.

Table 9.1. Types of antimicrobial synergy

Type	Mechanism	Example
Biochemical interaction	Sequential blockade Complementation	Trimethoprim–sulphonamides Mecillinam–cephalexin
Enhancement of permeability	Cell wall Cell membrane	β-lactam antibiotics Polymyxins
Protection	Enzyme inhibition	Clavulanic acid–amoxycillin
Differential population effects	Suppression of resistance	Antituberculosis drugs

Biochemical synergy

The clearest example of biochemical synergy is provided by the combination of trimethoprim and sulphonamides, which is most commonly used clinically as co-trimoxazole. Sulphonamides and diaminopyrimidines like trimethoprim interfere with sequential stages in bacterial folate synthesis. Sulphonamides cut off the folate supply at source, while trimethoprim stops regeneration of the biologically active form of the vitamin (tetrahydrofolate), which is oxidized in the course of the manufacture of thymidylic acid for nucleic acid synthesis. The complete shutting off of folate activity can be accomplished by concentrations of sulphonamides and trimethoprim which alone are ineffective or only feebly inhibitory.

Another type of double blockade occurs with some β-lactam antibiotics, typified by mecillinam, and cephalexin. These two agents induce distinct and characteristic morphological changes in susceptible Gram-negative bacilli, but together complement one another to elicit the spheroplast response which most other β-lactam agents evoke (see Fig. 1.5). The explanation of this is that mecillinam binds to a particular protein in the bacterial envelope (PBP 2; see Chapter 1) which has the effect of causing generalized surface changes in the cell wall. Cephalexin binds to a different protein (PBP 3) which is involved in bacterial division; the bacteria continue to grow, but fail to divide. When both processes are inhibited simultaneously, a region of cell wall weakness develops at the potential cleavage site as the bacteria grow, and a wall-deficient spheroplast starts to emerge at the incipient division point. Because the spheroplast is osmotically fragile it normally bursts unless osmotic protection is given, and the combination of mecillinam and cephalexin is consequently much more rapidly bactericidal than are the individual compounds. Most members of the β-lactam family do not exhibit this form of synergy simply because they are able alone to attack both the sites that mecillinam and cephalexin individually affect.

However, the potential for this sort of interaction may exist with other combinations. Imipenem and clavulanic acid, like mecillinam, bind preferentially to PBP 2 and several agents other than cephalexin (e.g. cephradine, aztreonam, and temocillin) bind almost exclusively to PBP 3. Moreover, low concentrations of most penicillins and cephalosporins have a cephalexin-like effect.

Enhancement of permeability

Many bacteria are antibiotic resistant, not because their intracellular target site is insusceptible to the drug, but because the cell manages to keep out the noxious agent. For example, the protein-synthesizing machinery of *Escherichia coli* is as susceptible to erythromycin as that of *Staphylococcus aureus*, but the drug penetrates the *Esch. coli* cell only with difficulty.

Those antibiotics which act at the level of the cell wall (e.g. β-lactam agents) or the cell membrane (e.g. polymyxins) may interfere with the cell's ability to exclude another agent. The most familiar example of this is provided by the interaction of penicillins and aminoglycosides acting against enterococci. Enterococci, like other streptococci, are resistant to aminoglycosides and the resistance is associated with failure of the drug to penetrate the cell wall. Penicillin alone, in sufficient concentration, kills enterococci relatively slowly and persisters survive prolonged exposure. In the presence of penicillins and aminoglycosides, however, the rate of killing is much increased and persisters are also killed. Studies with radioactive streptomycin have shown that this is associated with an increase in uptake of the aminoglycoside.

Aminoglycosides and β-lactam antibiotics act synergically against other species of bacteria, but the effect is not usually so dramatic as in the case of enterococci.

Protection

The resistance of bacteria to β-lactam antibiotics is generally due to bacterial enzymes (β-lactamases) which destroy the drug. This mode of resistance suggests the possibility, mooted many years ago, of using an enzyme inhibitor to allow the enzyme-labile drug to achieve its effect unscathed. Early attempts using penicillins like cloxacillin and nafcillin (which are β-lactamase stable, but have no useful activity against Gram-negative bacilli) in combination with ampicillin generally failed in the aim of overcoming the resistance of some Gram-negative bacilli. However, potent broad-spectrum enzyme inhibitors have since been developed which offer better prospects of success. One of the most active of these is the novel naturally occurring β-lactam compound, clavulanic acid, which is marketed in combination with amoxycillin or ticarcillin. Similar formulations include the penicillin sulphones, sulbactam (combined with ampicillin), and tazobactam (combined with piperacillin).

Sulbactam, which is poorly absorbed when given orally, has also been formulated as a linked ester with ampicillin to produce a so-called *mutual pro-drug*. This manoeuvre improves the oral absorption of both compounds in a similar manner to the various esters of ampicillin; as in the case of ampicillin pro-drugs (see Chapter 1), the two compounds are separated by tissue esterases as they are absorbed.

Although resistance to aminoglycosides and chloramphenicol may be mediated by enzymic mechanisms, the protection principle has not yet been applied outside the β-lactam field.

Differential population effects

If spontaneous mutation to resistance occurs with a high frequency, two or more antibiotics may be used together mutually to prevent the emergence of resistance. If the frequency of resistance is one in every million bacteria (one in 10^6) and if resistance is unlinked, the probability of double resistance occurring in a single bacterium is one in a million million (1 in 10^{12}). If three drugs are involved, the probability becomes 1 in 10^{18}. In order to contemplate this astronomical figure it might be useful to consider that this is equivalent to one triple mutant occurring in a solid mass of bacteria weighing 1000 kg.

All the major antituberculosis drugs suffer from mutational resistance problems and the mutual prevention of resistance principle has been widely and successfully used for many years in the chemotherapy of tuberculosis.

ANTAGONISM

Just as two antibacterial compounds can operate in a mutually beneficial way, they can also sometimes interfere with each other's activity.

Antagonism of bactericidal activity

The form of antagonism which has received most attention is that occurring between predominantly bacteristatic agents (such as tetracycline and chloramphenicol) and those bactericidal agents (pre-eminently, β-lactam antibiotics) which rely on cell growth to achieve their lethal effect. Clearly, if bacterial growth is rapidly halted, the bacteridical activity of such agents will be abolished.

Mutual antagonism

In most cases antagonism operates in one direction only: one substance interferes with another, but is itself unaffected. This means that if the interfering substance is the more active of a pair, its dominance will prevail and any antagonism will be undetectable.

An exception to the general one-way rule is provided by fusidic acid and some penicillins which when combined exhibit mutual antagonism against certain strains of staphylococci. Both fusidic acid and penicillin are usually bactericidal to *Staph. aureus*, but against some strains substantially less killing is observed with the combination than with either agent alone. What apparently happens is that fusidic acid prevents the growth of those cells that it does not kill and, as already stated, penicillins are unable to kill non-growing bacteria. Cell death mediated by fusidic acid is accompanied by collapse of the bacteria, suggesting a secondary effect on the bacterial cell wall following the primary inhibition of protein synthesis—perhaps because the auto-lytic/synthetic balance which occurs in normal wall growth is upset by the non-production of essential enzymes. Penicillin prevents this secondary effect on the bacterial cell wall and thus interferes with the bactericidal action of fusidic acid. It is probable that a similar interaction occurs between penicillins and other inhibitors of protein synthesis in *Staph. aureus*.

Despite the mutual antagonism that can be demonstrated in the test-tube, there is little evidence this this form of interaction has any therapeutic relevance.

Chemical interactions

Occasionally two drugs may interact chemically. Thus, in mixtures of relatively high concentrations of carbenicillin and gentamicin, the β-lactam ring of the penicillin and amino groups of the aminoglycoside interact chemically, so that both compounds are inactivated. This interaction probably has no significance at the concentrations achieved within the body, but penicillins and aminoglycosides should not be mixed together in intravenous infusions.

Some other examples of *in vitro* and *in vivo* incompatibilities are given in Chapter 18.

Dissociated resistance

An unusual form of antagonism is mediated by erythromycin in those erythromycin-resistant staphylococci that owe their resistance to an inducible methylation reaction occurring at the ribosomal binding site (see Chapter 12). Erythromycin is the specific inducer of the enzyme causing this reaction, and lincosamides and macrolides other than erythromycin do not trigger the effect. Consequently, erythromycin can antagonize these compounds by inducing resistance to them.

The phenomenon is readily shown by disc testing of staphylococci displaying dissociated resistance. A very similar reduction of the inhibi-tion zone produced by nalidixic acid and other quinolones can be caused by nitrofurantoin in some enterobacteria (Fig. 9.1), but in this case the mechanism of the antagonism is unknown.

Inducible resistance to β-lactam antibiotics, which is a feature exhib-ited by many strains of *Enterobacter* spp. and some other Gram-negative bacilli, may give rise to a similar phenomenon. Thus, potent inducers of chromosomal β-lactamases, such as cefoxitin, may cause resistance to poor inducers, such as cefotaxime.

METHODS FOR DEMONSTRATING ANTIBIOTIC INTERACTIONS

Chess-board titration

The most popular method used to detect antimicrobial interactions is the chess-board (or checker-board) titration test in which two drugs are cross-titrated against each other (Fig. 9.2). After incubation a so-called *isobologram* is constructed by plotting the inhibition of growth observed at each drug concentration on an arithmetic scale. The line of *additivity* joins the MICs of the individual drugs acting alone; a deviation of this line towards the axes of the graph suggests synergy (Fig. 9.3); a deviation away from the axes is often taken to indicate antagonism, although indifference may also produce this result. Alternatively, the summation of the *fractional inhibitory concentrations* (ΣFIC) can be calculated: if drugs A and B alone each inhibit growth at a concentration of 4 mg/l and the combination of the two inhibits growth in a mixture containing each drug at a concentration of 1 mg/l,

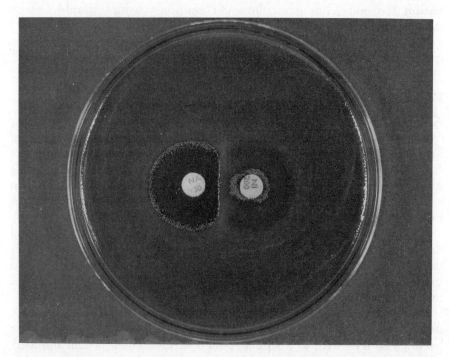

Fig. 9.1. Antagonism of nalidixic acid (NA 30) by nitrofurantoin (NI 200). [Photograph courtesy of George Sharp and Richard Edwards.]

then the ΣFIC $= \frac{1}{4} + \frac{1}{4} = \frac{1}{2}$. A ΣFIC of 1 clearly indicates simple additivity. Theoretically, a ΣFIC below 1 should indicate synergy, but in practice partial antibacterial effects below the MIC often cause apparent deviations from additivity when true synergy is absent. It is probably wise to ignore results which indicate less than a fourfold reduction in the MIC of at least one of the components.

It is often insufficiently appreciated that chess-board titrations detect only certain types of interaction. Those interactions in which it is bactericidal activity which is being potentiated or suppressed cannot usually be adequately investigated by this means. Such interactions can usually be demonstrated effectively only by carrying out viable counts at intervals and constructing killing curves. Bactericidal end-points can be measured in chess-board titrations, but this is usually unsatisfactory since it is often the rate of killing which is affected.

Agar diffusion tests

Antimicrobial synergy can often be demonstrated in agar diffusion tests as shown in Fig. 9.1 for nalidixic acid and nitrofurantoin.

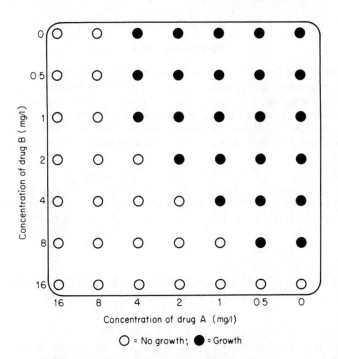

O = No growth; ● = Growth

Fig. 9.2. Chess-board titration of two drugs. The example shows synergy: the MIC of drug A alone is 8 mg/l and that of B is 16 mg/l; in combination 2 mg A plus 4 mg B per litre inhibit growth of the test organism.

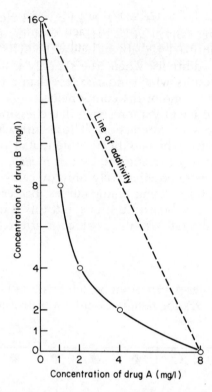

Fig. 9.3. Isobologram drawn from data presented in Fig. 9.2. The lowest concentrations of the two drugs to inhibit growth (alone and in combination) are plotted. Because the two drugs interact synergically, the resultant isobologram deviates from the line of additivity towards the axes of the graph. If the two drugs had displayed antagonism, the line would have deviated above the line of additivity. Note that, although the drugs are tested in $\log_2$ concentration steps, the results are plotted on an arithmetic scale.

   This type of test offers a visually satisfying method of demonstrating antibiotic interactions, but is insufficiently quantitative for most purposes.

THERAPEUTIC RELEVANCE OF ANTIBIOTIC INTERACTIONS

Demonstration of synergy or antagonism *in vitro* by no means guarantees that the interaction will have any relevance in treatment. Pharmacokinetic differences between agents may dictate that the compounds do not meet in the body in a ratio which has been shown to interact in the laboratory. Even when interacting compounds are carefully chosen to ensure comparable pharmacokinetics, crucial factors militating against the interaction may be overlooked. The synergy between trimethoprim and sulphonamides is so striking when tested in chess-board titrations that the possibility of using trimethoprim alone was scarcely considered for many years. It is now clear, however, that, in most clinical situations, trimethoprim alone is equally effective. In urinary tract infection, a major indication for co-trimoxazole therapy, the concentration of trimethoprim achieved in urine is so far above the minimum inhibitory concentration that the slower-acting sulphonamide gets no opportunity to act. In tissue infections, in which lower concentrations may be involved, differential partition of trimethoprim and sulphonamides into intra- and extracellular compartments may prevent their interaction.

In fact, only a few antimicrobial interactions have been proven to have therapeutic relevance. These include: the interaction between penicillin and aminoglycosides in enterococcal endocarditis, the avoidance of resistance by triple therapy in tuberculosis, the protection of β-lactam agents by β-lactamase inhibitors, and the antagonism between tetracycline and penicillin in pneumococcal meningitis.

10

Use of the laboratory

R. C. B. Slack

This book is about antimicrobial therapy and is not intended as a treatise on clinical laboratory microbiology. However, basic microbiological principles must be understood in order to appreciate the scope and limitations of laboratory control of antimicrobial therapy in the individual patient, and the object of this chapter is to fill in a little of this background.

There is still more art to the science of microbiology than to other branches of clinical pathology. There is, for example, more scope for singular methods of processing specimens and for individual interpretation of results in examining a specimen of sputum than in measuring plasma urea. Very often the methods used depend on the experience and preferences of the individual microbiologist. In some countries attempts have been made to bring about more standardization of microbiological methods (in particular antibiotic susceptibility testing), but standardization does not guarantee that the correct result is always obtained!

SPECIMEN COLLECTION

Clinical laboratories rely on the quality of the specimens they receive; none more so than microbiology departments where the 'result' of culture may depend on the degree of care observed in taking the specimen. A single extraneous bacterium introduced into a blood culture during collection may contaminate the culture, resulting in a false positive result. This is one of the many slips that can totally alter laboratory results and may, on occasion, be detrimental to the patient.

A few of the more common problems are listed.

1. *Inappropriate specimen*: saliva is submitted instead of sputum; a superficial skin swab is taken instead of a swab of pus (a specimen of pus in a sterile bottle is always preferable to a swab when possible).

2. *Inadequate specimen*: the specimen may be too small (especially fluids for culture for tubercle bacilli); rectal swabs are no substitute for faeces.

3. *Wrong timing*: specimens taken after the start of chemotherapy, when the causative organism may no longer be demonstrable, or after the patient has recovered—it is not uncommon for the laboratory to receive rock-hard faeces from patients with 'diarrhoea'.

4. *Wrong container*: blood for culture put in a plain (sometimes unsterile) bottle instead of the correct culture fluid; biopsies put into bactericidal fixatives.

5. *Clerical errors*: incorrect labelling; incomplete or misleading information on request forms.

SPECIMEN TRANSPORT

Not only must the specimen be collected properly, but it must also be received in the laboratory in good condition. Prompt transport to the laboratory is essential. Material submitted for culture is alive; any delay in reaching the optimal cultural conditions will result in loss of viability. With fastidious organisms such as gonococci or viruses this may result in failure to isolate the organism. The converse problem—overgrowth of pathogens by fast-growing commensals—also commonly occurs during the period between collection of the specimen and processing in the laboratory.

The ideal would be to eliminate transport problems by inoculating appropriate culture media at the bedside and incubating them immediately. This may be achieved in special units with laboratories attached, but is not practicable in most situations. An exception is blood culture where the counsel of perfection should apply.

The nearest approach to 'culture in transit' that has been widely adopted is the dip-culture method for culture of urine. For swabs, most laboratories recommend a form of suspended animation in which the specimen is placed in a special transport medium comprising soft buffered agar containing charcoal to inactivate any toxic substances.

Specimens from potential medical emergencies, such as bacterial meningitis or malaria, should be delivered to the laboratory immediately (and it should not be below the dignity of a doctor to do this!) and brought to the attention of a senior member of the laboratory staff.

SPECIMEN PROCESSING

The flow diagram (Fig. 10.1) outlines the three main steps which occur for every bacteriological request: microscopy, culture, identification and

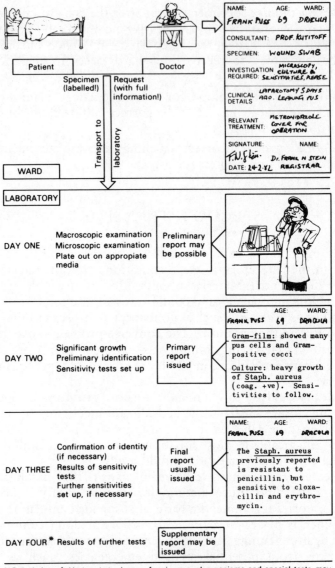

Patient — **Doctor**

Specimen (labelled!) | Request (with full information!)

Transport to laboratory

WARD

Request card:

NAME:	AGE:	WARD:
FRANK PUSS	69	DRACULA

CONSULTANT: PROF. KUTITOFF

SPECIMEN: WOUND SWAB

INVESTIGATION REQUIRED: MICROSCOPY, CULTURE & SENSITIVITIES, PLEASE

CLINICAL DETAILS: LAPAROTOMY 5 DAYS AGO. LEAKING PUS

RELEVANT TREATMENT: METRONIDAZOLE COVER FOR OPERATION

SIGNATURE: F.N.Stein. NAME: Dr. FRANK N STEIN

DATE: 24.2.82 REGISTRAR

LABORATORY

DAY ONE
Macroscopic examination
Microscopic examination
Plate out on appropiate media

Preliminary report may be possible

DAY TWO
Significant growth
Preliminary identification
Sensitivity tests set up

Primary report issued

NAME:	AGE:	WARD:
FRANK PUSS	69	DRACULA

<u>Gram-film:</u> showed many pus cells and Gram-positive cocci

<u>Culture:</u> heavy growth of <u>Staph.</u> aureus (coag. +ve). Sensitivities to follow.

DAY THREE
Confirmation of identity (if necessary)
Results of sensitivity tests
Further sensitivities set up, if necessary

Final report usually issued

NAME:	AGE:	WARD:
FRANK PUSS	69	DRACOLA

The <u>Staph. aureus</u> previously reported is resistant to penicillin, but sensitive to cloxacillin and erythromycin.

DAY FOUR * Results of further tests

Supplementary report may be issued

*N.B. isolation of *M.tuberculosis* viruses, fungi, unusual organisms and special tests may take longer

Fig. 10.1. Flow diagram showing the various steps between obtaining a specimen from a patient and the issue of the final report. Note the importance of the period before the specimen arrives in the laboratory: unless the specimen is properly taken and transported it may be useless and unless the request card is properly completed wrong tests may be done.

sensitivity testing. Even with the most rapidly growing bacteria and with improved methods, results of culture and sensitivity often take 48 hours. This may be further delayed if there is a mixture of organisms or if slowgrowing pathogens, such as *Mycobacterium tuberculosis* or viruses, are involved. Not all micro-organisms are readily cultivable and a report of 'Sterile' or 'No growth' does not definitively mean that the specimen contained no organisms, but that the laboratory was unable to isolate any from the specimen.

Because of the inevitable delay in obtaining culture results there is a need to inform clinicians of really important findings before the complete results are known. Microscopical findings are usually available on the same day as the specimen is received and in urgent cases can be reported within 1 hour or less. For example, a Gram-film of CSF can be done very quickly and may give the physician a reliable guide to primary therapy (which may be life saving) while waiting for cultural confirmation of the result. Similarly, positive blood cultures and other findings serious to the individual patient or his immediate contacts are usually telephoned directly to the doctor. Where the antibiotic sensitivity is predictable (e.g. *Streptococcus pyogenes* is always sensitive to penicillin) this advice may be given with the initial report. With many bacteria the report 'sensitivity to follow' is all that can be imparted before sensitivity testing, although a 'best guess' based on known patterns of resistance in the hospital or community may be suggested.

SIGNIFICANT ISOLATIONS

Although many diseases have a well-defined microbial aetiology, the information obtained about patients and the data accrued from the laboratory examination of their specimens are often too sparse to form a complete opinion as to the microbial cause in an individual case. Most patients with infection survive and many improve so rapidly that the significance of microbes isolated is never known. Thus, although we know from historical and epidemiological evidence that *Str. pyogenes* causes tonsillitis and is involved in the aetiology of rheumatic fever, when an individual patient presents with joint pains following a sore throat we cannot be absolutely sure that the *Str. pyogenes* in his throat is the cause of his illness, since we know, also on epidemiological evidence, that these bacteria are carried normally in the pharynx of about 5 per cent of the community, and sore throat is often due to other causes. In such situations, additional information (such as raised antistreptolysin O antibodies in the serum in this case) may be needed in order to establish a causal relationship.

The greatest difficulty is encountered with specimens from areas of the body which have a resident microbial flora which may sometimes assume a pathogenic role. Isolations from respiratory sources are often the most difficult to interpret. Demonstration of *M. tuberculosis* is always a significant finding and even in the absence of clinical disease the patient must be further examined and treated. This organism, a recognized cause of tuberculosis from the time of Koch, is a true human pathogen and is high on anyone's list of 'wanted bacteria'. On the other hand *Candida albicans* would often be thought of as a harmless commensal, although it can cause serious disease in immunocompromised patients. The ability of some organisms to strike whilst the host defences are down has given these the title *opportunist* pathogens. However, merely by looking at cultures of these opportunists, it is impossible to say in a particular case whether or not they are adopting a pathogenic role and laboratory personnel have to make an informed guess as to their significance based on ancillary findings (e.g. presence or absence of pus; numbers of organisms isolated) and clinical information provided on the request card. If the latter is absent, non-contributory or misleading, as it frequently is, the report may be valueless.

In the absence of adequate guidance, the laboratory can adopt one of two approaches: report any microbe isolated regardless of any possible significance or report only common pathogens and dismiss all the others as 'normal flora'.

The importance of this to ultimate laboratory control of antimicrobial therapy is that if the isolate is not considered 'significant', no further work, including sensitivity tests, will be carried out. The corollary is that many sensitivities may be tested and reported on organisms that have no role in the patient's disease. This occurs more commonly than is usually admitted. Many patients receive potentially toxic antimicrobials because commensal bacteria isolated from a badly taken specimen were considered significant and sensitivity tests reported. Sometimes a great deal of effort and expense is put into treating colonizing organisms which are merely filling a vacuum left by the normal flora and which would quietly disappear if antimicrobial chemotherapy were withheld.

Non-cultural methods

Rapid advances in immunological and molecular techniques have provided an array of antigen and DNA detection methods. Although these tests are not widely available at present for bacterial pathogens they are increasingly being used to make a viral diagnosis. If the only way to confirm a diagnosis is by finding non-viable microbial products it will not be possible to perform antimicrobial susceptibility tests. Specific treatment will be based on general principles and guesswork. However, the sequences of many genes conferring antibiotic resistance in human pathogens have been characterized and 'probes' made which can recognize, for example, the different TEM β-lactamases (see Chapter 12). New or unusual mechanisms of resistance cannot be detected by these methods; nor is it possible to be certain that any gene found is expressed *in vivo*.

WHAT THE LABORATORY REPORTS

The final report reaching the clinician must be self-explanatory, even dogmatic. It is not practicable, or desirable, to test each organism isolated against all antibiotics. What usually happens is that a restricted range of antimicrobials is tested against isolates considered significant with a different selection for Gram-positive and Gram-negative bacteria. Primary testing can often be restricted to a few old and well-tried agents that are perfectly adequate for most common infections (Table 10.1). More extensive testing, particularly of expensive, broad-spectrum agents, should be reserved for resistant isolates or bacteria from patients with serious infections that are presenting problems of management. Usually, only two or three of the sensitivities tested are reported even if more are performed. Restricted reporting has the important function of reinforcing local antibiotic policies and of discouraging clinicians from using inappropriate agents. Additional tests carried out, but not reported, are often useful if the patient fails to respond to the chosen agent or is hypersensitive to it. Testing many agents also provides useful epidemiological information of trends of antimicrobial susceptibility in the community and of clusters of multiply resistant bacteria, indicating cross-infection or spread from a common source.

Most infections are caused by a single organism, often a well-known pathogen. In these cases there is usually no problem in deciding what to test and report. However, some specimens (e.g. those from abdominal wounds) are often infected with mixtures of organisms and each must be individually identified and tested against appropriate antimicrobials.

The choice of antibiotic tested varies with the site of infection and the pharmacological properties of the drug. Some agents, such as nitrofurantoin and nalidixic acid, achieve therapeutic concentrations only in urine and are of no value in other infections. Information about the individual patient may alter drug testing; if the patient is allergic to penicillins alternatives will be sought; in pregnancy, sulphonamides and trimethoprim should be avoided if possible because of the risk of folate deficiency; tetracyclines should not be used in late pregnancy or in young children owing to deposition in teeth. These limitations of sensitivity testing can be taken into account by

Table 10.1. Examples of a restricted range of antimicrobial agents selected for primary sensitivity testing of some common pathogens

Organism	Antimicrobial agents tested
Staphylococcus aureus	Benzylpenicillin Flucloxacillin (methicillin) Erythromycin
Streptococcus pyogenes (and other streptococci)	Benzylpenicillin Erythromycin
Anaerobes	Benzylpenicillin Clindamycin Metronidazole
Escherichia coli (and other enterobacteria)	Ampicillin (amoxycillin) Trimethoprim Cephalosporins* Gentamicin
Pseudomonas aeruginosa	Azlocillin (ticarcillin) Gentamicin (tobramycin) Ciprofloxacin (ofloxacin)
Urinary isolates	Ampicillin (amoxycillin) Trimethoprim Sulphonamides Nalidixic acid Nitrofurantoin

*A representative of the earlier cephalosporins, such as cephalexin is usually chosen for primary testing.

the laboratory only if the appropriate information is given on the request card.

Restrictions imposed by the large number of available antibiotics may be approached in various ways. Some groups of agents, such as sulphonamides or tetracyclines, are so similar in terms of their antibacterial spectrum that only one representative of each needs to be tested. With other drugs where there is differential susceptibility of bacteria to different members of the group, such a decision is less easy. An organism sensitive to cephalexin, one of the earliest cephalosporins, is also usually sensitive to all subsequent members of that group and this is often used as a screen for cephalosporin-sensitive bacteria. However, the converse is not true; an organism resistant to cephalexin may be sensitive to later cephalosporins and a definitive statement in this regard can be made only by testing the appropriate compound. The same principle applies to nalidixic acid and newer, more active quinolones.

INTERPRETING SENSITIVITY REPORTS

The report to the clinician shown in Fig. 10.1 tells him that *Staphylococcus aureus* is the likely causative organism of the wound infection and that penicillin would be inappropriate, but that erythromycin or cloxacillin would be useful. The statement 'this organism is resistant to penicillin' means that penicillin would not influence the outcome. The infection may well improve due to host defences or to adequate drainage of pus, but since penicillin-resistant staphylococci are invariably β-lactamase producers any penicillin which reached the wound would be rapidly destroyed. Such a statement is based on sound laboratory and clinical evidence. On the other hand, with bacteria of relatively low-level resistance (i.e. where disc testing shows inhibition of growth which is less than that produced using a sensitive control organism) the statement of resistance is more difficult to determine and depends on such factors as site of infection and drug penetration. The laboratory will try to weigh up the evidence and score the result as *sensitive* or *resistant*, or may play safe by using the rather unsatisfactory phrase *reduced* or *intermediate sensitivity*.

The statement 'this organism is sensitive to cloxacillin' implies that use of this antibiotic (or a related β-lactamase-stable penicillin) would influence the outcome. This is more difficult to support than a statement about resistance. Treatment with the antibiotic may elicit little response in the patient because insufficient drug may have penetrated into a large collection of pus. More importantly (although unlikely in the present example, since *Staph. aureus* is commonly incriminated in infected wounds) the wrong organism may have been tested. One crucial limitation of the report to the clinician is that the innocent bystander was picked from a collection of bacteria isolated.

Assuming the correct organism and antimicrobials were tested and the results as good as possible in the laboratory, there is still a large gap between saying the isolate is sensitive and saying that the patient will recover from the infection. Many of the host factors influencing the outcome will be described in Chapter 15.

CONCLUSION

The use of the laboratory requires a brain at both ends: thought in the request and in the collection of specimens and thought in the processing of the specimens and in the production of the end report in the laboratory. The final synthesis of interpretation and action based on the report depends on cooperation between clinicians and microbiologists, so that each knows what the other requires. Microbiological expertise is available in most centres to advise on antimicrobial therapy and it is in the interests of the patients to use it. Many laboratories have virology departments and many of the points on specimen collection also apply to virus investigations. When in doubt, the laboratory should be consulted. For unusual diseases and problem cases it is often possible to seek help from specialized units such as tropical hospitals and institutes. In some countries reference laboratories are available which provide expertise in particular areas. In the UK many of these operate under the aegis of the Public Health Laboratory Service at Colindale. Worldwide, the Centers for Disease Control (CDC) Atlanta, Georgia, USA, offer a service for the diagnosis and therapy of unusual infectious diseases.

Part III

Resistance to antimicrobial agents

11

The problem of resistance

K. J. Towner

DEFINITION OF RESISTANCE

Bacterial isolates have been labelled *sensitive* or *resistant* to antimicrobial agents ever since such agents were brought into use. Some of the criteria on which this categorization has been based have been discussed already in Chapter 7, where the concepts of the minimum inhibitory and minimum bactericidal concentrations (MIC and MBC) of an antibiotic have also been described. The decision as to whether a given bacterial isolate should be labelled sensitive or resistant depends ultimately on the likelihood that an infection with that organism can be expected to respond to treatment with a given drug, but microbiologists and clinicians have become accustomed to the idea that an organism is 'resistant' when it is inhibited *in vitro* by an antibiotic concentration which is greater than that achievable *in vivo*. Unfortunately, making a true judgement is somewhat less straightforward than this traditional working definition, since there is usually no simple relationship between the MIC (or MBC) of an antibiotic and clinical response. Therapeutic success depends not only on the activity of the antimicrobial agent against the infecting organisms, but relies also on the drug reaching the site of infection in sufficient concentration (i.e. its pharmacokinetic behaviour) and the contribution that the host's own defences are able to make towards clearance of the offending microbes.

INTRINSIC RESISTANCE

If whole bacterial species are considered, rather than individual isolates, it is apparent immediately that bacterial species are not all intrinsically sensitive to all antibiotics (Table 11.1). Species vary widely in this respect and, for example, a coliform infection would not be treated with erythromycin, or a streptococcal infection with an aminoglycoside, since the organisms are intrinsically resistant to these drugs. Similarly, *Pseudomonas aeruginosa* and *Mycobacterium tuberculosis* are intrinsically resistant to most of the agents used to treat more tractable infections. Such intrinsically resistant organisms are

Table 11.1. Effective antimicrobial spectrum of some of the most commonly used antibacterial agents

Organism	Penicillins	Cephalosporins	Aminoglycosides	Tetracyclines	Macrolides	Chloramphenicol	Quinolones*	Sulphonamides	Trimethoprim	Metronidazole	Glycopeptides
Gram-positive bacteria											
Staph. aureus	V	S	(S)	(S)	(S)	S	V	(S)	(S)	R	S
Str. pyogenes	S	S	R	(S)	S	S	V	(S)	S	R	S
Other streptococci	V	S	R	(S)	S	S	V	(S)	S	R	S
Enterococci	S	R	R	(S)	S	S	V	(S)	(S)	R	(S)
Clostridium spp.	S	S	R	S	S	S	R	(S)	R	S	S
Gram-negative bacteria											
Esch. coli	V	V	(S)	(S)	R	(S)	S	(S)	(S)	R	R
Other enterobacteria	V	V	(S)	(S)	R	(S)	S	(S)	(S)	R	R
Ps. aeruginosa	V	V	V	R	R	R	S	R	R	R	R
H. influenzae	V	V	R	(S)	S	S	S	(S)	(S)	R	R
Neisseria spp.	V	S	R	(S)	S	S	S	(S)	R	R	R
Bacteroides spp.	R	V	R	(S)	S	S	R	(S)	R	S	R
Other organisms											
Mycobacteria	R	R	V	R	R	R	S	R	R	R	R
Chlamydia	R	R	R	S	S	S	S	S	R	R	R
Mycoplasmas	R	R	R	S	S	S	S	R	R	R	R
Fungi	R	R	R	R	R	R	R	R	R	R	R

S = usually considered sensitive; R = usually considered resistant; (S) = strain variation in sensitivity; V = variation among related drugs and/or strains.
*Refers to newer fluoroquinolones such as ciprofloxacin etc., not to nalidixic acid and earlier congeners.

sometimes termed *insensitive*, with the term *resistant* reserved for variants of normally susceptible species that acquire the protection of resistance traits.

The most obvious determinant of bacterial response to an antibiotic, and hence intrinsic resistance, is the presence or absence of the target for the drug's action. Thus polyene antibiotics, such as amphotericin B, kill fungi by binding tightly to the sterols in the fungal cell membrane and altering the permeability of the fungal cell. Since bacterial membranes do not contain sterols, bacteria are intrinsically resistant to this class of antibiotics. Similarly, the lipopolysaccharide outer envelope of Gram-negative bacteria is important in determining sensitivity patterns, since many antibiotics cannot penetrate this barrier to reach their intracellular target.

Fortunately, intrinsic resistance is often predictable in a clinical situation, and should not pose problems provided that an informed and judicious choice is made of appropriate antimicrobial therapy. Of greater concern is the acquisition or emergence of resistance in previously sensitive bacterial species, sometimes during the course of therapy itself.

ACQUIRED RESISTANCE

Introduction of clinically effective antimicrobial agents has been followed invariably by the rapid emergence of resistant strains of bacteria belonging to species that would normally be considered to be sensitive. This phenomenon of initial success followed by the emergence of resistance has been repeated many times. Acquisition of resistance has seriously reduced the therapeutic value of many important antibiotics, but is also a major stimulus to the pharmaceutical industry in its constant search for new and more effective antimicrobial drugs.

The first systematic observations of acquired drug resistance were made by Paul Ehrlich between 1902 and 1909 while using azo dyes, organic arsenicals, and triphenylmethane derivatives to treat mice infected experimentally with trypanosomes. However, antibacterial chemotherapy really started with the introduction into clinical practice of sulphonamides in 1935 and penicillin in 1941. Within a very few years, micro-organisms described originally as being susceptible to these agents were found to have acquired resistance. *Neisseria gonorrhoeae* is an outstanding example. In 1938 almost all strains of this organism were susceptible to sulphonamides, but by 1948 less than 20 per cent of clinical isolates retained susceptibility and, as a consequence, sulphonamides were no longer used regularly in the treatment of gonorrhoea. Less dramatic increases in sulphonamide resistance were also observed with haemolytic streptococci, pneumococci, coliforms, and many other bacteria.

Similarly, when penicillin came into use in the early 1940s, less than 1 per cent of all strains of *Staphylococcus aureus* were resistant to its action. By 1946, under the selective pressure of this antibiotic, the proportion of penicillin-resistant strains found in hospitals had risen to 14 per cent. A year later, 38 per cent were resistant, and today resistance is found in more than 90 per cent of all strains of *Staph. aureus*. In contrast, over the same period, an equally important pathogen, *Streptococcus pyogenes*, has remained more or less uniformly sensitive, although there is no guarantee that resistance will not spread to *Str. pyogenes* in future years.

There is no easy explanation for the marked observed differences in the acquisition of resistance between different species, but it is clear that simple possession of the genetic capacity for resistance does not always explain its prevalence in a particular species. Even when selection pressures are similar, the end result may not be the same. Thus, although about 90 per cent of all strains of *Staph. aureus* are now resistant to penicillin, the same has not happened to sulphonamide or ampicillin resistance in *Escherichia coli* under ostensibly similar selection pressure. At the present time, apart from localized outbreaks involving epidemic strains, about 30–40 per cent of *Esch. coli* strains are resistant to sulphonamides or ampicillin, and this level has remained more or less steady for a number of years. However, since an increasing incidence of resistance is at least partly a consequence of selective pressure, it is not surprising that the withdrawal of an antibiotic from clinical use may often, but not always, result in a slow reduction in the number of resistant strains encountered in a particular environment.

The introduction of new antibiotics has also resulted in changes to the predominant spectrum of organisms responsible for infections. Thus the 1960s saw the introduction of the semi-synthetic 'β-lactamase stable' penicillins and cephalosporins which temporarily solved the problem of staphylococcal infections. Unfortunately, Gram-negative bacteria then became the major pathogens found in hospitals, and rapidly acquired resistance to multiple antibiotics in the succeeding years. In the 1970s the pendulum swung the other way with the first outbreaks of hospital infection with multi-resistant staphylococci, which can be resistant to nearly all antistaphylococcal agents. Outbreaks of infection caused by such organisms have occurred subsequently all over the world.

Use of vancomycin in response to this problem provides an excellent illustration of the way in which extensive use of a drug can be a major factor in the spread of resistance. Vancomycin was used infrequently for at least 30 years (partly because it was too toxic in its original impure form) without the development of any significant resistance. Less toxic preparations are now available and the use of vancomycin has increased dramatically. It is thus no great surprise that resistance to vancomycin has now emerged in enterococci, with the potential for spread to *Staph. aureus* and coagulase-negative staphylococci.

Types of acquired resistance

Two main types of acquired resistance may be encountered in bacterial species that would normally be considered sensitive to a particular antibacterial agent.

Mutational resistance
In any large population of bacterial cells a very few individual cells may spontaneously become resistant (see Chapter 13). Such resistant cells have no particular survival advantage in the absence of antibiotic, but

following the introduction of antibiotic treatment all sensitive bacterial cells will be killed, so that the (initially) very few resistant cells can proliferate until they eventually form a wholly resistant population. Many antimicrobial agents have been shown to select, both *in vitro* and *in vivo*, for this type of acquired resistance in many different bacterial species. The problem has been recognized as being of particular importance in the long-term treatment of tuberculosis with antituberculous drugs.

Transmissible resistance

A more spectacular type of acquired resistance occurs when genes conferring antibiotic resistance transfer from a resistant bacterial cell to a sensitive one. The simultaneous transfer of resistance to several unrelated antimicrobial agents can be demonstrated readily, both in the laboratory and in the patient. Exponential transfer and spread of existing resistance genes through a previously sensitive bacterial population is a much more efficient mechanism of acquiring resistance than is the development of resistance by mutation of individual sensitive cells.

Mechanisms by which transfer of resistance genes takes place are discussed in Chapter 13. Here it is sufficient to stress that, however resistance appears in a hitherto sensitive bacterial cell or population, it will only become widespread under the selective pressures produced by the presence of appropriate antibiotics. Also, the development of resistant cells does not have to happen often or on a large scale. A single mutation or transfer event can, if the appropriate selective pressures are operating, lead to the replacement of a sensitive population by a resistant one. Without selective pressure, antibiotic resistance may be a handicap rather than an asset to a bacterium.

CROSS-RESISTANCE AND MULTIPLE RESISTANCE

These terms are often confused. *Cross-resistance* involves resistance to a number of different members of a group of chemically related agents which are affected alike by the same resistance mechanism. For instance, there is almost complete cross-resistance between the different tetracyclines since tetracycline resistance results largely from an efflux mechanism which affects all members of the group. The situation is more complex in other antibiotic groups. Thus, resistance to aminoglycosides may be mediated by any one of a number of different drug-inactivating enzymes (see Chapter 12) with different substrate specificities, and the range of aminoglycosides to which the organism is resistant will depend on which enzyme it produces. Cross-resistance can also be observed occasionally between unrelated antibiotics. For example, a change in the outer membrane structure of Gram-negative bacilli may concomitantly deny access of unrelated compounds to their target sites.

In contrast, *multiple drug resistance* involves a bacterium becoming resistant to several unrelated antibiotics by different resistance mechanisms. For example, if a staphylococcus is resistant to penicillin, gentamicin, and tetracycline, the resistances must have arisen independently, since the strain destroys the penicillin with a β-lactamase, inactivates gentamicin with an aminoglycoside-modifying enzyme, and excludes tetracycline from the cell by an active efflux mechanism.

It is not always clear whether cross-resistance or multiple resistance is being observed. Genes conferring resistance to several unrelated agents can be transferred *en bloc* from one bacterial cell to another on plasmids (see Chapter 13), thereby giving the appearance of cross-resistance. In such cases, detailed biochemical and genetical analysis may be required to prove that the resistance mechanisms are distinct (multiple resistance), although the genes conferring resistance are linked and transferred together on one plasmid.

THE CLINICAL PROBLEM OF DRUG RESISTANCE

There is concern that antibiotic resistance is becoming so commonplace that the next century will resemble the pre-antibiotic era. However, it is important not to overstate the problem: most infections are still readily treatable with old and reliable agents. None the less, the problem is global and is becoming more serious; in future years there is a real possibility that physicians will be faced increasingly with infections for which effective treatment is not available.

Enterobacteria

The prevalence of resistance in hospital strains of Enterobacteriaceae has been increasing steadily for the past 20 years, particularly in large units, and although cephalosporins, quinolones, and aminoglycosides have been developed to cope with the problem, resistance to these newer compounds is already starting to emerge. Epidemics of diarrhoeal disease caused by multi-resistant strains of intestinal pathogens, including *Vibrio cholerae*, shigellae, salmonellae, and toxin-producing strains of *Esch. coli*, have occurred around the world, especially in South East Asia and Africa. Widespread resistance is a particular problem in less-developed areas of the world where heavy and indiscriminate use of antibiotics may combine with a high prevalence of drug-resistant bacteria in the faecal flora, poor standards of sanitation, and a high incidence of diarrhoeal disease to encourage the rapid emergence and spread of multi-resistant strains of enteric bacteria.

Staphylococci and enterococci

So far as developed countries are concerned, methicillin-resistant *Staph. aureus* (MRSA) continue to to cause outbreaks in some hospitals and are endemic in others. Coagulase-negative staphylococci and enterococci are gaining importance as multi-resistant pathogens causing infections that are difficult to treat. A combination of antibiotics may be required to treat serious enterococcal infections, but the emergence of high-level aminoglycoside resistance may seriously limit this option. Enterococci carrying genes conferring resistance to glycopeptide antibiotics have also been reported, and it may be only a matter of time before such resistance genes find their way into staphylococci.

Pneumococci

Another major problem concerns the emergence of resistance in *Streptococcus pneumoniae*, a common cause of community-acquired pneumonia and other forms of sepsis. This organism was, until recently, combated easily by treatment with penicillin and its derivatives. Unfortunately, *Str. pneumoniae* isolates with resistance to most antibiotics can now be found, albeit infrequently, in most countries of the world. In some countries the situation is serious. Such infections are presently treatable with vancomycin and broad-spectrum cephalosporins, but the range of alternative treatments is narrowing.

Haemophilus and *Neisseria*

Resistance is also becoming a problem with the two other major causative organisms of bacterial meningitis. Strains of *Haemophilus influenzae* with resistance to ampicillin and chloramphenicol (or both) have been reported from a number of countries. The frequency of resistance is increasing gradually, but with explosive increases in resistance being reported from some countries. Thus, in Barcelona, Spain, more than half of the strains of *H. influenzae* isolated from patients with meningitis have been reported to be resistant to both ampicillin and chloramphenicol. Decreased susceptibility to penicillin in isolates of *Neisseria meningitidis* has also been a particular problem in Spain (20 per cent of isolates in 1987–9), but is also occasionally encountered in other countries, including the UK. The emergence of resistance to these long-term mainstays of therapy has important implications, since life-threatening infections caused by these organisms need immediate treatment.

Tuberculosis

A further emergent resistance problem involves strains of *M. tuberculosis* that are multi-resistant to isoniazid, ethambutol, rifampicin, and streptomycin. Infections caused by such strains have been seen mainly with HIV-infected patients, but transmission to health-care workers has also occurred. This problem can be expected to grow because of the general susceptibility to tuberculosis in certain populations, the difficulty of ensuring compliance with treatment regimens, and the ineffectiveness of conventional prophylaxis against resistant strains.

Problems of 'blind' therapy

In most situations in which antimicrobial agents need to be used, treatment must be started, and is often completed, without the benefit of laboratory help. This is true both in domiciliary practice, where access to the laboratory may be limited, and also in hospitals, where severe infections need treatment urgently and there is often no time to wait for culture (and sensitivity) results from the specimens taken. Even if the infecting organism is recognized to be multi-resistant and therapy is chosen accordingly, treatment failures may still occur simply because such infections tend to be associated with critically ill patients who have impaired host defences or have been subjected to invasive procedures. Such patients have often already received antibiotics, are older, or have already been confined to hospital for prolonged periods.

Drug resistance is a significant clinical problem because it limits the number of therapeutically effective agents, puts constraints on those which can be used, and sometimes forces the use of more expensive, more toxic, or otherwise more difficult agents than would be chosen normally. In any clinical situation there is therefore a need for knowledge of local resistance trends. Indeed, under circumstances where access to a microbiology laboratory is difficult or ruled out because of time constraints, such information is vital for a judicious and informed choice of appropriate antimicrobial therapy. It is also of paramount importance that the development and spread of resistance should be contained by sensible prescribing and by the implementation of agreed control of infection policies. Many hospitals now have Control of Infection teams of doctors (normally microbiologists) and nurses who have a roving commission to investigate outbreaks of infection. Such intervention is crucial in the containment of the spread of antibiotic resistance and in the preservation of the effectiveness of the antimicrobial agents remaining in the armamentarium (see Chapter 14).

12

Mechanisms of acquired resistance

K. J. Towner

Three conditions must be met in order that a particular antimicrobial agent can inhibit sensitive bacteria.

1. A vital target susceptible to the action of a low concentration of the antibiotic must exist in the bacterial cell.
2. The antibiotic must be able to reach the target.
3. The antibiotic must not be inactivated before binding to the target.

The targets of individual antibiotics are often enzymes or other essential proteins. Most antimicrobial agents have to pass through the cell wall and outer membranes to reach their target, and many are carried into the cell by active transport mechanisms that are occupied more normally in transporting sugars and other beneficial substances. Almost alone among the clinically useful antibacterial agents, polymyxins exert their effects at the cell surface by disrupting the cell membranes from the outside in a way which resembles the action of some detergents.

Some of the differences in susceptibility of bacterial species are related to differences in cell wall structure. For example, the cell envelope of Gram-negative bacteria is a more complex structure than the Gram-positive cell wall and offers a relatively greater barrier to many antibiotics, including penicillins and macrolides, while polymyxins attack the Gram-negative outer membrane which is not present in Gram-positive cells.

Resistant bacteria were classified originally into two groups: those able to grow in the presence of levels of unmodified antibiotic lethal to sensitive cells, and those able to destroy or otherwise inactivate the drug. It is now considered more useful to subdivide the mechanisms by which resistance can arise into four major groups. These are:

(1) destruction or inactivation of the antibiotic;
(2) an alteration of the target site to reduce or eliminate binding of the antibiotic to the target;
(3) a reduction in cell surface permeability or blockage of the mechanism by which the antibiotic enters the cell;

Table 12.1. Important known resistance mechanisms for the major groups of antibiotics

Inactivation or modification	Altered target site	Reduced permeability or access	Metabolic by-pass
β-Lactam antibiotics	β-Lactam antibiotics	Tetracyclines*	Trimethoprim
Chloramphenicol	Streptomycin	β-Lactam antibiotics	Sulphonamides
Aminoglycosides†	Chloramphenicol Erythromycin‡ Fusidic acid Quinolones Rifampicin Glycopeptides‡	Chloramphenicol Quinolones	

* Resulting from an increased efflux.
† Resulting in reduced drug uptake.
‡ Resulting from enzymic modification.

(4) acquisition of a replacement for the metabolic step inhibited by the antibiotic.

It is worth emphasizing that certain resistance mechanisms overlap within these groups. Some of the known mechanisms of resistance to different antibiotics are summarized in Table 12.1

INACTIVATION OR MODIFICATION MECHANISMS

These are probably the most important resistance mechanisms to be met in clinical practice since they include the common modes of resistance to penicillins and cephalosporins, the therapeutic agents of widest use.

β-Lactam antibiotics

There are many different agents in this group (see Chapter 1) and a correspondingly large number of *β-lactamases* which catalyse hydrolysis of the β-lactam ring to form an inactive product (Fig. 12.1). In addition, varying levels of β-lactamase production, as well as differences in permeability of the Gram-negative cell envelope, play a considerable part in determining the differential susceptibilities of bacteria to this group of antibiotics.

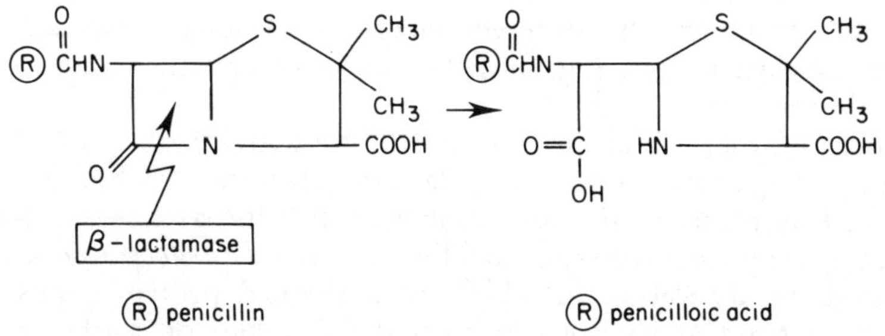

Fig. 12.1. β-lactamase hydrolysis of penicillin to form the corresponding penicilloic acid, which is antibacterially inactive. Cephalosporins may be attacked in a similar fashion, but the resultant cephalosporoic acid is usually unstable and disintegrates into smaller fragments.

To begin with, all bacteria appear to contain enzymes capable of hydrolysing β-lactam antibiotics. Indeed, it has been suggested that the normal function and evolutionary origin of β-lactamases is to break a β-lactam structure that is a transitory intermediate in cell wall synthesis. These inherent enzymes are encoded by the chromosome, and are normally bound closely to the cell membrane. In general, they are produced only in small amounts, they attack cephalosporins more readily than penicillins, and they act relatively slowly. It is doubtful whether these enzymes have any clinical significance in most cases, but in certain organisms, notably *Enterobacter* spp., *Citrobacter* spp., and *Pseudomonas aeruginosa*, gross overproduction of these chromosomal enzymes has been associated with treatment failures, even with ostensibly 'β-lactamase-stable' cephalosporins.

From a clinical point of view, most interest centres on the large number of *plasmid-encoded enzymes* which are the major cause of bacterial resistance to penicillins and cephalosporins in clinical isolates. However, the picture is complicated by *transposons* (described more fully in Chapter 13), which allow movement of genes between plasmids and the chromosome, so that the distinction between plasmid-encoded and chromosomally encoded enzymes can sometimes become blurred.

Among Gram-positive cocci, the only plasmid-encoded β-lactamases of major clinical significance are found in staphylococci. These enzymes rapidly hydrolyse benzylpenicillin, ampicillin, and most other penicillins, but are less active against 'antistaphylococcal penicillins' and cephalosporins. Staphylococcal β-lactamases are inducible exoenzymes conforming to a few biochemical types which are probably related closely. In streptococci, β-lactamases are usually absent, and these bacteria have consequently remained, with few exceptions, susceptible to benzylpenicillin. In contrast, the plasmid-encoded β-lactamases of Gram-negative bacilli embrace a wide variety of types which are physico-chemically quite distinct. A number of characters have been used to distinguish the different enzymes. Among these, substrate profile, isoelectric focusing, and the action of enzyme inhibitors are probably the most useful.

Substrate profile refers to the hydrolytic activity of a β-lactamase preparation against a number of β-lactam substrates. Profiles are often expressed as ratios related to a value of 100 for a chosen reference substrate, frequently benzylpenicillin. *Analytical isoelectric focusing* is a method of separation in which an individual protein aligns itself as a sharp band at its isoelectric point (pI value) on a pH gradient produced electrophoretically in a polyacrylamide gel. The position of a β-lactamase in the gel can be detected with a special cephalosporin substrate, nitrocefin, which changes colour from orange to red when hydrolysed by the enzyme. The technique is sufficiently sensitive to detect β-lactamases in strains thought previously to lack any such enzyme, and two or more β-lactamases produced by a single strain can be separated clearly. *Inhibitors* of β-lactamase activity include the isoxazolylpenicillins, the sulphydryl inhibitor *p*-chloromercuribenzoate, and β-lactam compounds such as clavulanic acid which, though exhibiting poor antibacterial activity themselves, are potent inhibitors of certain types of β-lactamase.

By these and other techniques, it has been possible to distinguish more than thirty different plasmid-encoded β-lactamases in Gram-negative bacteria, and many more probably remain to be characterized. The most widely distributed of these enzymes is TEM-1, which is encoded by numerous different plasmids and transposons (see Chapter 13). This no doubt explains its wide distribution, which includes many enterobacteria, *Ps. aeruginosa*, *Haemophilus influenzae*, and *Neisseria gonorrhoeae*. Other types of β-lactamase that are encountered in Gram-negative bacilli include: numerous variants of TEM-1 (some of which may exhibit an altered substrate spectrum); SHV-1 (common in *Klebsiella* spp.); the OXA group of enzymes, which are capable of hydrolysing methicillin and isoxazolylpenicillins; and the PSE group, which hydrolyse carbenicillin at least as fast as benzylpenicillin, and which were thought originally to be confined to *Ps. aeruginosa*.

The clinical importance of staphylococcal β-lactamase has been much reduced by the availability of cloxacillin and other β-lactamase-stable penicillins. Progress has also been made towards the control of resistance caused by β-lactamases of Gram-negative organisms with the introduction of 'β-lactamase-stable' cephalosporins and novel β-lactam combinations that include a β-lactamase inhibitor, such as clavulanic acid. However, novel plasmid-encoded β-lactamases have now been described that inactivate even the newer 'β-lactamase-stable' β-lactam agents. Many of these novel enzymes seem to be derived by mutation from the widely distributed TEM-1 and SHV-1 β-lactamases.

Fortunately, strains that elaborate such enzymes are still relatively uncommon, although they are now being reported with increasing frequency from many different countries.

Aminoglycosides

Resistance to aminoglycosides results largely from interference with the drug transport mechanism following modification of the antibiotic by one or more of a series of enzymes produced by the resistant bacteria. Such *aminoglycoside-modifying enzymes* are often plasmid encoded, but have been associated increasingly with the presence of transposons and integrons (see Chapter 13). They are classified according to the precise type of modification performed and by the site of modification on the aminoglycoside molecule. At the time of writing, over thirty such modifying enzymes and their variants have been identified, and these can be divided into three main groups: aminoglycoside acetylating enzymes (AAC), aminoglycoside adenylating enzymes (AAD), and aminoglycoside phosphorylating enzymes (APH).

The acetylating enzymes, of which there are at least sixteen identified types, catalyse the transfer of acetate from acetyl coenzyme A to an amino group on the aminoglycoside molecule. These enzymes modify only deoxystreptamine-containing aminoglycosides and are, therefore, without effect on streptomycin or spectinomycin. Aminoglycoside adenylating enzymes are nucleotidyl transferases that use ATP or other nucleotides as substrates and attach the nucleotide to exposed hydroxyl groups; phosphotransferases also modify hydroxyl groups, but by attachment of a phosphate molecule. Examples of the most widely distributed enzymes are listed in Table 12.2.

It is apparent from Table 12.2 that a variety of patterns of cross-resistance can be shown by bacteria elaborating different enzymes, but the pattern is complicated further because many clinical isolates produce more than one enzyme at any one time. It can therefore be difficult to predict which enzymes are present simply from a consideration of the substrate range. A more practical consideration is that sensitivity or resistance to any one agent cannot be predicted reliably from results with another, and sensitivity tests must therefore be performed against any of these agents which are considered for use in treatment.

Fig.12.2 shows the structure of kanamycin A, a typical aminoglycoside, and indicates the various sites at which modification can take place. Clearly, the presence or absence of available amino or hydroxyl groupings will affect the susceptibility to various enzymes, and this is the basis of variability within the aminoglycoside group. The steric configuration of the groupings is also important: thus the semi-synthetic aminoglycoside amikacin is, structurally, related closely to kanamycin A, but is much less susceptible to enzymic modification

Table 12.2. Examples of some of the most common aminoglycoside-modifying enzymes

Enzyme	Typical substrates	Bacterial distribution	
		Gram-positive	Gram-negative
Acetyl transferases			
AAC(3)-I	Gen	−	+
AAC(3)-II	Gen, Tob, Net	−	+
AAC(2′)	Gen, Tob	−	+
AAC(6′)-I	Tob, Amk, Net	+	+
AAC(6′)-II	Gen, Tob, Net	−	+
Nucleotidyl transferases			
AAD(6)	Str	+	−
AAD(4′) (4″)	Tob, Amk	+	−
AAD(2″)	Gen, Tob	−	+
AAD(3″)(9)	Str, Spc	−	+
AAD(9)	Spc	+	−
Phosphotransferases			
APH(6)	Str	−	+
APH(3′)	Neo, Kan	+	+
APH(2″)	Gen	+	−
APH(3″)	Str	+	+

Amk, amikacin; Gen, gentamicin; Kan, kanamycin; Neo, neomycin; Net, netilmicin; Spc, spectinomycin; Str, streptomycin; Tob, tobramycin.

The figure in brackets indicates the site of modification according to the internationally accepted numbering system for the various parts of the complex aminoglycoside molecule (see Fig. 12.2).

because of a hydroxy-aminobutyric acid side-chain which alters the steric configuration of the molecule fundamentally.

When the aminoglycoside-modifying enzymes were first described, they were considered to be examples of drug-inactivating enzymes analogous to those responsible for resistance to β-lactams and chloramphenicol. However, aminoglycoside-modifying enzymes mediate resistance by modifying only small amounts of antibiotic. These enzymes are strategically placed near the inner cytoplasmic membrane where they are accessible to acetyl coenzyme A and ATP. As soon as a few molecules of drug are modified, all further transport of drug into the cell becomes blocked.

An additional minor mechanism of resistance to aminoglycosides, unrelated to modifying enzymes but also involving reduced permeability, has been associated with alterations in outer membrane proteins that result in reduced transfer of the antibiotic into the cell.

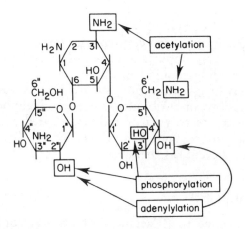

Fig. 12.2. Structure of kanamycin A, showing the sites at which enzymic modification can occur.

Chloramphenicol

Resistance to chloramphenicol is another example of drug inactivation; in both Gram-positive and Gram-negative bacteria, such resistance is normally associated with production of an enzyme, chloramphenicol acetyl transferase, which converts the drug to either the monoacetate or diacetate. The acetylated drug is unable to bind to the bacterial ribosome and is therefore without effect on protein synthesis. A number of different acetyl transferases have been described. Some appear to be genus and species specific; others, usually plasmid associated, have achieved a wider distribution. This variety is a little surprising since chloramphenicol has been used less widely than many other antibiotics because of its rare, but serious, toxic side effects. The selective pressures on the evolution of diverse inactivating enzymes must therefore have been correspondingly less than with, for example, the penicillins.

ALTERATION OF THE TARGET SITE

This type of resistance has been described for many antibiotics, including β-lactam agents, streptomycin, erythromycin, chloramphenicol, fusidic acid, quinolones, rifampicin, and glycopeptides. In many cases, resistance arises from the selection of rare, pre-existent mutants from within an otherwise sensitive bacterial population. Such mutations may affect the structure of the target site directly or may result in modification of the target site by an indirect mechanism involving an enzymic activity (see below).

The emergence of resistance involving target site alterations during therapy may be an important cause of treatment failure with certain drugs, including rifampicin, quinolones, fusidic acid, and various antituberculous drugs. Clinically, such resistance can be prevented by using combinations of antibiotics, since the likelihood of independent resistance mutations to two or more unrelated antibiotics appearing simultaneously in the same cell is very small; this strategy has been crucial in antituberculosis therapy.

β-Lactam antibiotics

So far as resistance to β-lactam antibiotics is concerned, the major clinical mechanism of resistance involves the enzymic inactivation of the β-lactam by a β-lactamase (see above). However, other resistance mechanisms involving target site modification have been reported. Thus, strains of *Streptococcus pneumoniae* with reduced susceptibility to penicillin have been shown to exhibit alterations in the target penicillin-binding proteins (PBPs) that result in reduced ability to bind penicillin. Similarly, methicillin resistance in *Staphylococcus aureus* is associated with the synthesis of a modified PBP which exhibits decreased affinity for methicillin and other β-lactam antibiotics. Low-level resistance to penicillin in *N. gonorrhoeae* has also been associated with alterations to PBPs. Such resistance appears to have developed by rare mutational events and to have become disseminated as a result of considerable antibiotic selection pressure.

Streptomycin

Streptomycin binds to a particular protein, designated S12, in the smaller (30S) ribosomal subunit in bacteria. A mutation resulting in a single amino acid change in the structure of this protein can prevent the binding of streptomycin entirely and endow the bacteria with resistance to very high concentrations of the drug. This is a very specific alteration since other aminoglycosides which are assumed to have an identical mode of action, such as kanamycin and gentamicin, are unaffected by this change.

Erythromycin and chloramphenicol

Changes in the proteins of the larger (50S) ribosomal subunit have been implicated in resistance to chloramphenicol and macrolides such as erythromycin. However, erythromycin resistance in staphylococci and streptococci isolated from human infections results more usually from methylation of the 23S ribosomal RNA subunit by an inducible plasmid-encoded enzyme. Methylation of the ribosomal RNA renders the bacteria resistant not only to other macrolides, but also to lincomycin and clindamycin by reducing ribosomal binding of these drugs. However, since erythromycin is a specific inducer of the methylating enzyme, bacteria carrying a plasmid encoding this property are resistant to the other drugs only in the presence of erythromycin. This phenomenon is known as *dissociated resistance*.

Fusidic acid

Fusidic acid inhibits translocation of the growing polypeptide chain. Mutations altering the structure of the protein involved (elongation factor G) result in the cell becoming resistant to the action of this antibiotic.

Quinolones

The DNA gyrase (DNA topoisomerase II) target of quinolone antibiotics is essential for bacterial DNA replication. Most resistance to both the older (e.g. nalidixic acid) and newer (e.g. ciprofloxacin) quinolone antibiotics is caused by structural alterations to one of the subunits of DNA gyrase, although mutations resulting in altered permeability to quinolones are also known to occur.

Rifampicin

Resistance to rifampicin is invariably the result of a structural alteration to the β-subunit of RNA polymerase (involved in the transcription of DNA to messenger RNA) that reduces its binding affinity for rifampicin.

Glycopeptides

Resistance in enterococci to the glycopeptide antibiotics vancomycin and teicoplanin represents a particularly interesting example of target site alteration. Glycopeptides bind to the D-alanyl–D-alanine terminus of the peptidoglycan pentapeptide (see Chapter 1). Enterococci that exhibit high-level resistance to glycopeptides produce two new enzymes, a ligase and a dehydrogenase, with formation of a new depsipeptide terminus, D-alanyl–D-lactate, to the pentapeptide. This substitution allows cell wall synthesis to continue in the presence of the antibiotic.

INTERFERENCE WITH DRUG TRANSPORT AND ACCUMULATION

Variants exhibiting low levels of resistance to almost any antibiotic can be isolated readily from most bacteria, and such variants often result from changes in permeability of the bacterial cell envelope. Such resistance can increase in a stepwise fashion, and is usually accompanied by other phenotypic changes (e.g.slower growth rate, colonial variation on solid media, reduced virulence) which become more marked as the degree of resistance increases. The clinical significance of this type of resistance has never been assessed properly, but it is likely that the slight shift in penicillin susceptibility of gonococci which has been observed over the years may result from such changes.

In addition to reduced drug accumulation resulting from enzymic modification of aminoglycosides (see above), interference with transport of drugs into the bacterial cell is of proven importance in clinical isolates as a cause of resistance to members of the tetracycline and β-lactam groups of antibiotics.

Tetracyclines

Uptake of tetracyclines into normal cells involves an active transport mechanism that uses energy and results in accumulation of drug inside the cell.

Plasmid-mediated resistance to tetracyclines is common in both Gram-positive and Gram-negative bacteria. Generally, there is complete cross-resistance in that a strain resistant to one tetracycline is resistant to all the others, although exceptions may be found with minocycline and some investigational compounds. The precise mechanism of resistance is a complex phenomenon, but is often associated with the synthesis of an additional membrane protein that mediates rapid efflux of tetracyclines from resistant cells by an active mechanism, so that drug entering the cell is removed almost simultaneously and never reaches an inhibitory level. Such resistance is normally inducible, and full expression of resistance is obtained only after cells have been exposed to sub-inhibitory concentrations of the drug. There is no evidence for enzymic inactivation of tetracycline by clinical isolates of bacteria, or for modification of the ribosomal target. However, some strains of bacteria produce a cytoplasmic protein which appears to have the function of protecting ribosomes from tetracycline attack.

β-Lactam antibiotics

The outer membranes of Gram-negative bacilli vary greatly in permeability to various penicillins and cephalosporins. Most β-lactams reach their targets in Gram-negative bacilli by passing through the water-filled pores (*porins*) that extend across the outer membrane bilayer. Studies have shown that the rate of permeation is governed largely by the physical size of a particular β-lactam molecule in comparison with the size of the porin, but ionic charge also plays a part. In some bacteria, resistance can result from changes to the size or function of the porins, so that passage of the antibiotic is prevented. In a few instances, non-specific changes in cell permeability to β-lactam antibiotics are encoded by genes carried on plasmids; these changes seem to affect the overall outer membrane structure of the cell and are related directly to plasmid carriage.

Chloramphenicol

A few strains of chloramphenicol-resistant Gram-negative bacilli possess a plasmid that appears to confer the property of impermeability to chloramphenicol upon the host cell.

Quinolones

Quinolone-resistant strains of *Escherichia coli* have been described in which resistance is caused by impermeability associated with a decrease in the amount of the OmpF outer membrane porin protein. Such strains may simultaneously acquire resistance to β-lactam antibiotics and some other agents that gain access through the OmpF porin.

METABOLIC BYPASS

Most common resistance mechanisms can be accommodated in one or other of the three major groups described already. However, there are two known examples in which a plasmid provides the cell with an entirely new and drug-resistant enzyme that can bypass the sensitive chromosomal enzyme which is also present unaltered in the cell.

Sulphonamides

Sulphonamides exert their bacteriostatic effect by competitive inhibition of dihydropteroate synthetase, an enzyme which links *p*-aminobenzoic acid and pteridine to form dihydropteroate. Sulphonamide-resistant strains of Gram-negative bacilli synthesize an additional plasmid or transposon-encoded (see Chapter 13) dihydropteroate synthetase that is unaffected by sulphonamides. The additional enzyme allows continued functioning of the threatened metabolic pathway in the presence of the drug. At least two such sulphonamide-insensitive enzymes are widespread in Gram-negative bacilli throughout the world.

Trimethoprim

Trimethoprim blocks a later step in the same metabolic pathway by inhibiting the dihydrofolate reductase enzymes of susceptible bacteria. Resistant strains synthesize a new, trimethoprim-insensitive, plasmid or transposon-encoded dihydrofolate reductase as well as the normal drug-sensitive chromosomal enzyme. At least twelve groups of trimethoprim-insusceptible dihydrofolate reductases have been described for Gram-negative bacilli, and a further example is found in multi-resistant isolates of *Staph. aureus*.

Elucidation of the mechanisms of drug resistance has resulted in the development of new or modified antimicrobial agents designed to circumvent the problem. However, any attempt to limit the spread of drug resistance requires not only a knowledge of the resistance mechanisms themselves, but also an understanding of the genetic factors that control their emergence and continued evolution. These factors are the subject of the next chapter.

13

The genetics of resistance

K. J. Towner

All the properties of a microbial cell, including those of medical importance such as antibiotic resistance and virulence determinants, are determined ultimately by the microbial *genome*, which in turn comprises the three sources of genetic information in the cell: the chromosome, plasmids, and bacteriophages. Resistance of bacteria to antimicrobial agents may be either intrinsic or acquired (see Chapter 11). Intrinsic resistance is the 'natural' resistance possessed by a bacterial species and is usually specified by chromosomal genes. An example of a bacterial species with a high degree of intrinsic resistance is *Pseudomonas aeruginosa*. In contrast to intrinsic resistance, acquired resistance occurs in sensitive cells, either following alterations to the existing genome or by transfer of genetic information between cells. Thus a fundamental knowledge of microbial genetics is essential for an understanding of the development and spread of resistance to antimicrobial drugs.

The heritable information which specifies a bacterial cell, and which passes to daughter cells at cell division, is carried in bacteria, as in all living cells, as an ordered sequence of nucleotide pairs along molecules of DNA. The process of *transcription* of this information into messenger RNA, and its subsequent *translation* into functioning proteins by ribosomes, is also similar in bacteria and in other cells.

THE BACTERIAL CHROMOSOME

The main source of genetic information in a bacterial cell is the chromosome. Each bacterial cell has a single chromosome which, in the vast majority of cases, is known to form a single closed circular DNA molecule. In *Escherichia coli*, the organism studied most intensively, this single DNA molecule comprises about 4×10^3 kb (kilobases) and is about 1.4 mm in length. The chromosome is coiled and looped into a compact bundle in the cytoplasm of the cell, but it is not separated from the cytoplasm by any form of nuclear membrane. Transcription of the DNA and translation of the resulting messenger RNA can therefore proceed simultaneously. Most bacterial chromosomes contain sufficient DNA to encode for 1000–3000 different genes. Not all of these genes are required to be expressed at any one time, and indeed it would be energetically wasteful for the cell to do so. Gene regulation is therefore necessary, and this can occur at either the transcriptional or translational level.

Chromosomal mutations to antibiotic resistance

Mutations result from rare mistakes in the DNA replication process and occur between 10^{-4} and 10^{-10} per cell division. They usually involve deletion, substitution or addition of one or only a few base pairs, which causes an alteration in the amino acid composition of a particular peptide product. Such mistakes are random and spontaneous. They occur continuously in all the genes of a cell and are independent of the presence or absence of a particular antibiotic. The vast majority of mutations are repaired by the cell without any noticeable effect. The only influence that an antibiotic has is to *select* for the occasional spontaneous antibiotic-resistant mutant that may be present in a large sensitive population. In such a situation, the sensitive cells will be killed by the antibiotic while the resistant mutant will survive and proliferate to become the predominant type. Most chromosomal resistance mutations result in alterations to permeability or specific antibiotic target sites, but some result in enhanced production of an inactivating enzyme or bypass mechanism. The latter type are mutations at the transcriptional or translational level in gene regulatory mechanisms.

Chromosomal mutations to antibiotic resistance can be divided into *single-step* and *multi-step types*.

Single large-step mutations

With these mutations, a single mutational change results in a large increase in the minimum inhibitory concentration (MIC) of a particular antibiotic. Single-step mutations affecting the target sites of nalidixic acid, rifampicin, fusidic acid, or streptomycin arise spontaneously and may lead to treatment failure when these drugs are used alone. In some Gram-negative bacilli, mutations in the genetic regulatory system for the normally low-level chromosomal β-lactamase may result in a vast over-production of this enzyme and slow hydrolysis of compounds such as cefotaxime and ceftazidime that are considered under normal circumstances to be β-lactamase stable.

Multi-step mutations

These are sequential mutations that result in cumulative gradual stepwise increases in the MIC of a particular antibiotic. They are clinically quite common, especially in situations in which only low concentrations of antibiotic can be delivered to the site of an infection.

Since spontaneous mutations to unrelated antibiotics are normally independent, combined therapy with two or more antibiotics will often circumvent potential clinical problems arising from chromosomal mutations to resistance.

PLASMIDS

The bacterial chromosome carries all the genes necessary for the survival and replication of the bacterial cell under most circumstances. Many, perhaps all, bacteria also carry additional molecules of DNA (usually between 2 and 200 kb in size) known as plasmids, which are separate from, and normally replicate independently of, the bacterial chromosome. Plasmids can carry genes which confer a wide range of properties on the cells which carry them. In general, these are properties that are not essential for the survival of the cell under normal circumstances, but which offer the cells a survival advantage in unusual or adverse conditions. Examples of such properties are:

(1) fertility—the ability to conjugate with and transfer genetic information into other bacteria (see later).

(2) resistance to antibiotics—most antibiotic resistance encountered clinically is associated with plasmids.

(3) ability to produce bacteriocins—proteins inhibitory to other bacteria which may be ecological competitors.

(4) toxin production;

(5) immunity to some bacteriophages;

(6) ability to use unusual sugars and other substrates as foods.

Plasmid incompatibility

Many different kinds of plasmid have been described. Plasmids differ in size, DNA base composition, in the DNA fragments that can be recognized after treatment with restriction endonucleases ('plasmid fingerprints'), and in their incompatibility behaviour. Compatible plasmids can coexist in the same host cell, while incompatible plasmids cannot, and so tend to be unstable and displace one another. There are at least twenty *incompatibility (Inc) groups* within the plasmids found in Enterobacteriaceae, and similar incompatibility schemes are used to subdivide staphylococcal plasmids and those found in *Pseudomonas* spp. The mechanism of incompatibility appears to be related functionally to plasmid genes involved in control of replication and copy number in the host cell. Although only a few genes are involved directly, plasmids belonging to the same Inc group often share greater DNA homology and show other similarities of structure and function compared with plasmids belonging to different Inc groups.

BACTERIOPHAGES

The third possible source of genetic information in a bacterial cell is a bacteriophage. Bacteriophages (phages) are viruses which infect bacteria. Most phages will attack only a relatively small number of strains of related bacteria—they have a narrow and specific host range. Phages can be divided into two main types:

virulent phages that inevitably destroy by lysis any bacteria that they infect, with the release of numerous new phage particles from each lysed cell;

temperate (lysogenic) phages that may either lyse or *lysogenize* infected bacterial cells. In the state of lysogeny, the phage nucleic acid is replicated in a stable and dormant fashion within the infected cell, often following insertion into the host cell chromosome. Such a dormant phage is known as a *prophage*. However, while in the prophage state, some prophage genes may be expressed and may confer additional properties on the cell. Once in every few thousand cell divisions, a prophage becomes released from the dormant state and enters the lytic cycle, with subsequent destruction of its host cell and release of new phage particles into the surrounding medium.

TRANSFER OF GENETIC INFORMATION

There are three ways in which genetic information can be transferred from one bacterial cell into another: transformation, transduction, and conjugation.

Transformation involves lysis of a bacterial cell and the release of naked DNA into the surrounding medium. Under certain circumstances, some of this DNA can be acquired by intact bacterial cells in the vicinity. This process has been much studied in the laboratory, but there are few convincing demonstrations of its occurrence *in vivo*. The process depends crucially on the ability of the recipient cells to be *competent* for uptake of free DNA.

Transduction involves the accidental incorporation of bacterial DNA, from either the chromosome or a plasmid, into a bacteriophage particle during the phage lytic cycle. The phage particle then acts as a vector and transfers the bacterial DNA to the next cell which it infects.

Conjugation involves physical contact between two bacterial cells. The cells adhere to one another and DNA passes unidirectionally from one cell, termed the donor, into the other, the recipient. Ability to conjugate depends on carriage of an appropriate plasmid or transposon (see later) by the host cell.

The existence of these transfer mechanisms means that bacteria do not have to rely solely on a process of mutation and selection for their evolution. By such mechanisms they can acquire and express blocks of genetic information that have evolved and been refined elsewhere. A bacterial cell can, for example, acquire by conjugation a plasmid which carries genes conferring resistance to several different antibiotics, and, as a result, within a very short time following the receipt of such a plasmid by a sensitive cell, the organisms in a given niche may change from a state in which they are all sensitive to a state in which it is very difficult to find an antibiotic that is effective against them. Of course, the ability to transfer genes in this way does not eliminate the need to evolve them in the first place but, once they have evolved, it ensures their eventual widespread dissemination under appropriate selection pressures.

EVOLUTION OF NEW RESISTANCE GENE COMBINATIONS

The distinction between chromosomal and plasmid genes is not absolute. Where appropriate regions of DNA homology exist, classic ('normal') recombination can occur, both between different plasmids and between plasmids and the chromosome. Although this process can lead to the formation of new antibiotic resistance gene combinations, it is relatively uncommon in bacteria because there are few regions of sequence homology between the bacterial chromosome and plasmids which can be exploited for this purpose. A more important mechanism by which antibiotic resistance genes can pass from one bacterial replicon to another is the 'illegitimate' recombination process known as *transposition*.

Transposons

Transposition depends on the existence of specific genetic elements termed *transposons*. These elements are discrete sequences of DNA capable of translocation (transposition) from one replicon (plasmid or chromosome) to another. Unlike classic ('normal') recombination, transposons do not share extensive regions of homology with the replicon into which they insert. In many cases, transposons consist of individual resistance genes, or groups of genes, bounded by DNA sequences called either *direct* or *inverted repeats*—a sequence of bases at one end of the transposon which also appears, either in direct or reverse order, at the other end. These repeats may be relatively short, often of the order of 40 bp, but longer examples have been identified. It is likely that these DNA sequences provide highly specific recognition sites for certain enzymes (*transposases*) that catalyse the movement of transposons from one replicon to another without the need for extensive regions of sequence homology. Depending upon the transposon involved, insertion may occur at only a few or at many different sites on the host replicon. Transposons may carry genes conferring resistance to many different antibiotics, as well as other metabolic properties, and their existence helps to explain how a single antibiotic resistance gene can become disseminated over a wide range of unrelated replicons.

Isolated DNA sequences analogous to the terminal sequences of transposons can also move from one replicon to another, or be inserted in any region of any DNA molecule. Such *insertion sequences* contain no known genes unrelated to insertion functions but, in principle at least, two similar insertion sequences could bracket any assemblage of genes and convert it into a transposon. Thus, theoretically, all replicons are accessible to transposition and all genes are potentially transposable. This is of crucial evolutionary importance since it explains how genes of appropriate function can accumulate on a single replicon under the impact of selection pressure. Transposons and insertion sequences therefore play a vital part in plasmid evolution.

Integrons

Transposons may contain combinations of genes conferring resistance to various different antibiotics. An important question concerns the mechanism by which new combinations of antibiotic resistance genes can be formed. It is now apparent that special molecular structures, termed *integrons*, may enable the formation of new combinations of resistance genes within a bacterial cell, either on a plasmid or within a transposon, in response to selection pressures.

Integrons appear to consist of two conserved segments of DNA located either side of inserted antibiotic resistance genes. Individual resistance genes seem to be capable of insertion or removal as 'cassettes' between these conserved structures. The cassettes can be found inserted in different orders and combinations. Integrons also act as an expression vector for 'foreign' antibiotic resistance genes by supplying a promoter for transcription of cassettes derived originally from completely unrelated organisms. Integrons lack many of the features associated with transposons, including direct or inverted repeats and functions required for transposition. They do, however, possess site-specific integration functions, notably a special enzyme termed an *integrase*.

The precise role of integrons in the evolution and spread of antibiotic resistance genes remains to be determined, but at least three potential mechanisms of spread exist:

(1) the potential mobility of an integron itself by site-specific insertion;

(2) spread following insertion of an integron into a transposon;

(3) horizontal transfer of integrons on plasmids.

The process of evolution and spread of antibiotic resistance genes is still continuing. The origin of resistance genes carried by integrons, transposons or plasmids, or even the origin of these elements themselves, is not known, but it has been possible to observe a steady increase in the numbers of resistant bacterial strains following the introduction of successive chemotherapeutic agents into clinical use. It is clear that transposition of resistance determinants is involved in the spread of these determinants. For example, a transposon encoding TEM-type β-lactamase production in enteric bacteria has been able to cross generic boundaries to cause penicillin resistance in gonococci and ampicillin resistance in *Haemophilus influenzae* by insertion into plasmids indigenous to these organisms. There are many other examples, and the evolutionary process is a continuous event.

GENOTYPIC RESISTANCE

To summarize the earlier discussion, genes conferring resistance to antibiotics are often found inserted into integrons, and may either be part of the bacterial chromosome or be carried on plasmids, transposons, or as part of a phage genome. The distribution of these genes between the chromosome and other elements reflects to some extent the biochemical mechanisms involved. For example, resistance which results from mutational alteration of an existing target protein will normally be chromosomal in location and will not be integron associated, while resistance genes for entirely new enzymes, such as the aminoglycoside-modifying enzymes, novel β-lactamases, or trimethoprim-resistant dihydrofolate reductases, are commonly carried on plasmids and transposons as part of integrons. This reflects the fact that the evolution of any new enzyme is likely to be a very long process, while the occurrence of the genes for such enzymes on plasmids, transposons, and integrons enables spread of these genes between different strains, species, and genera rather than requiring evolution of the genes afresh by each bacterial strain for itself.

Chromosomal and plasmid-mediated types of resistance may be equally important in the management of an individual patient. However, the plasmid-encoded variety has achieved greater notoriety because of the spectacular fashion in which bacteria may acquire resistance to a number of unrelated agents by a single genetic event. Certainly, it has been plasmid-encoded resistance which has caused most problems in the highly selective environment of the hospital. Nevertheless, mutational resistance involving the bacterial chromosome is a common cause of treatment failure with some compounds, and it is strange but true that antibacterial agents for which resistance is not known to be encoded on plasmids (e.g. nalidixic acid and rifampicin) generally suffer from mutational resistance problems instead.

PHENOTYPIC RESISTANCE

So far as is known, phenotypic resistance to antibacterial agents is rare, although it is not always possible to be sure that phenotypic changes brought about in the microenvironment of a lesion do not contribute to insusceptibility of bacteria in the infected host. In the laboratory, phenotypic resistance can sometimes be induced; for example, the outer envelope of *Ps. aeruginosa* can be altered by varying the conditions of growth, and this affects susceptibility to polymyxins.

Another example is the failure of penicillins and cephalosporins to kill *persisters* (those cells in a bacterial population that survive exposure to concentrations of β-lactam agents lethal to the rest of the culture). This does not result from a genetic event since the resistance is not heritable, and it is probable that the 'resistant' bacteria are caught in a particular metabolic state at the time of first encounter with the drug.

A peculiar form of phenotypic resistance is observed with mecillinam, a β-lactam antibiotic which, unusually among β-lactam agents, does not affect bacterial cell division. Mecillinam induces surface changes in susceptible Gram-negative bacilli which generally lead to death of the bacteria by osmotic rupture once sufficient damage has been incurred. However, those bacterial cells in the population which happen to have a low internal osmolarity will survive and, since mecillinam lacks the ability to prevent growth and division, such bacteria continue to grow in a morphologically altered form. On withdrawal of the drug, the bacteria resume their normal shape and, in due course, revert to the same mixed susceptibility as the original parent culture.

THE INFLUENCE OF ANTIBIOTIC SELECTION PRESSURE

Antibiotic resistance genes, and the genetic elements which carry them, existed before the introduction of antibiotics into human medicine. It has become established beyond doubt that the emergence and survival of predominantly resistant bacterial populations is a result of the selective pressure associated with the widespread use of antibiotics. Resistant cells survive in a given niche at the expense of sensitive cells of the same or other species. However, drug resistance, whether chromosomal or plasmid encoded, often carries metabolic penalties for the cell. If the selective pressures of antibiotic use are withdrawn, there is sometimes a gradual return to sensitivity in the population. Individual cells may lose their plasmids and chromosomal mutations may revert to sensitivity. The implications of this process for efforts to control and limit the spread of bacterial drug resistance are discussed in the next chapter.

14

Control of the spread of resistance

A. M. Emmerson

Almost fifty years of antibiotic use have brought great benefits to humans and animals. Foremost among these is the saving of life and relief of suffering by therapeutic use. Many of the killing bacterial diseases which were rife in the early years of this century have been successfully combated almost to the point of extinction. Pneumococcal pneumonia, tuberculosis, and streptococcal puerperal sepsis, for example, used to kill many hundreds of young people every year. Deaths from these and many other bacterial diseases are now rare in young adults, at least in developed countries, although this may change.

Substantial amounts of antibiotics are also used outside normal therapy for prophylaxis and growth promotion in animal husbandry, and even in plant protection in agriculture. These wider uses have been very important in controlling losses due to infectious disease and in helping to meet growing demands for animal protein for food. The economic benefits of antibiotic use in food production are very large indeed.

Compared with most other drugs of similar potency, antibiotics are remarkably safe, and they are also remarkably effective. This has inevitably led to liberal, even lavish use, and concern has frequently been expressed that excessive and inappropriate use of these agents is the chief cause of the widespread emergence of resistant organisms which threatens the continued effectiveness of antimicrobial therapy (see Chapter 11).

Attention has repeatedly been drawn to the world-wide public health problem of the spread and persistence of drug-resistant organisms, and there have been frequent calls for regulation to curb the unnecesary use and flagrant misuse of antimicrobial drugs in some countries. The following practices have been clearly identified as largely contributing to the present situation: dispensing antibiotics without prescription; using clinically useful antibiotics as growth promoters in animal feeds and on agricultural crops; prescribing antibiotics for ailments for which they are ineffective; misleading consumers by advertising antibiotics as 'wonder drugs', especially in areas where dispensing is not regulated; and using different labelling and advertising to sell the same product in different parts of the world. Consumers, prescribers, dispensers, manufacturers, and government regulatory agencies are all involved in different ways, and all need to be convinced of the vital importance of prudent antibiotic use.

AVAILABILITY OF ANTIBIOTICS

In the UK, successive Acts of Parliament have provided a comprehensive system of control of the manufacture, importation, distribution, sale, supply, and description of medicinal products, including antibiotics, for human and veterinary use. The intention of this legislation is to give Health and Agriculture Ministers powers that will ensure that all medicinal products offered for sale or supply in the UK are adequately tested for safety, quality, and efficacy, and enable them to prohibit the retail sale or supply of medicinal products except on the prescription of a doctor, dentist, or veterinarian. The ministers are advised by authoritative advisory committees and individuals, and exercise their powers by a comprehensive, but flexible system of Product Licences (see Chapter 33). There is, however, at present no body charged with advising specifically on antibiotics and antibiotic use, and there probably should be. There is no other example in therapeutics in which local misuse of an effective agent brings about a general diminution in its effectiveness.

Similar legislation covers much of Continental Europe and the USA. Indeed, the American Federal Authorities have been more often criticized for delaying the introduction or restricting the use of valuable agents than for permitting their indiscriminate use. In the rich, developed world the sale and distribution of antibiotics are fairly tightly controlled, while the poorer, but numerically much larger, developing world provides a much bigger market in which the sale and distribution of these agents are largely unrestricted.

Paradoxically, the use of antibiotics in the Third World needs extending, not restricting, if standards of health are to be brought up to those of the developed world. However, this clearly needs to be done in a controlled manner, and over-the-counter availability of antimicrobial drugs is, in the end, going to create more problems than it solves. It was no great surprise that chloramphenicol-resistant typhoid bacilli first emerged in South America and penicillin-resistant gonococci in South East Asia.

The onus of providing the necessary legislation obviously rests with individual governments, with the advice and support of international agencies such as the World Health Organization. However, pharmaceutical houses also have a part to play in ensuring that their products are advertised and marketed to the same standards as those they apply in the countries of the developed world.

THE USE OF ANTIBIOTICS IN AGRICULTURE

Antibiotic-resistant bacterial populations arise in humans and animals by the use of antibiotics, whether for therapy, prophylaxis, or growth promotion. The non-therapeutic uses have come under heavy criticism by those concerned in the treatment of infectious disease, despite their immense value in animal husbandry and food production. The extent to which resistant organisms in animals contribute to resistant organisms in humans, as opposed to the recycling by cross-infection of resistant organisms within the human population, is still much in dispute. Accurate figures on antibiotic usage are hard to come by, but current overall use of antibiotics in human medicine is probably at least four times that in animal husbandry and veterinary medicine per unit of body weight. It is likely therefore that human medical use contributes more to the human resistant bacterial population than does non-human use. Nevertheless, it has been shown conclusively that resistant bacteria, both commensal and pathogenic, arising in animal populations do pass to human hosts, and this source of human resistant bacteria cannot be ignored.

The Swann Report

The use of certain antibiotics in restricted amounts to promote growth in livestock, mainly pigs and poultry, is common practice, and concern about dangers resulting from the reported increase in resistant bacteria has been voiced by both medical and veterinary professions. In the UK this concern led to the setting up in 1968 of the Joint Committee on the use of Antibiotics in Animal Husbandry and Veterinary Medicine under the Chairmanship of Professor M. M. Swann, and the production a year later of what has come to be known as the 'Swann Report'. This report presented a masterly analysis of the whole problem of the use of antibiotics in animal husbandry, and made several recommendations, the most important of which were:

(1) that permission to supply and use drugs without prescription in animal feeds should be restricted to antibiotics shown to be effective for this purpose, of little or no use for treatment of infections in humans or animals, and not likely to cause resistance against therapeutic agents in general use;

(2) that therapeutic antibiotics should be available for use in animals only when prescribed by a member of the veterinary profession;

(3) that a single committee should be set up with overall responsibility for the whole field of use of antibiotics and related

substances whether in humans, animals, food preservation, or for other purposes.

There were more than twenty further cogent recommendations, some of which were implemented.

In the decade following the publication of the *Swann Report* efforts were made to follow its recommendations and intentions, but with limited success. The direct commercial use of therapeutically useful antibiotics as growth promoters has been stopped, but the boundaries between feed additives for growth promotion, antibiotics prescribed prophylactically, and antibiotics used to treat sick animals have always been blurred. There has been widespread diversion of antibiotics properly prescribed for treatment of sick animals into feeds intended for well animals. Antibiotics have been readily available without prescription on an illicit but extensive black market. Also, it has always been unclear how much the use of feed additives contributed to the resistance problem, compared with the equally extensive therapeutic use of antibiotics in veterinary medicine, which there was little attempt to control.

IRRATIONAL USE OF ANTIBIOTICS

Whatever the contribution to the human load of resistant bacteria from the use of antibiotics in animal husbandry, the major selective pressure leading to resistant bacteria in humans is the use of antibiotics in human medicine. Often this use is inappropriate and unsupported by laboratory cultures. Several surveys of the use of antibiotics have found that inappropriate prescribing is widespread. Studies in the mid-1970s indicated that 25–30 per cent of patients received antibiotics while in hospital although the reason for such high usage was often obscure. At this time, there was great uncertainty among prescribers on how to use antibiotics for prophylaxis of infection.

A national survey of infection in forty-three hospitals in the UK confirmed that nearly a quarter of hospital patients received antibiotics; this ranged from 8 per cent in obstetric patients to more than 60 per cent of those in intensive care units. However, less than 50 per cent of those patients who were prescribed antibiotics showed any evidence of infection. Another study indicated that most patients receiving antibiotics were treated without bacteriological evidence of the infecting agent; doctors prescribing antibiotics for these patients were unable to specify the pathogen against which treatment was intended in half of the cases. This study also emphasized that only 7 per cent of antibiotics prescribed for conventional surgical prophylaxis fulfilled all the criteria used to assess the suitability of choice of drug and the method and timing of its administration.

Much of the irrational prescribing of antibiotics stems from lack of information on likely infecting pathogens. Delays in diagnosis occur through poor or non-existing sampling techniques, delay in transport, slow and laborious laboratory techniques, and unsatisfactory reporting methods. Antibiotic prescribers need rapid, accurate information, and near-patient testing is not yet available in microbiology. A rapid slide test for *Streptococcus pyogenes* in a throat swab at the bed side would negate the need for antibiotic use in many patients with viral sore throats. Unfortunately those rapid methods presently available have poor specificity or poor sensitivity.

One of the major problems in dealing with patients in whom an infection is suspected is distinguishing between infection and colonization. Patients with an undiagnosed fever may well be colonized with potentially pathogenic micro-organisms, but may not be infected. The distinction is not always obvious, and under these circumstances it is understandable for a clinician to prescribe antibiotics. However, good practice dictates that all relevant samples for culture should be collected before treatment.

RATIONAL USE OF ANTIBIOTICS

Each prescribing doctor has the responsibility to provide the best possible treatment for the patient, taking into account the risks of adverse effects. The widespread use of antibiotics has led to a marked increase in antibiotic resistance of many hospital-associated pathogens and there is ample evidence of the ways in which antibiotic resistance has imposed serious limitations on the treatment of most of the important bacterial infections.

Every attempt should be made to establish a clinical and microbiological cause of any infection; it is not rational to treat patients merely because they have a raised temperature. Where possible, all appropriate samples should be collected before treatment. The initial choice of antimicrobial therapy will depend on the most likely infection, the severity of the illness, and the type of the patient. If the identity of the organism is known then treatment can be specific and a single, narrow-spectrum antibiotic used. If the infecting organism can be targeted then broad-spectrum antibiotics do not need to be used, thus leaving much of the body's normal flora undisturbed.

Successful empirical therapy is based on good surveillance and prompt guidance from clinical laboratory staff. Initial therapy is subsequently modified according to the results of pre-treatment samples. The duration of therapy will depend on the type and severity of the illness and the patient's response. Potentially toxic drugs should be monitored accordingly. Infection control staff should be contacted for specialized advice if the patient is infected with contagious pathogens such as methicillin-resistant *Staphylococcus aureus* (MRSA) or *Str. pyogenes*.

CONTROL OF ANTIBIOTIC USE

The principles which should be followed in deciding which antibiotic, if any, to use in a given situation are discussed in Chapter 15. However, even in relatively straightforward clinical situations there are often several equally effective agents which might be used. Choice may then be determined by a locally agreed set of guidelines for the rational use of antibiotics.

Antibiotic policies

Clinicians do not take kindly to ill-informed interference, least of all with their prescribing habits, but all would agree that a rational approach to prescribing is the basis of medical practice. Guidance on the most appropriate use of antibiotics should not be too restrictive, should reflect local needs, and should be formulated with the agreement of the local users. The basis of most antibiotic policies is education and communication. The aims of an antibiotic policy are to offer guidelines for the rational use of antimicrobial agents in an attempt to prevent or delay the emergence of resistance micro-organisms. Advice should also include the most effective treatment for the individual patient. The basis of all sound antibiotic policies is good microbiology laboratory surveillance, which is required to detect important change in bacterial resistance. The policy chosen should be monitored by a clinical microbiologist or by a small enthusiastic sub-group of the drugs and therapeutics sub-committee. Day-to-day control of antibiotic usage can be monitored by the pharmacy department and ward pharmacists, but good communication within the hospital or health area is of the utmost importance.

Clinicians need to be aware of the local and changing patterns of infection and resistance in their locality. Information about new agents, together with some assessment of their likely place in the antimicrobial armoury; concerned discussion with colleagues to reach a consensus on appropriate usage; involvement of pharmacist and microbiologist as well as clinician—all these need to be brought into play. It may be that the most important function of an antibiotic policy is to provide a vehicle for ensuring that regular discussion amongst all those concerned in antibiotic prescribing does take place.

Blind faith in a restrictive antibiotic policy is *not* the answer to control of antibiotic usage since bacterial resistance patterns change due to selective pressure, and therefore a flexible system should be used. It is essential that an active infection control programme is also in place, so that patients harbouring multiply antibiotic-resistant bacteria are appropriately treated.

Monitoring antibiotic policies

Although most policies are based on the release of restricted antibiotic sensitivity reports, full clinical advice is usually available from the microbiology department. Policies may be tailor-made for individual units, and ward stocks restricted to agents named in the formulary. Ward pharmacists, if they are available, should maintain up-to-date records and maintain stocks; unused drugs should be returned to the pharmacy. Restricted drugs may be available in the emergency cupboard, but a record of all antibiotics removed should be kept. Antibiotics used for surgical prophylaxis should be prescribed for 1 day or less, and treatment courses re-prescribed every 5 days if necessary. Overall scrutiny of antibiotic usage by ward, unit or hospital can be carried out by the drugs and therapeutics sub-committee. Computer print-outs can be readily scrutinized and aberrant prescriptions followed up. The policy is based on consensus and voluntary agreement. Cross-sectional surveys are easy to carry out and should be performed at regular intervals once a month on selected wards. Special attention should be paid to the use of antibiotics for surgical prophylaxis, their use should be the subject of regular audit.

Antibiotic audit should not be a policing exercise and should not imply a threat to the clinician's freedom to prescribe as he or she thinks best. Rather, it should serve as a reminder of the need to justify selection of antimicrobials in the light of critical analysis.

Benefits of monitoring antibiotic use

Formularies are a way of ensuring that drug therapy is cost effective and cost beneficial. Monitoring antibiotic usage should provide ward, unit, and hospital-wide information on prescribing patterns. This should prove useful for trend analysis and allow discrepancies to be identified. Such information lends itself to detailed scrutiny to differentiate between rational, questionable, and irrational antibiotic usage. Clinical efficacy and adverse side-effects can be evaluated. Correlations between antibiotic usage and antimicrobial resistance can be sought, and changes can be made. Prospective, controlled trials on new antibiotics can be made and cost–benefit analyses undertaken.

Table 14.1. Audit of antibiotic prescribing

---

1 What is the most likely anatomical site of the infection?
2 What clinical, radiological evidence, and laboratory findings support the evidence of infection?
3 Have bacteriological investigations been requested?
4 Has the organism responsible for the infection been isolated?
5 If not, what is the suspected organism?
6 Are there any recognized underlying or predisposing conditions relevant to the diagnosis of infection?
7 Was the diagnosis, confirmed, doubtful or unknown?
8 Should the patient have received an antibiotic?
9 Was the antibiotic an appropriate choice?
10 Was the dose appropriate?
11 Was its frequency of dosage appropriate?
12 Was the route of administration appropriate?
13 Was the course of treatment of suitable duration?

Although there are many benefits of monitoring antibiotic use, such a strategy costs money. Few studies have attempted to cost the total resource put into preparing and monitoring a formulary. The effect (or outcome) of drug utilization review studies is unknown. It is not enough simply to count the total cost of antibiotic consumption; there are too many variables. Although a 'defined daily dose' can be used as a standard unit of measurement, the case mix of different wards is so variable that direct comparisons are difficult. Nevertheless, without information on antibiotic prescribing habits it is impossible to control the use of antibiotics effectively.

The next stage on from monitoring antibiotic usage is antibiotic audit, thereby closing the loop (see Table 14.1).

CONTROL OF THE EMERGENCE OF RESISTANCE

All antibiotic use creates selective pressures which lead to the emergence of resistant bacterial strains. Antibiotics are vital to the practice of modern medicine; we cannot abandon them, or even unreasonably restrict their use. Resistant bacteria will continue to appear, and to cause problems in the treatment of the infections they cause. Surveillance of the use of antibiotics —locally, nationally, and internationally— coupled with the monitoring of emerging patterns of bacterial resistance will help to influence prescribing practice and the development of meaningful antibiotic policies, as long as the people collecting the information ensure that it is passed on to the people who use the drugs. Few will recklessly continue to prescribe antibiotics to which local resistance is common, as long as they know that local resistance *is* common. The dissemination of accurate, up-to-date information is vital in establishing the appropriate use of antibiotics which, together with control of infection measures, is the best protection against the unrestricted spread of drug resistance.

Part IV

General principles of usage of antimicrobial agents

15

General principles of the treatment of infection

R. G. Finch

Antimicrobial agents are among the most commonly prescribed drugs. Their use has had a major impact on the control of most bacterial infections in humans and to a lesser, although constantly increasing, degree, is affecting the outcome of many fungal, viral, protozoal, and helminthic infections. The principles governing the use of antimicrobial agents to be discussed in this chapter apply specifically to the management of bacterial infections, although the overall approach is similar when selecting treatment for other microbial diseases.

Antimicrobial therapy demands an initial *clinical evaluation* of the nature and extent of the infective process and knowledge of the likely causative pathogen(s). This assessment should be supported, whenever practical, by laboratory investigation aimed at establishing the microbial aetiology and its susceptibility to antimicrobial agents appropriate for the treatment of the infection. The choice of drug, its dose, route, and frequency of administration are also dependent upon an appreciation of the pharmacological and pharmacokinetic features of a particular agent. Furthermore, the range and predictability of adverse reactions of a particular compound should be kept in mind.

CLINICAL ASSESSMENT

The clinical evaluation should define the anatomical location and severity of the infective process. The history and examination frequently determine such infective states as meningitis, arthritis, pneumonia, and cellulitis. Although such diseases may be caused by a wide variety of organisms, the range of pathogens is usually limited, and the pattern of susceptibility reasonably predictable. This, therefore, permits a rational selection of chemotherapy in the initial management of such infections.

The anatomical location is not only critical from the point of view of the most likely pathogen and the most suitable choice of drug, but also determines the *route of administration*. Superficial infections of the skin, such as impetigo which is caused by *Streptococcus pyogenes*, or infection of the mucous membranes such as oral or vaginal candidiasis, caused by *Candida albicans*, respond well to topical application. However, if infection is caused by the microbial invasion of tissues or the bloodstream, adequate tissue concentrations of a drug may be achieved only by either intramuscular or intravenous administration.

Other clues as to the nature of the infection are gleaned from epidemiological considerations such as the age, sex, and occupation of the patient. In tropical countries, diseases such as malaria, amoebiasis, and salmonellosis (including typhoid fever) are prime suspects in the investigation of fever and diarrhoea, and local knowledge about the prevalence of diseases like filariasis, schistosomiasis, and trypanosomiasis, which are circumscribed in distribution, may be used to advantage. In countries free from these diseases as indigenous problems, a history of overseas travel should alert the physician to consider exotic infections.

Pre-existing medical problems may predispose to infection; such conditions include valvular heart disease, underlying malignant disease, or the presence of prosthetic devices such as artificial hip joints, heart valves, or intravascular cannulae.

Under some circumstances the invading pathogen may be part of the host's normal flora. The normal host defences may be breached in a variety of ways. For example, the skin or mucous membranes, which are normally a most effective barrier against infection, may permit access of pathogenic organisms to the deeper tissues when traumatized by a surgical incision or by accident. Similarly, burns can denude large areas of the body with subsequent infection by bacteria, notably *Pseudomonas aeruginosa*, *Staphylococcus aureus*, and *Str. pyogenes*, which may be acquired from contact with patients or staff within the hospital.

The circulating and tissue phagocytes provide an important defence against infection. Therefore, an absolute or relative deficiency of circulating polymorphonuclear leucocytes is commonly associated with recurrent, frequently serious, infection. In patients with acute leukaemia, cytotoxic chemotherapy often depresses the circulating leucocytes to low levels for several days or weeks. Such patients are extremely vulnerable to serious episodes of infection, particularly Gram-negative bacillary bacteraemia, which carries a high mortality if untreated.

LABORATORY ASSESSMENT

Few infective conditions present such a typical picture that both a definitive clinical and microbiological diagnosis can be made without recourse to the laboratory. Therefore, whenever possible, a clinical diagnosis should be supported by laboratory confirmation. Such confirmation makes both the diagnosis and the management, in particular the selection of antimicrobial chemotherapy, more certain and allows for a more sound assessment of the likely prognosis. However, when infection is obvious or strongly suspected on clinical grounds, therapy should be instituted as soon as appropriate specimens for laboratory investigation have been taken. In some cases (e.g. pneumococcal meningitis) the patient's chances of survival are directly related to the promptitude with which therapy is started. Furthermore, laboratory reports are not always contributory and several days may be lost trying to establish a microbiological diagnosis, during which time the patient's condition may deteriorate.

Serological tests which demonstrate antibody against specific microbial antigens are important in the diagnosis of more persistent infections such as syphilis, brucellosis, and Q fever. Tests to demonstrate the presence of microbial antigens are also valuable in the diagnosis of selected infections. For example, fluorescent antibody reagents can detect *Pneumocystis carinii* in sputum or bronchial lavage material, while pneumococcal antigen is often present in sputum, serum, and urine of patients with pneumococcal pneumonia.

SELECTION OF ANTIMICROBIAL CHEMOTHERAPY

In vitro susceptibility

In vitro testing of drugs provides indirect evidence of the likely clinical response of a particular pathogen to a specific drug or drugs. Confirmation of clinical efficacy can be determined only *in vivo* and, hence, the importance of clinical evaluation of all new antimicrobial agents. Controlled experimental evidence gained from the treatment of artificial infections in animals provides only indirect evidence of the likely clinical efficacy. Occasionally *in vitro* evidence of activity is not borne out by *in vivo* evidence of success. For example, *Salmonella typhi* is susceptible *in vitro* to many drugs active against Gram-negative bacilli, including gentamicin; however, typhoid fever responds clinically only to a limited range of drugs, including chloramphenicol, amoxycillin, and co-trimoxazole. This may in part be due to the intracellular location of *S.typhi* in this disease.

Bacteristatic or bactericidal agents

Antibacterial agents are often separated into either bactericidal or bacteristatic agents according to their ability to kill or inhibit bacterial growth. This separation is somewhat artificial since some bacteristatic drugs may be bactericidal either in higher concentrations or against different bacterial species. Bacteristatic agents must rely on host defences, in particular the phagocytic cells, to finally eliminate the infection, since if the drug is withdrawn bacteria have the opportunity to recover. Under most circumstances the choice between a cidal or a static agent is not critical. This is not the case in the treatment of infective endocarditis. Here bacteria are protected against phagocytic activity within the vegetations present on the deformed or prosthetic heart valve or adjacent endocardium. Under these circumstances it is important to use a bactericidal drug or combination of drugs which penetrate the vegetations and thus eradicate the infection. Similarly, patients with neutropenia from cytotoxic chemotherapy or other causes of bone marrow aplasia are extremely vulnerable to infection. Bacteristatic drugs are inappropriate in these cases and bactericidal agents should be selected.

Pharmacokinetic factors

The aim of chemotherapy is to eliminate an infection as rapidly as possible. To achieve this a sufficient concentration of the drug or drugs selected must reach the site of infection. The choice of agent is, therefore, as much dependent upon the pharmacological and pharmacokinetic features of the drugs, which determine absorption, distribution, metabolism, and excretion, as upon its antimicrobial properties. These aspects are discussed in more detail in Chapter 16.

In general, drugs are administered either topically, by mouth, or by intravenous or intramuscular injection. Oral absorption is most erratic. Drugs must first negotiate the acid condition of the stomach before being absorbed, usually from the proximal small bowel. This occurs most readily when the stomach is empty and it is generally advised that they be swallowed approximately 30 minutes before a meal.

Absorption can be increased by protecting a drug from acid inactivation by a coating (so-called *enteric coating*) which subsequently breaks down once the tablet is beyond the stomach. Alternatively, the drug may be modified chemically to produce a more acid-stable formulation (see Chapter 16). For most minor infections, including skin, soft-tissue, respiratory tract, and lower urinary tract infection, oral therapy is appropriate.

In contrast to oral administration, intravenous administration avoids the vagaries of gastrointestinal absorption, and achieves rapid therapeutic blood and tissue concentrations. Intramuscular administration requires absorption through the tissue capillaries and is generally rapid except in conditions of cardiovascular collapse and shock when tissue perfusion is impaired. Relatively avascular sites such as the aqueous, and in particular the vitreous, humour of the eye, are difficult sites in which to achieve adequate concentrations of drugs. In contrast, the presence of inflammation increases the permeability of many natural barriers such as the meninges and in this situation allows higher concentrations of certain drugs, such as the penicillins, to be achieved within the CSF. Other drugs, most notably chloramphenicol, are little influenced by such inflammatory changes.

CHOICE OF ANTIMICROBIAL REGIMENS

Drug dosing

There are no universally applicable guidelines for drug dosing, which is frequently determined by factors such as tolerability and toxicity as well as the activity of a particular drug against a particular infecting organism. Some agents, most notably the penicillins, have such a wide margin of safety that enormous doses are frequently prescribed. Only in a few cases (e.g. treatment of *Ps. aeruginosa* infection with ticarcillin) does such antimicrobial overkill have a microbiologically rational basis. In an attempt to provide a rule of thumb in devising dosage schedules some authors suggest that blood levels four or eight times higher than the MIC of the organism are most likely to produce therapeutic tissue concentrations. However, for practical purposes, dosages are based on experience gained from the treatment of a wide variety of infections. Guidance can sometimes be obtained by back titration of the patient's serum against the infecting organism (see Chapter 8). A serum bactericidal titre of 8 or more obtained about 1 hour after a parenteral dose usually indicates adequate therapy in patients with infective endocarditis.

Length of therapy

Treatment should continue until all micro-organisms are eliminated from the tissues or the infection has been sufficiently controlled for the normal host defences to eradicate it. This end-point is in general determined by clinical observation and evidence of the resolution of the inflammatory process such as the return of body temperature and white cell count to normal.

Many infections come under control within a few days and 7 days' treatment is often sufficient. Uncomplicated urinary tract infections usually respond very rapidly to chemotherapy. Selection of the least dose compatible with complete resolution is desirable (see Chapter 21). In contrast, patients with pulmonary tuberculosis require 6–9 months' treatment with isoniazid and rifampicin if relapse is to be prevented (see Chapter 26). Furthermore, 10 days' penicillin treatment is necessary to eradicate *Str. pyogenes* from the throat in patients with streptococcal tonsillitis, although symptomatic improvement occurs within a few days. There is no universally 'correct' duration of chemotherapy and each problem should be judged on its merits based on the clinical response to treatment.

ADVERSE REACTIONS

Antimicrobial agents, like all other therapeutic substances, have the potential to produce adverse reactions. These vary widely in their nature, frequency, and severity. Many reactions, such as gastrointestinal intolerance, are minor and short lived but others may be serious, life threatening, and occasionally fatal. Drug reactions are unfortunately a common cause of prolonged hospitalization or may precipitate hospitalization. Drug reactions may be predictable and dose dependent, for example nephrotoxicity associated with the use of the antifungal agent, amphotericin B. However, many adverse reactions are unpredictable. The subject is discussed more fully in Chapter 18.

COMBINED THERAPY

In general, single-drug therapy of established infections is preferred whenever possible. Such an approach is known to be effective and reduces the risks of adverse reactions and drug interactions that may accompany multiple-drug prescribing. None the less, there are a few situations where combined chemotherapy has definite advantages over single drug therapy.

Initial therapy

In the management of acute and potentially life-threatening infections combined chemotherapy covering all likely pathogens is often used until the cause of the infection is established. It is common practice to combine flucloxacillin with an aminoglycoside, such as tobramycin or gentamicin, in the initial treatment of serious infections. However, should there be evidence that the infection has arisen in association with mucosal surfaces, such as the gut or female genital tract, then metronidazole or clindamycin is frequently added to meet the possibility of a mixed anaerobic and aerobic bacterial infection. Once a definitive diagnosis is established it is important to adjust the therapeutic regimen to one that is most appropriate.

Synergy

Under some circumstances combined chemotherapy is selected for its known synergic effect on a pathogenic organism. This increased ability to inhibit or kill the pathogen may speed resolution or reduce the risk of relapse when treating difficult infections. One of the commonest requirements for synergic therapy is the treatment of infective endocarditis caused by enterococci and occasionally by oral streptococci. The combination of two bactericidal drugs, penicillin and gentamicin (or streptomycin), is synergic both *in vitro* and *in vivo* and is associated with a more favourable response to treatment than is single-drug therapy.

Antagonism

Some drugs may have an opposite effect and be antagonistic. For example, shortly after penicillin and tetracycline became available, it was shown that the two drugs together produced a worse clinical result in the treatment of pneumococcal meningitis than did either drug alone. In this situation a bacteristatic agent (tetracycline) prevents penicillin from achieving its bactericidal effect on the cell wall, which is dependent on bacterial growth.

Prevention of drug resistance

It is uncommon for the bacterium causative of an infection to become resistant during treatment, although some drugs including streptomycin, rifampicin, fusidic acid, and nalidixic acid encourage the rapid emergence of resistant bacteria. These bacteria do not develop resistance in response to treatment, but small numbers of pre-existent resistant mutants proliferate when the sensitive population is suppressed.

In the treatment of tuberculosis combined chemotherapy is used specifically to prevent the emergence of resistant variants present in the tuberculous tissues.

COST

Antimicrobial drugs vary widely in their cost. In general, generic drugs cost less than proprietary preparations, whilst well established, widely used agents tend to be less expensive. Injectable preparations are usually more expensive than oral preparations, and syrups and drops are usually more expensive than tablets and capsules.

The use of very high dosage also escalates the cost. Sometimes this is unavoidable, as in the treatment of *Ps. aeruginosa* infections with large doses of expensive antipseudomonal agents, but, in general, high dosage should not be used without justification.

Among the most expensive antimicrobial agents are the parenteral cephalosporins, and quinolones, all antipseudomonal compounds, intravenous metronidazole, and most antiviral agents. It is, therefore, apparent that whenever drugs which are both equally effective and tolerated are available then it is reasonable to select the cheaper agent. This is a most important consideration in some developing countries where drug costs can account for 20 per cent of an already meagre health budget. The *British National Formulary* provides a useful approximate guide to the cost of drugs for doctors in the UK.

In addition to the unit cost of a drug, other direct costs include the use of disposable materials for drug administration, staff time in preparation and administration, and assay costs to ensure adequate and safe dosaging. Comparative cure and relapse rates are also currently under scrutiny since the need for further treatment entails additional expense.

FAILURE OF ANTIMICROBIAL CHEMOTHERAPY

Patients with established infection may fail to respond to antimicrobial therapy for a variety of reasons.

Choice of therapy

Firstly, the choice of drug may be inappropriate for the infecting strain. This stresses the need to establish a microbiological diagnosis whenever possible so that the *in vitro* susceptibility of the pathogen can be confirmed. On the other hand, some infections are caused by intracellular pathogens, as in brucellosis, chlamydial disease, and typhoid fever. For treatment to be successful, sufficient antibiotic must penetrate the cell; this limits the number of agents which are clinically effective. Failure may also result if the drug is inadequately concentrated at the site of the infection; this may occur if the dose is insufficient or the route inappropriate. By changing to the parenteral route or increasing the dose, therapeutic success may follow.

The route of excretion also requires consideration. For instance, in renal failure, drugs normally excreted by the kidneys may fail to reach therapeutic concentrations in the urine so that treatment of a urinary tract infection with drugs such as nalidixic acid and nitrofurantoin may be unsuccessful.

Presence of necrotic material

Treatment may also fail because of the presence of necrotic material, an eschar, or abscess. Antibiotic penetration of such avascular material is poor, so surgical debridement of necrotic material or drainage of pus should be carried out early. Antibiotic treatment under these circumstances is an adjunct to such surgical management.

Presence of foreign material

Infection that occurs in association with bladder catheters, intravascular devices, hip prostheses, or inanimate foreign material which gains access to the tissues following surgical or traumatic injuries may fail to respond to antimicrobial chomotherapy. Under these circumstances, total eradication of infection is rarely achieved until the foreign material is removed.

If antimicrobial therapy is to be successful these drugs can only exhibit their full power as 'magic bullets' if used intelligently and if full recognition is paid to the need to individualize each course of treatment to both the patient and the pathogen.

16

Pharmacokinetics

D. Greenwood

Ehrlich's 'magic bullet' notion of chemotherapy foresaw substances which when given as a single dose would localize in the sites of infection and destroy the organisms there. Despite the enormous advances made in the development of antimicrobial compounds none exhibits the remarkable properties Ehrlich visualized. The great majority of antimicrobial agents are widely distributed in the body in response to forces which have nothing to do with infection and may, in fact, result in the concentrations of the agent being least in the sites where they are most needed.

Among the many properties that must be exhibited by therapeutically useful chemotherapeutic agents, the ability to achieve effective concentrations, and act in the complex environment of the infected lesion is essential. When antibiotics are given systemically the delivery and maintenance of effective concentrations at the site of infection are determined by the concentrations achieved in the blood, which are in turn determined by the absorption, metabolism, and excretion of the drug and by the way in which the blood-borne drug is distributed to the tissues. From serial measurements of the concentration of the agent in the serum, it is possible to calculate both its rates of absorption and elimination and the volume in which the drug is distributed. The *volume of distribution* indicates whether it is largely confined within the vascular compartment or spreads out into the extracellular fluid—the site of most infections—or penetrates into cells where some organisms, for example mycobacteria and brucella, multiply. The rates of transfer, volume of distribution, and other key properties can be given numerical values which provide succinct and quantitative statements of the drug *pharmacokinetics*. For the present purpose, it is necessary only to examine in turn each stage of movement of the drug from absorption to delivery to the infected site and the factors which influence each of the stages.

ABSORPTION

Many antibiotics do not produce adequate plasma levels when given by mouth and are available only as injectable preparations. In some countries, injections are favoured over oral therapy, but this has more to do with cultural differences and traditions than with proven therapeutic benefit. In the UK, the convenience of the oral route, particularly in domiciliary practice, means that antibiotics are given by mouth whenever possible. In some cases, as with cefuroxime and cefuroxime axetil, considerable effort is put into the preparation of oral derivatives of the original compound. The need for properties such as stability in solution means that pharmaceutical preparations (injections, capsules, tablets, syrups, etc.) can contain different derivatives of the drug, sometimes with distinct properties.

Oral administration

The degree to which compounds are absorbed when given orally differs greatly. Chloramphenicol is so well absorbed that there is no place for an injectable form of the drug except in patients who cannot swallow. However, the drug is so bitter that it cannot be given as a syrup; hence a tasteless derivative is used for such preparations which is microbiologically inactive until it is hydrolysed in the gut with the liberation into the plasma of the active form. This device of producing derivatives which have some particularly desirable property but act in the body by the liberation of the parent drug is widely used; such preparations are collectively called *pro-drugs*.

Antibiotic esters

Erythromycin is irregularly absorbed and often produces low plasma concentrations. Several derivatives have been produced in an attempt to overcome this difficulty, including erythromycin estolate which, like the tasteless chloramphenicol preparation, is microbiologically inactive, but is much more lipid soluble than the parent drug and much better absorbed in the small intestine, where non-specific esterases liberate the active erythromycin into the portal vein. Esterification as the means of improving the oral absorption of drugs has been fairly widely used, other examples being the esters of ampicillin, such as pivampicillin, talampicillin, and bacampicillin.

Generally, esters show another important benefit in addition to the increased plasma levels obtained: their absorption, unlike that of the parent compound, is much less affected by the presence of food in the stomach. If patients are to take drugs at regular intervals it is very difficult to separate the administration of all doses from meal times and it is a great advantage in a drug to be unaffected by such influences. A further advantage of such pro-drugs is that they are not degraded by the bowel flora and, being microbiologically inactive, the fraction of the drug which is not absorbed does not disturb the gut flora as do active antibiotics—an effect believed to lessen the chances of post-antibiotic diarrhoea and of superinfection with resistant organisms.

Interference with absorption

The original tetracycline, chlortetracycline, is a good example of an oral agent which is not well absorbed. Moreover, its naturally low absorption is further depressed by the simultaneous administration of food, especially substances such as milk which contain high concentrations of calcium or magnesium, with which tetracycline forms stable insoluble chelates. The unabsorbed compound is active and it powerfully disturbs the bowel flora—an effect that most probably underlies the bowel disturbances which commonly follow its use.

Attempts in the past to minimize these side-effects by the administration of the drug with milk or alkali secured any desirable effect they may have had in limiting the gastrointestinal symptoms at the expense of drug absorption.

Parenteral administration

Intravenous injection

The most direct way of ensuring adequate concentrations of antibiotic in the blood is by intravenous injection. The highest instantaneous concentrations are, of course, achieved by a single rapid intravenous injection, but any benefit of this may be offset by rapid excretion, and many agents are given by infusion over 15 or 20 minutes. It was common practice at one time to add antibiotics to drip infusions, but this should be avoided since the slow rate of administration results in low plasma levels of the drug. Sometimes degradation of the drug in solution can occur over the prolonged period of administration, particularly if administration is combined with glucose. Certain combinations of penicillin and aminoglycosides mutually inactivate each other when mixed in intravenous solutions.

Rapid injection or infusion results in high concentration of the drug, which then declines rapidly as the drug diffuses into the extracellular space and into the cells if they are accessible to it. There follows a period during which the concentration of drug falls more or less rapidly, depending on the rate at which it is metabolized and excreted (Fig.16.1).

Plasma half-life

This phase principally determines the period for which active drug is available to the body; the time required for the concentration of drug in the plasma to fall by half is called the *plasma half-life*. Half-lives of different antibiotics vary considerably. That of benzylpenicillin, for example, is only 30 min. while that of fusidic acid is 12 h. Drug distributed into the tissues may be bound there and this drug, as distinct from that in the plasma, may be relatively slowly remobilized and excreted. When a drug behaves in this way the rate of elimination may be very slow and the *terminal half-life* very much greater than that during the main excretory phase.

Drug accumulation

If large doses are given or the half-life of the drug is such that complete elimination has not occurred before the next dose is administered, the concentration of drug in the plasma will progressively rise. The excretion phase being logarithmic, the rate of elimination rises as the concentration of drug rises; eventually excretion proceeds as fast as the accumulation and the drug reaches a steady state (Fig. 16.2). This

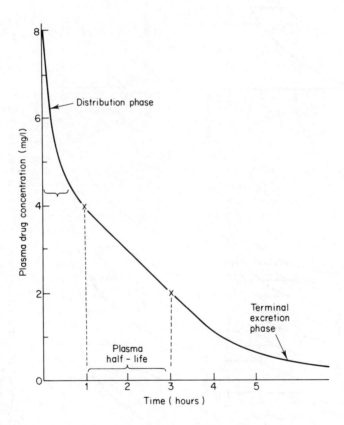

Fig. 16.1. Decline in plasma concentration of a drug after its intravenous injection. Three phases may be distinguished: an initial rapid fall as the drug is distributed from the plasma; a less rapid fall during the main period of excretion and metabolism; and a terminal slow decline representing, for example, the release of the drug from binding sites.

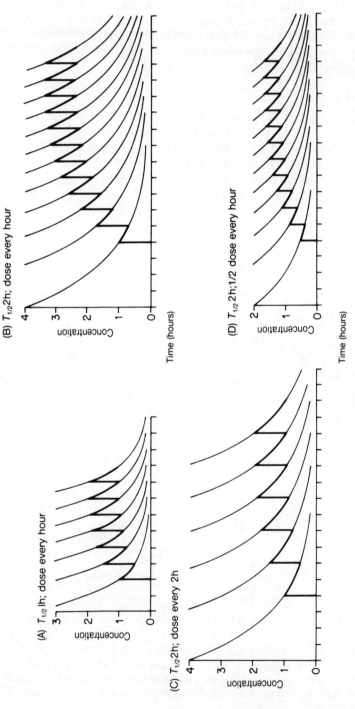

Fig. 16.2. Steady-state concentrations on various drug regimens. The thin lines are identical curves showing the fall in concentration of an agent with the half-life ($T_{1/2}$) shown. The thick lines indicate the concentrations achieved by doses given at intervals of (A, C) every half-life, and (B, D) twice every half-life. In each case a steady state is eventually reached, but the time taken to achieve steady state and the concentration achieved depend on the conditions. [From F. O'Grady (1971). *British Medical Bulletin* **27**, 142–7.]

may be beneficial in achieving a constant exposure of the infecting organism to the agent, but it can also be hazardous if the agent is toxic. The possibility of accumulation and its consequences must be considered when an agent with a long half-life is administered or the patient's capacity to eliminate the agent is known or thought likely to be impaired.

Intramuscular injection

When all the drug is delivered directly into the plasma within a short time the plasma half-life is determined solely by the rate of elimination. When, however, uptake into the plasma is much slower then the persistence of the drug will depend not only on the rate at which it is eliminated but also on the rate at which it is added. Absorption from intramuscular sites is usually rapid, but special *depot preparations* of drugs such as procaine penicillin have been developed which possess the property that absorption from the injection site is slow and the plasma level correspondingly prolonged (Fig. 16.3).

DISTRIBUTION

Protein binding

Compounds in the plasma generally reach the tissues by diffusion, but in some cases there is active secretion, as in the saliva, the bile, and the

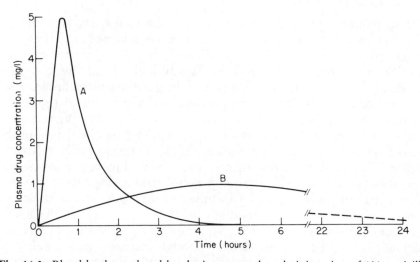

Fig. 16.3. Blood levels produced by the intramuscular administration of (A) penicillin and (B) procaine penicillin.

urine. One important factor affecting the diffusibility of compounds is the degree to which they are bound to plasma proteins, mostly albumin. With some drugs, such as cloxacillin, ceftriaxone, or fusidic acid, more than 90 per cent of the drug is bound and is antibacterially inactive. Only the diffusible fraction of the drug reaches the tissues and only this fraction exerts any antimicrobial effect. As the unbound fraction diffuses away, more of the plasma-bound drug dissociates and the equilibrium between the bound and the free compound is maintained. Because of this effect in limiting the activity and diffusibility of the drug, high degrees of protein binding have been held to be highly disadvantageous.

Two things have to be considered. The first is that, in order to be therapeutically effective, adequate concentrations of free drug must be achieved at the site of infection. That this occurs with the compounds mentioned, despite high degrees of protein binding, is clear from their clinical efficacy. The second is that bound drug will go wherever the protein goes and that includes the protein poured into the infected sites with inflammatory exudate. To this extent, protein-bound drug may be looked upon as a pro-drug with the valuable property of 'homing in' on to sites of inflammation. Once in the site, as far as is known, the concentration of free and active drug is still defined by the equilibrium between free and bound drug.

Another important aspect of protein binding is that protein-drugs compete for binding sites and it is possible to displace one with another of higher affinity, resulting in increased concentration and possibly toxic effects of the liberated drug (see Chapter 18).

Access to infected sites

The main interest in the distribution of antimicrobial agents is in the area which is least easy to study: the concentration achieved at the infected target. Some sites can be sampled directly, important examples being the CSF or the bronchial secretions. The difficulty is that there is good reason to believe that the distribution of drug in the subarachnoid space and the bronchi is far from homogeneous, and a comprehensive view of the behaviour of the drug in these sites is hard to obtain. What is clear is that the specialized tissues which separate the drug circulating in the plasma from these important sites of infection are normally relatively impermeable to all but a few agents. Macrolides, fluoroquinolones, and trimethoprim appear to be unusually well-distributed agents, lipid solubility apparently playing a part in this, and it is claimed that the more lipid-soluble tetracycline derivatives develop higher concentrations in the bronchi than do the traditional compounds. Most drugs enter the infected site in high concentrations through increased permeability of the vascular endothelium produced by the inflammatory process, and an important result of this is that as the drug exerts its antibacterial effect and the inflammation subsides the drug is progressively excluded again. In some cases of meningitis treated with high doses of ampicillin, for example, exclusion of the drug as inflammation subsides may lead to a recrudescence of infection.

Tissue concentrations

One of the most difficult areas to study is soft-tissue infection. Some tissues, such as the tonsil, are accessible, and by homogenizing samples of such tissue in suitable fluid the 'tissue' concentration of antibiotics can be measured. If this concentration is significantly higher than that of the blood the result is helpful, although there is no way of knowing where precisely the drug is located in anatomical terms. If the concentration is less than that of the blood the measurements may represent simply the effect of diluting the drug present in the tissue blood vessels. This cannot be overcome by washing out the blood since this may artificially lower the tissue concentration by encouraging the diffusion of agent.

Attempts have been made to assess the antibiotic concentrations present in extracellular fluid by the creation of artificial collections of fluid which can be repeatedly sampled. In animals this has been achieved by implanting a sterile mesh into the subcutaneous tissue or muscle and allowing it to fill with fluid. In human, blisters can be raised on the skin by application of vesiculating agents such as cantharides. In general, the concentration of antibacterial agents rises and falls very much less rapidly in these spaces than it does in the plasma, and the concentrations achieved are considerably lower and more prolonged.

How closely these spaces mimic normal tissue spaces and particularly infected tissue spaces in their composition and fluid dynamics is much disputed. Interesting differences can be demonstrated in them in the behaviour of various antibacterial agents, but these do not appear to be decidedly reflected in differences of therapeutic performance. Perhaps the most extraordinary feature of antimicrobial pharmacokinetics is that, after 50 years of intensive clinical and experimental study, we still do not know what shape of drug concentration/time curve is needed at the site of infection to secure optimum antimicrobial effects. If we knew that we would be one step (of several required) towards more rationally based dosage schedules.

METABOLISM

Many antibiotics are modified in the body; the resulting metabolites are important for two reasons. Firstly, they are generally, though not always, less active microbiologically than is the parent compound. Some metabolites show not only different degrees, but different spectra, of activity. The generation of such compounds can considerably complicate the microbiological assay of the drug, and progress in understanding the more complicated situations of this kind has relied heavily on the development of such methods of drug measurement as high-pressure liquid chromatography. The second importance of the metabolites is that they may differ from the parent compounds in toxicity. If they are relatively inactive and more toxic, conventional microbiological assay of the drug will give very poor guidance as to the toxic hazard.

EXCRETION

The major route of excretion for most antibiotics is via the urine, in which very high concentrations may be achieved. Many drugs excreted in this way are active against the organisms commonly responsible for urinary tract infections and the high concentrations of drug achieved in the urine play an important part in their elimination. Excretion is by glomerular filtration or tubular secretion, and sometimes both. Metabolites and parent drugs may be handled differently by the kidney. In pyelonephritis the principal site of infection is in the peritubular areas of the medulla. Drug can reach this space by diffusion from the plasma, but high concentrations can also be achieved by non-ionic back-diffusion. As the urine becomes more concentrated in its progress towards the collecting tubule, the concentration of drug rises markedly so that a large concentration gradient develops between the tubular contents and the interstitial space where organisms multiply. Only un-ionized species of drug are diffusible; the delivery of high tubular concentrations of the drug into the infected site therefore depends on the proportion of drug un-ionized at the pH of the tubular content. Nitrofurantoin, for example, is a weak acid and in renal tubular contents the greater part of the drug will be un-ionized and free to diffuse into the peritubular space.

Tubular secretion

The principal compounds excreted in the urine by active tubular secretion are the penicillins and cephalosporins. This process is so effective as to clear the blood of most of the drug during its passage through the kidney and plays a major part in determining the short half-life of compounds excreted in this way. The period for which inhibitory levels of rapidly excreted agents like benzylpenicillin are present in the blood can be increased by either increasing the frequency of administration or reducing the drug's tubular secretion. Many agents share the tubular route of excretion and will compete with one another for the active transport mechanism. The oral uricosuric agent, probenecid, is a potent competitor in this regard; its administration in conjuction with penicillins reduces the renal excretion and so prolongs the plasma half-life.

Some cells in other parts of the body behave in a way analogous to those of the proximal renal tubules. It is, for example, believed that active secretion of drug by cells of the choroid plexus is responsible for the rapid fall in CSF penicillin levels that is seen in patients treated for bacterial meningitis. It is likely that the same mechanism is responsible for the fall in CSF glucose levels, at one time attributed to metabolism of the sugar by the infecting bacteria. Probenecid can be used to slow the active secretion of pencillin via the choroid plexus, but little use has been made of this method of conserving drug levels in the CSF.

Biliary excretion and enterohepatic recirculation

Some antibiotics, for example erythromycin, produce very low and sometimes undetectable levels in the urine. Many such compounds are excreted in the bile, and metabolites produced in the liver may also follow this route. When the bile enters the small intestine a significant proportion of the drug may be reabsorbed and, if so, enterohepatic recirculation can play a significant part in maintaining plasma levels of the drug. Because of its relative inaccessibility, it is difficult in practice to obtain entirely satisfactory figures for the concentration of drugs excreted in the bile. Most studies are done on bile obtained at operation or post-operatively, when the bile is draining through a T-tube and conditions are plainly not physiological. Nevertheless, there is good evidence that some agents achieve unusually high biliary levels and are, therefore, valuable in the treatment of bacterial cholangitis. Naturally, this route of excretion ceases when the biliary tract is obstructed or hepatic function deranged, and it is plainly prudent to avoid administering to such patients agents for which this is a major route of elimination.

17

Prescribing in the young and the elderly

R. G. Finch

Children are no longer considered to be small adults for the purposes of prescribing. The former practice of scaling down an adult dose on a weight basis may result in either subtherapeutic or toxic concentrations and this is no longer readily accepted. This applies to the prescribing of all drugs in childhood, not only antimicrobial agents.

Similarly, the risks of adverse reactions increase significantly in elderly patients, especially if liver and kidney function is impaired by age or disease. The evaluation of new drugs in paediatric and elderly patients presents particular problems and is extremely important, since the pharmacological handling of the drugs and their unwanted effects may differ considerably in infants, young children, the elderly, and normal adults.

PAEDIATRIC PRESCRIBING

In childhood, pharmacokinetic and pharmacodynamic factors often differ markedly from those in the adult, hence, dosages may be adjusted according to surface area, which is more closely related to the ability to metabolize drugs. However, in infancy and early childhood the surface area is larger, relative to the older child and adult, hence there is a risk of overdosing when using such a system.

To arrive at a safe yet effective concentration of a drug is not without difficulties. In fact, for many drugs the dosages have not been accurately determined, even in adults. In the case of new antimicrobial agents, pharmacological and toxicological investigations are more commonly carried out in an adult population, so that information in children and particularly in infants and neonates may be extremely limited. Lack of such information may preclude the widespread use of a potentially useful agent in childhood.

To derive the necessary information in childhood requires painstaking and careful observations in sick children since pharmacokinetic information is not available from healthy children for ethical reasons.

Furthermore, owing to physiological differences, information in the preterm or low-birthweight infant cannot necessarily be applied to heavier or full-term infants. Very few centres have the expertise to carry out such exacting work.

Age-related epidemiology of infections

When selecting antimicrobial therapy, knowledge of age-related infections is important in the initial management, before laboratory information is available. Many infections, although not entirely peculiar to infancy and childhood, are none the less much more frequently encountered in this age group. For example, the classic viral exanthems of rubella, measles, and varicella are primarily diseases of childhood. Such age-related infections reflect the ready transmission of these agents and the susceptibility of a relatively non-immune population. Certain bacterial infections are also much more common in the very young. Neonatal meningitis is primarily caused by *Escherichia coli* and group B streptococci, whilst in the pre-school child *Haemophilus influenzae* is more frequent. Meningococcal infection is largely a disease of childhood.

Upper respiratory tract infections are extremely common in childhood. Many are caused by viruses, but infection is often complicated by secondary bacterial invasion with *Streptococcus pneumoniae* or *H. influenzae*.

Cystic fibrosis is largely a disease of children, although careful management is seeing an increasing number of sufferers survive into adult life. A major complication of this disease is recurrent lower respiratory tract infection in which *Staphylococcus aureus* and *Pseudomonas aeruginosa* predominate. Such infections are difficult to control and it is often impossible to eliminate *Ps. aeruginosa* completely from the sputum.

Physiological considerations

Paediatric prescribing recognizes the fact that growth and development, including organ function and metabolism are frequently undergoing change in childhood. This is particularly so for the neonatal period in which both chronological age, gestational age, and body weight are important considerations. Dosages of many drugs, including antimicrobial agents, vary on account of the state of flux of various physiological functions.

Gastric pH is neutral at birth, but falls to adult levels by age 2–3 years. Acid labile drugs, such as the oral penicillins, are absorbed more efficiently than in the older child or adult.

Transdermal absorption is markedly increased and has been associated with hearing loss after the application of polymyxin, and methaemoglobinaemia following topical mafenide acetate.

Protein binding also varies with age, being lower in the neonate and infant. Reduced binding can increase the apparent volume of distribution of a drug, with an effect on peak and trough concentrations of certain agents. This is rarely of therapeutic importance. Variation in renal maturity, differences in the extracellular, fluid volume, and the immaturity of various enzyme systems are important determinants of drug disposition, excretion, and metabolism. In the neonate, renal function is less efficient than in the older child since glomerular and tubular functions continue to mature. The creatinine clearance rate in the neonate is approximately one-third that in the older child. However, most infants achieve an adult glomerular filtration rate by the age of 12 months. Hence, drugs excreted by the kidneys may require dose modification if toxicity is to be avoided.

Kidney function is not the only consideration. The volume of distribution of antibiotics is important in determining the dose that is necessary to achieve a therapeutic concentration at the site of infection. Agents which are essentially confined to the extracellular fluid, such as the aminoglycosides, are affected by the proportionally larger extracellular fluid volume in the neonate compared with the older child and the adult. The extracellular fluid volume is approximately one-third of the body weight in the newborn.

To consider a specific example, the guidelines for prescribing the aminoglycoside gentamicin vary according to body weight, and also the chronological age, against which the drug's half-life varies inversely. This takes into consideration the immaturity of renal function, the different clearance rates, and the differing volumes of distribution. For example, the mean half-life of gentamicin in neonates less than a week old is about 4–5 h, whereas for infants older than 1 month the half-life decreases to 2–5 h. In order to ensure safe, yet therapeutic, drug concentrations in infants weighing less than 2000 g, the daily dosage of gentamicin is 5 mg per kg, 12 hourly, compared with 7.5 mg per kg, 12 hourly, in larger infants.

Metabolic considerations

Many drugs, including antimicrobial agents, undergo metabolic bio-transformation prior to their elimination from the body. Such transformation is effected by a variety of enzyme systems, many of which are present in the liver. In the neonate this organ and its enzymes are still maturing. For example, glucuronidation of chloramphenicol may be delayed in the neonate so that toxic blood and tissue concentrations develop. This can result in hypotension, cardiovascular collapse, and death if unrecognized. The syndrome has been graphically described as the *grey baby syndrome*. Tetracyclines administered to children under 8 years of age may be deposited in the bones and teeth. In addition to producing dental staining, enamel hypoplasia may also result. Other problems of drug toxicity and drug interactions are not peculiar to childhood and are discussed in Chapter 18.

Placental passage of antimicrobial agents

Drugs, including antibiotics, are frequently prescribed to pregnant women— although following the thalidomide disaster there is a more critical approach to prescribing in pregnancy. Antimicrobial agents are prescribed in pregnancy for various reasons, but most commonly for maternal urinary and respiratory tract infections. Such drugs may also be prescribed to the mother to treat intra-uterine infections such as amnionitis, when further pharmacological considerations will determine the success or failure of therapy.

Pregnancy frequently alters the pharmacokinetic behaviour of drugs, including anti-infective agents. Plasma concentrations of ampicillin are 50 percent of those observed in the non-pregnant state, as a result of increased plasma clearance. The same applies to many cephalosporins.

The placenta is not only an important defence against fetal infection, but also largely determines the concentration of a drug in fetal tissues. The transplacental passage of drugs may be by simple diffusion, or by an active transport system. As in other membrane situations, molecular weight, ionizability, lipid solubility and blood flow are all important considerations. Small molecular weight drugs below 1000 daltons tend to cross readily.

Antimicrobial agents which achieve good concentrations in fetal tissues include ampicillin, penicillin G, sulphonamides, chloramphenicol, metronidazole, and nitrofurantoin. The aminoglycosides cross moderately well and have occasionally been associated with fetal ototoxicity. The cephalosporins and clindamycin cross less readily, whilst erythromycin is particularly poor in this respect.

The general caution restricting all unnecessary prescribing in pregnancy, in particular during the first 3 months when organogenesis is maximal, also applies to antimicrobial drugs. For example, the antifolate properties of trimethoprim and the sulphonamides carry a theoretical risk of inducing fetal abnormalities. However, of more importance is the complication of hyperbilirubinaemia that can result from the use of sulphonamides in the latter few weeks of pregnancy or during the neonatal period. Displacement of protein-bound bilirubin by sulphonamide may result in toxic concentrations of bilirubin and the risk of kernicterus.

Excretion of antimicrobial agents into breast milk

In common with other drugs, antimicrobial agents can enter human breast milk and therefore may potentially affect the suckling infant.

The secretory process may either be active or passive and the final concentration is determined by factors such as molecular weight, lipid or water solubility, the degree of protein binding and, of course, maternal serum concentrations. Breast milk has a neutral pH, and drugs which ionize more readily tend to be weak bases.

There are few antimicrobial drugs which readily pass into breast milk and achieve concentrations similar to those in maternal blood. However, isoniazid and some sulphonamides do so. Tetracycline achieves moderate concentrations and could possibly cause discoloration of primary dentition and enamel hypoplasia. Chloramphenicol and erythromycin are found in concentrations approximately half those present in maternal blood. The penicillins and cephalosporins are generally poorly excreted into human breast milk.

In general, such concentrations are more of theoretical than of practical significance. There have been occasional reports of dapsone and nalidixic acid associated drug toxicity in children with glucose-6-phosphate dehydrogenase deficiency. Disturbance of the bowel flora has been reported with ampicillin; use of clindamycin has resulted in bloody diarrhoea. Under most circumstances, the short-term administration of antimicrobial agents to lactating mothers need not interfere with breast feeding.

Patient compliance

Of particular importance in paediatric prescribing is the acceptability of the medication to the patient. Injections are understandably unpopular with children and their anxious parents and oral preparations are preferred whenever possible, provided their use does not compromise the likely success of therapy. In some cases antibiotics that are otherwise poorly absorbed when given by the oral route are available as esters or salts which exhibit greatly improved oral absorption, as for example with erythromycin. Similarly, chloramphenicol is extremely bitter; however, chloramphenicol palmitate is much more palatable. The need to make preparations palatable with syrup and flavourings is important if compliance is to be observed. Children generally find tablet and capsule preparations difficult to swallow—hence the popularity of flavoured syrup suspensions. One word of caution is necessary since some preparations contain high concentrations of sucrose which may encourage caries formation. This applies essentially to children on long-term preparations, which for the most part will be drugs other than antimicrobial agents.

In addition to palatability, compliance is increased by making the prescribing instructions clear and least disruptive to the normal daily routine. Unnecessary disturbance of sleep patterns is a sure way to reduce compliance.

An important aspect of all prescribing, particularly with paediatric formulations which may be attractively coloured and sweet tasting, is the need to warn parents that any residual medication should be discarded. Accidental self poisoning in childhood may occasionally be life threatening.

PRESCRIBING IN THE ELDERLY

As with most therapeutic agents, use of antibiotics is greatest in old age. This reflects the increased susceptibility to microbial disease in this age group, since the host response to infection is often impaired, as a result either of involution or the immunosuppressive effects of disease or drugs. Moreover, the inflammatory response is often dampened and this may lead to more serious infective states, which can have a profound effect on major organ function and thus modify response to antimicrobial therapy.

Age-related infection

Infection is an important cause of morbidity, and occasionally mortality, in the elderly. The classic infections of childhood (measles, mumps, chickenpox, etc.) have little impact in old age, whereas infections of the respiratory tract, urinary tract, and skin structures become more common as one grows older. For example, the lower respiratory tract, often compromised by life long exposure to cigarette smoke and atmospheric pollution, is an important target for infections that require medical consultation, hospital admission, and the administration of antibiotics.

Urinary tract infections increase substantially beyond the age of 50. In the male this is largely related to benign or malignant enlargement of the prostate; in the female it may have various causes, including sphincter disturbance, uterine prolapse, pelvic neoplasms, and poor hygiene compounded by periods of immobility.

Intra-abdominal infection may complicate gall bladder disease, diverticulosis, and malignancy of the bowel, while metabolic disorders, notably diabetes mellitus, predispose to infection of the urinary tract and septicaemia, as well as infected ischaemic or neuropathic ulcers of the feet.

Physiological changes in the elderly

In contrast to the situation in childhood, prescribing in the elderly must take account of the involution of many physiological systems.

Host defences become progressively less efficient with age, and simultaneous degenerative, neoplastic, and metabolic disorders predispose to infection. Gastric acid output often falls, with a rise in gastric pH; reduced blood flow to the gut and liver may lower first-pass extraction leading to increased oral bioavailability. Changes in lean body mass and body water may lower the apparent volume of distribution. Changes in the functional integrity of the kidneys and liver, which are the major organs of drug excretion and metabolism; can substantially alter drug disposition and elimination; superimposed disease can further aggravate the natural decline in function.

These changes may have the advantage of allowing higher concentrations of drug to be achieved, but the risk of toxicity may also increase. Loss of glomerular function is a normal concomitant of advancing years and may be clinically inapparent. For this reason all drugs should be used with caution in the elderly, especially those compounds for which the route of excretion is primarily renal. Use of aminoglycosides in the older patient requires careful attention to dosage and monitoring of serum concentrations to ensure therapeutic, yet non-toxic, levels.

Adverse reactions

Unwanted effects of antimicrobial drugs are more common in the elderly. This partly follows from the increased frequency of drug prescription in this group, as well as the impaired efficiency of the excretory organs. However, certain drug reactions cannot be explained by such considerations as, for example, the increased frequency and severity of serious adverse reactions to co-trimoxazole seen in the elderly. Here rashes, including the Stevens–Johnson syndrome with extensive skin and mucous membrane ulceration, and major blood dyscrasias are more common in the elderly. The effect is almost certainly related to the sulphonamide component of this drug.

Elderly patients are often prescribed multiple drugs and such polypharmacy raises important issues of drug interactions which may affect pharmacological activity, as well as increasing the risks of side-effects. Examples include the chelation of tetracyclines by antacids and the effect of H_2-antagonists on the activity of drugs such as the quinolones that are affected by alterations in pH. Likewise, the co-administration of theophyllines and quinolones, such as ciprofloxacin and enoxacin, or macrolides, such as erythromycin, can result in toxic concentrations of the former leading to agitation, confusion, and even seizures.

The principles of antimicrobial prescribing are common to all age groups, but greater attention to issues of drug distribution, excretion, and potential for adverse reactions is necessary in patients at the extremes of age. The burden of infection falls most heavily on the very young and the very old, and antibiotic prescribing is correspondingly more common in these age groups. In the treatment of infection in the young and the elderly it is essential, therefore, to choose the safest and most effective agent, and to use it in appropriate dosage for the shortest time necessary.

18

Adverse reactions to antibiotics

R. G. Finch

No antimicrobial agent is totally free from unwanted side-effects, and about 5 per cent of patients prescribed antimicrobial therapy will develop an adverse reaction of some sort. Most are trivial; some merely inconvenient. Others may require admission to hospital for specialist management, while a few are life threatening or fatal. Due caution should always be exercised before a patient is placed on antimicrobial therapy, to see whether there is an identifiable contra-indication to the use of the agent. Unnecessary or inappropriate prescribing is to be deplored for several reasons, but in particular for unjustifiably running the risk of avoidable adverse reactions.

Adverse reactions range from the allergic to the toxic. Others are unpredictable and defined as idiosyncratic, while alterations to the microbial flora can result in complicating disease. However, it is important to keep a proper perspective on the relative frequency of adverse events and this is indicated in Table 18.1.

DETERMINANTS OF TOXICITY

Genetic

A few adverse reactions are genetically determined. For example, patients deficient in the enzyme glucose-6-phosphate dehydrogenase are at risk of developing acute haemolysis when prescribed drugs such as the sulphonamides, nitrofurantoin, and the antimalarial primaquine. Occasionally, the use of chloramphenicol, or nalidixic acid, may be similarly complicated. This reaction may be avoided by screening for this X-linked erythrocyte enzyme defect, which is more commonly found among persons of Mediterranean, Far Eastern, or African stock. Similarly, the ability to acetylate the antituberculous drug, isoniazid, is genetically determined. In slow acetylators, isoniazid toxicity may occur.

Chemical

Many intravenously administered drugs, including antimicrobial agents, produce local irritation and frank phlebitis. To overcome this it may

Table 18.1. Relative frequency of selected adverse reactions to antimicrobial agents

Antimicrobial agent	Frequent	Infrequent
Aminoglycosides	Ototoxicity Nephrotoxicity	Rashes
Cephalosporins	Hypersensitivity rashes *Candida* overgrowth	Nephrotoxicity (cephaloridine) Anaphylaxis Haematological toxicity
Chloramphenicol	Dose-related marrow toxicity	Aplastic anaemia Grey baby syndrome Optic neuritis
Clindamycin	Rash Diarrhoea	Hepatitis Pseudomembranous colitis
Co-trimoxazole and sulphonamides	Rashes (sulphonamide)	Megaloblastic anaemia
Erythromycin	Gastrointestinal intolerance	Cholestatic jaundice Deafness
Fusidic acid	Gastrointestinal intolerance (oral)	Hepatotoxicity (intravenous)
Nalidixic acid and other quinolones	Gastrointestinal intolerance Rashes	Confusion/convulsions Photosensitivity
Nitrofurantoin	Gastrointestinal intolerance	Hypersensitivity pneumonitis Haemolysis Peripheral neuropathy Rashes
Penicillins	Hypersensitivity reactions—mainly rashes	Haematological toxicity Encephalopathy Interstitial nephritis
Rifampicin	Hepatotoxicity Liver enzyme induction	Hypersensitivity 'Influenza syndrome' (intermittent treatment) Haematological toxicity
Tetracyclines	Gastrointestinal intolerance Candidiasis Dental staining and hypoplasia in childhood	Photosensitivity Nephrotoxicity Staphylococcal enterocolitis
Vancomycin	'Red man' syndrome	Nephrotoxicity

be necessary to adjust the pH of an intravenous infusion by suitable buffering. In like manner, pain may accompany the intramuscular injection of a drug. For example, cefoxitin is given with a local anaesthetic, lignocaine, to counter the pain at the injection site.

Many drugs may produce gastrointestinal discomfort due to a local chemical irritation of the gastric and intestinal mucosa. Here, again, suitable buffering, enteric coating, or slow-release formulations may diminish these symptoms and increase the acceptability of a drug.

Metabolic

Drug accumulation

Drugs may be excreted unchanged, but this is unusual. More usually, they undergo oxidation, reduction, hydrolysis, or conjugation to a greater or lesser degree before excretion. The liver is the major site of this metabolization, although other organs such as the kidneys are also involved. When disease impairs renal or hepatic function there is the risk of accumulation of the drug, or a metabolite, which may reach toxic concentrations in the tissues.

Similarly, in the premature or full-term neonate, both renal and hepatic functions are physiologically immature so that some adjustments of dosaging may have to be made (see Chapter 17).

Enzyme induction

Certain drugs may cause hepatic enzyme induction or the synthesis of a new enzyme. This is well known for barbiturates, where it may have therapeutic effects. Occasionally enzyme induction may be undesirable. Rifampicin is a powerful inducer, decreasing the half-lives of many drugs such as prednisone, warfarin, digoxin, ketoconazole, and the sulphonylureas. Women simultaneously prescribed rifampicin and the contraceptive pill may conceive owing to inadequate circulating hormone concentrations that result from the induction of hepatic enzymes by rifampicin. Likewise, simultaneous administration of certain quinolones (e.g. enoxacin or ciprofloxacin) may result in the accumulation of toxic concentrations of theophyllines.

Electrolyte overload

Certain antibiotics such as carbenicillin, being relatively inactive, are prescribed in large doses. Each 1 g of carbenicillin contains 5.4 mmol sodium. This can result in sodium overloading and congestive cardiac failure, particularly in patients who also have impaired renal function.

Dental staining

Tetracyclines are taken up by developing bones and teeth. In the former there are no significant long-term complications. However, staining of the dentition is unsightly and ranges from patchy cream to extensive brown deposits. Enamel hypoplasia may also result. This ability to produce dental staining varies among the tetracyclines, being least with oxytetracycline. However, avoidance of all tetracyclines in children under 8 years of age will prevent such staining of the permanent dentition.

Histamine release

Too-rapid infusion of vancomycin can result in the release of histamine, which, in turn, can produce acute flushing, tachycardia, and hypotension—a reaction known as 'red man' syndrome.

Drug interaction

Drugs may interact with other agents *in vitro* when mixed before administration, or *in vivo* once the drugs are ingested or injected. The study of drug interactions has become increasingly important and complex as new therapeutic agents become available. In general, incompatibilities can be avoided by mixing the agents separately and administering them by a different route or at different times.

In vitro incompatibilities

Table 18.2 indicates the variety of *in vitro* incompatibilities associated with antimicrobial agents. This list is far from complete, and pharmaceutical advice should be sought whenever there is doubt concerning drug compatibility.

In vivo interactions

In vivo drug interactions include competition for plasma protein-binding sites and inhibition or induction of liver enzymes, thus interfering with or potentiating other therapeutic effects. Table 18.3 indicates the

Table 18.2. *In vitro* incompatibilities of selected antimicrobial agents

Antimicrobial agent	Agents with which incompatibility exists
Penicillin G	Ascorbic acid, tetracyclines, vancomycin, amphotericin B
Methicillin	Tetracyclines
Cephalothin	Erythromycin, tetracyclines, calcium gluconate, or chloride
Chloramphenicol	Tetracyclines, vancomycin, hydrocortisone, vitamin B complex preparations
Vancomycin	Chloramphenicol, hydrocortisone, heparin
Gentamicin	Carbenicillin

Table 18.3. *In vivo* incompatibilities of selected antimicrobial agents

Antibiotic(s)	Interacting agent(s)	Adverse reaction
Aminoglycosides	Curare-like agents	Neuromuscular blockade
Chloramphenicol Sulphonamides Isoniazid }	Phenytoin	Phenytoin toxicity
Enoxacin Ciprofloxacin Erythromycin }	Theophylline	Agitation, convulsions
Griseofulvin	Warfarin	Decreased anticoagulation
Ketoconazole	Oral antacids and H$_2$ antagonists	Decreased ketoconazole absorption
Ketoconazole	Cyclosporin A	Competitive inhibition and cyclosporin nephrotoxicity
Metronidazole	Alcohol	Nausea and vomiting (disulfiram effect)
Rifampicin	Oral contraceptives	Decreased efficacy
Sulphonamides Nalidixic acid }	Anticoagulants	Increased anticoagulation
Tetracyclines	Oral antacid preparations and oral iron	Decreased tetracycline absorption

variety of effects that have been described. Among the more important is interference with anticoagulant drugs, a problem that is commonly, but not exclusively, caused by antimicrobial agents. For example, rifampicin and griseofulvin impair anticoagulation by enzyme induction, while sulphonamides, chloramphenicol, co-trimoxazole, erythromycin, metronidazole, and the azole antifungals increase anticoagulation by enzyme inhibition, so that bleeding may occur.

Hypersensitivity

Among the antibiotics the β-lactam compounds have the greatest potential to produce hypersensitivity reactions. Because of the similar structure of the penicillins, hypersensitivity to one agent is usually accompanied by hypersensitivity to the whole group. Moreover, the structural similarities between the cephalosporin antibiotics and the penicillins are accompanied by a degree of cross-hypersensitivity between the two groups. About 10 per cent of patients who are hypersensitive to the penicillins show cross-hypersensitivity to the cephalosporins. This is much more likely to occur in patients experiencing a previous anaphylactic response to a penicillin when the subsequent use of all β-lactam antibiotics must be avoided. The monobactam compounds, of which aztreonam is the only one presently available, appear to be less allergenic and may be administered to patients with a history of hypersensitivity to other β-lactam antibiotics. This suggests that the sensitizing moiety of these drugs is not the β-lactam ring.

Immediate reactions

Immediate hypersensitivity reactions to the penicillins and cephalosporins can occur within minutes and produce nausea and vomiting, pruritus, urticaria, wheezing, laryngeal oedema, and cardiovascular collapse. In extreme cases the patient may die unless the attack is controlled with adrenaline and attention to the integrity of the airway. The estimated frequency for anaphylaxis is 1–5 for every 10 000 courses of penicillin prescribed.

Delayed reactions

Other hypersensitivity reactions tend to be delayed, and include drug fever, erythema nodosum, and a serum-sickness-like syndrome. Hypersensitivity rashes are particularly common with the semi-synthetic penicillins such as ampicillin and its analogues and the cephalosporins. The rashes are usually maculopapular and pruritic but they may also be vesicular, bullous, urticarial, or scarlatiniform.

The use of ampicillin is associated with a generalized maculopapular eruption in more than 90 per cent of patients suffering from infectious mononucleosis (glandular fever) and, less frequently, in association with cytomegalovirus infection. The exact reason for these hypersensitivity rashes in association with such viral infections is uncertain although both infections are characterized by intense polyclonal immunological responses. However, the response is short lived and does not reflect long-lasting penicillin hypersensitivity, so that future use of penicillins is not contraindicated in these patients.

Other antimicrobial agents that commonly produce hypersensitivity drug rashes are the sulphonamides and clindamycin. The sulphonamides and co-trimoxazole are responsible for a wide variety of eruptions which range from urticarial to maculopapular to erythema multiforme and its more severe variant, the Stevens–Johnson syndrome, in which there is both cutaneous and mucous membrane involvement and a significant mortality rate.

Hypersensitivity reactions may also involve individual organs. For example, the penicillins occasionally produce an interstitial nephritis. Nitrofurantoin may affect the lungs, and erythromycin estolate is associated with hypersensitivity cholestasis. Haemolytic anaemia, neutropenia, and thrombocytopenia may occasionally occur with the penicillins, cephalosporins, and sulphonamides.

Predicting hypersensitivity

This is difficult. Some individuals have a strong family history of drug allergy or of allergic disease such as asthma or eczema. Skin testing is occasionally carried out, but is unfortunately poorly predictive. It is therefore imperative to inquire about any previous episodes of hypersensitivity. When reactions occur they should be carefully documented and explained to the patient, so that serious hypersensitivity reactions can be avoided in the future.

Altered microbial flora

Antimicrobial drugs cannot distinguish between pathogenic organisms and those that make up the normal flora of the host. Even so-called 'narrow-spectrum' antibiotics like penicillin have a profound effect on the normal flora of the mouth and gut to eliminate or suppress penicillin-sensitive strains of streptococci and anaerobic bacteria. As a rule this alteration of the normal flora is without clinical consequence and is rapidly reversed on stopping treatment.

Some agents have a greater potential to suppress the normal flora, which may be complicated by the overgrowth of drug-resistant organisms which in turn may give rise to superinfection. In general, the worst culprits are broad-spectrum antibiotics such as the tetracyclines, ampicillin, and cephalosporins. Their use is occasionally associated with the overgrowth of yeasts, particularly within the oral cavity or in the vagina, where they may result in candidiasis,(monilia or thrush).

In the past, hospitalized patients receiving tetracycline and other broad-spectrum drugs, such as chloramphenicol, also experienced overgrowth with antibiotic-resistant strains of *Staphylococcus aureus* with a resultant enterocolitis. This was much feared, particularly in the post-operative patient, where mortality rates were high. For reasons that are not entirely clear this complication is nowadays seldom seen.

Of greater importance is the syndrome of antibiotic-associated colitis caused by toxin-producing strains of *Clostridium difficile*. This may follow the use of various agents, although clindamycin, ampicillin, and the cephalosporins are most commonly incriminated. It is thought, but not proven, that antibiotic use selectively favours proliferation of the causative organism. The colitis caused by the toxin may be severe, even life threatening. Oral vancomycin or metronidazole are successfully used to control the condition when it arises.

Finally, patients treated with antimicrobial agents are at risk of acquiring organisms from the environment. Because of the intensive selection pressure operating in many hospital units, organisms acquired in hospital are often more virulent and frequently exhibit resistance to a variety of antibiotics, putting the patient at increased risk.

TISSUE AND ORGAN-SPECIFIC TOXICITY

Gastrointestinal tract

Antimicrobial agents are commonly administered orally provided that absorption from the bowel is satisfactory. It is scarcely surprising therefore that a variety of gastrointestinal side-effects are associated with their use. Nausea, vomiting, and increased bowel movement, sometimes amounting to diarrhoea, are common, but are generally of minor inconvenience and do not interrupt treatment. Diarrhoea occurs in approximately 5–10 per cent of patients taking oral ampicillin or clindamycin. However, the most serious gastrointestinal complications are overgrowth of *Candida*, *Staph. aureus*, or toxin-producing strains of *Cl. difficile* (see above).

Skin

Skin rashes are among the more frequent adverse reactions caused by antimicrobial drugs. Most reactions are caused by hypersensitivity, as already described, but a wide variety of other eruptions may occur, including maculopapular, vesicular, and bullous eruptions, exfoliation, and erythema multiforme. Delayed hypersensitivity reactions with sulphonamides may result in erythema nodosum, which may be part of a serum-sickness-like syndrome with drug fever and arthralgia.

Photosensitivity eruptions occur with long-acting sulphonamides, the tetracyclines, particularly demeclocycline, and quinolones. The skin becomes red, oedematous, and vesicular. This side-effect is more common in hot climates.

Finally, a lupus syndrome is occasionally seen with the penicillins and sulphonamides. The eruption primarily affects the skin and, although the blood is positive for anti-nuclear factor, the phenomenon is rarely associated with severe systemic disease. Cessation of therapy is associated with resolution of the condition, although this may take some time.

Respiratory tract

Hypersensitivity reactions manifested by bronchial asthma and pulmonary eosinophilia may occur, usually in sensitized individuals. Asthmatic reactions are most likely in those who have an underlying bronchospastic tendency. Nitrofurantoin, *p*-aminosalicylic acid, the sulphonamides and β-lactam antibiotics may produce such reactions. Long-term use of nitrofurantoin has also been associated with a chronic interstitial pneumonitis progressing to fibrosis. The changes may be only partially reversible on stopping the drugs.

An indirect side-effect of antibiotic therapy is opportunistic lung infection. This usually occurs in patients with underlying malignant disease and those receiving cytotoxic or immunosuppressive therapy. Patients who are artificially ventilated are particularly vulnerable. The normal flora becomes modified and opportunistic pulmonary infection occurs.

Liver

The liver is a major organ of drug metabolism and excretion, and is consequently vulnerable to a variety of adverse effects. Antibiotics may affect the liver to produce an acute hepatitis or cholestasis. Such reactions are often unpredictable, although pre-existing liver disease suggests caution in prescribing potentially hepatotoxic drugs.

Several antimicrobial drugs, including carbenicillin, clindamycin, and *p*-aminosalicylic acid, may produce minor elevations of liver enzymes which uncommonly progress to a frank hepatitis with nausea, vomiting, and a tender enlarged liver. Cholestasis may be seen in association with nitrofurantion and erythromycin derivatives.

Isoniazid is a frequent cause of hepatitis which is uncommon below the age of 20 years, but increases significantly in persons of middle age and beyond. Symptoms usually develop within the first 2 months of treatment and subside on stopping treatment. Transient asymptomatic elevation of liver enzymes is common but of little significance. Routine testing of liver function is not justified unless symptoms develop.

Rifampicin may also produce elevation of liver enzymes, although when used in combination with isoniazid, as it may be in the treatment of tuberculosis, clinical hepatotoxicity appears to be no more frequent than when isoniazid is used alone.

A more serious variety of liver toxicity may follow the use of intravenous tetracycline in patients with pre-existing liver disease or during pregnancy. Under these circumstances liver necrosis may prove fatal.

Neurological system

Central nervous system

Ototoxicity is an important side-effect of the aminoglycoside antibiotics. However, their individual potential for either vestibulotoxicity or cochleotoxicity varies and is least for tobramycin. Vestibulotoxicity is recognized by unsteadiness of gait and nystagmus, whilst cochleotoxicity is recognized by a hearing loss which initially affects high frequencies that may only be detected by audiography. Deafness may also occasionally complicate the use of intravenous erythromycin in doses exceeding 4 g per day.

Although penicillins are (setting aside penicillin allergy) the least toxic of antibiotics, encephalitic reactions may occur with massive parenteral doses of penicillin G of 20 million units (12 g) or more per day. There is no conceivable therapeutic benefit in such heroic doses, which should be avoided. If intrathecal therapy with penicillin is contemplated the adult dose should not exceed 20 000 units because of the risk of convulsions, but intrathecal use is best avoided. Other β-lactam antibiotics such as the cephalosporins and imipenem may also be associated with convulsions and encephalopathy when given in high doses. High doses of quinolones may also produce convulsions. The phenomenon of benign intracranial hypertension may follow the use of nalidixic acid, tetracycline, and, occasionally, penicillin. This effect is reversible on stopping treatment. Optic neuritis is a rare complication of the use of chloramphenicol, whilst ethambutol is also associated with dose-related optic nerve damage and retinopathy.

Peripheral nervous system

Several agents may be associated with a peripheral neuropathy, although the mechanisms are not well understood. Isoniazid is known to interfere with pyridoxine metabolism. Nitrofurantoin competes with thiamine pyrophosphate and thus interferes with pyruvate oxidation. Metronidazole may produce a reversible peripheral neuropathy with prolonged use. The nucleoside analogues: zidovudine, didanosine, and zalcitabine used in the treatment of HIV disease have all been associated with peripheral neuropathy.

Neuromuscular blockade, although rare, is a potentially serious adverse reaction and occurs in association with the use of the aminoglycosides, polymyxins, tetracyclines, and lincomycin. The aminoglycosides produce neuromuscular blockade by a curare-like anticholinesterase effect and by competing with calcium; this is more likely to be seen following the use of muscle relaxants during anaesthesia.

Kidneys

Owing to the fact that the kidneys are the major route of drug excretion, it is not surprising that nephrotoxicity is relatively frequent. It is often dose related and is more common either in those with pre-existing renal failure or in those who are receiving other nephrotoxic agents.

Sulphonamides

Some of the early sulphonamides, which were rapidly excreted and poorly soluble, were prone to deposit crystals within the urinary tract, sometimes causing tubular damage and ureteric obstruction.

This complication is uncommon with modern sulphonamides, which are generally more soluble and more slowly excreted.

Penicillins
Benzylpenicillin and, occasionally, other penicillins may produce a hypersensitivity interstitial nephritis. This is recognized by haematuria, proteineuria, and such features as pyrexia and eosinophilia.

Cephalosporins
These vary in their nephrotoxic potential. Cephaloridine (no longer available in the UK) is nephrotoxic when more than 6 g per day is prescribed, particularly if prescribed in combination with a diuretic such as frusemide or ethacrynic acid. The evidence in favour of other cephalosporins being nephrotoxic is equivocal, although cephalosporins may potentiate aminoglycoside toxicity.

Tetracyclines
These may occasionally be nephrotoxic. This applies particularly to patients with pre-existing renal insufficiency and the elderly with physiological impairment of renal function. The degree of renal failure produced varies, but is usually reversible. An explanation of the phenomenon may lie in the anti-anabolic effect of tetracyclines. Outdated (time-expired) preparations of tetracyclines have caused tubulotoxicity with consequent electrolyte and amino acid loss.

A specific effect of demeclocycline is the production of nephrogenic diabetes insipidus, a phenomenon that has been put to therapeutic advantage in the management of the syndrome of inappropriate anti-diuretic hormone secretion.

Among tetracyclines, doxycycline is unique in being devoid of nephrotoxicity, reflecting its primary hepatobiliary route of excretion.

Aminoglycosides
These are the antibiotics most frequently associated with nephrotoxicity. Their nephrotoxic potential varies and nephrotoxicity occurs in decreasing order of frequency with kanamycin, gentamicin, tobramycin, amikacin, and netilmicin. Nephrotoxicity is potentiated by pre-existing renal disease, prolonged or repeated courses of treatment, or the simultaneous administration of other nephrotoxic agents. In many instances, the renal insufficiency produced is reversible, although permanent impairment including renal failure does occur.

Amphotericin B
Nephrotoxicity is the leading complication of the use of amphotericin B. This results from a combination of a reduction in glomerular filtration, renal tubular acidosis, and decreased concentrating ability.

Careful monitoring of renal function is a prerequisite to the use of this agent.

Haematological toxicity

Bone marrow toxicity may either be selective and affect one cell line, or be unselective and produce pancytopenia and marrow aplasia. Furthermore, immune-mediated haemolysis may occur in which Coombs' antibodies are detected. Bleeding may occur from platelet dysfunction or from thrombocytopenia. Eosinophilia may represent a hypersensitivity reaction.

β-Lactam antibiotics

The penicillins may rarely produce a primary haemolytic anaemia and also Coombs' antibody positive disease. In addition, a selective white cell depression has been described with ampicillin, flucloxacillin, and carbenicillin; the latter may also produce bleeding due to drug-induced platelet dysfunction or interference with fibrin formation. This may be important in the seriously ill patient with bone marrow suppression. Similarly, the cephalosporins may be associated with a positive Coombs' test, although frank haemolysis is uncommon. Eosinophilia occurs with variable frequency, as does the selective depression of white cells, and occasionally platelets, following the development of platelet antibodies. A vitamin K-dependent bleeding disorder has been associated with certain cephalosporins which possess a methyl-thiotetrazole side-chain. These include cephamandole, cefotetan, cefoperazone, and latamoxef. Although uncommon, bleeding has been identified largely in elderly or malnourished patients undergoing major surgery. It is both treated and prevented by the administration of vitamin K.

Sulphonamides

Among the more important groups of agents to produce haematological side-effects are the sulphonamides and sulphonamide-containing mixtures such as co-trimoxazole. Marrow toxicity may result in aplastic anaemia, or a selective neutropenia, or thrombocytopenia. In addition, haemolysis may be either primary or related to glucose-6-phosphate dehydrogenase deficiency. Co-trimoxazole may produce megaloblastic bone marrow changes or, less commonly, a peripheral megaloblastic anaemia. This tends to occur with prolonged therapy and is related to the joint antifolate action of the two components of co-trimoxazole.

Chloramphenicol

This has achieved notoriety for inducing marrow depression which is manifested in two ways. The more common dose-related bone marrow depression is seen when the daily dose exceeds 4 g. There is a progressive anaemia, neutropenia, and sometimes thrombocytopenia which is reversible on either discontinuing treatment or reducing the dosage. A more serious reaction is that of total bone marrow depression and aplastic anaemia. This is unpredictable but is estimated to occur with a frequency of 1 in 24 000–1 in 40 000 treatment courses. Mortality from aplastic anaemia is in excess of 50 per cent. Thiamphenicol, a derivative of chloramphenicol, available in some parts of the world, appears to be devoid of the irreversible toxic effects on the bone marrow.

PREVENTION OF ADVERSE REACTIONS

There are major difficulties in preventing adverse drug reactions. Patients frequently respond idiosyncratically to antimicrobial agents as to other drugs and the chief problem, especially with the rarer side-effects, is their unpredictability. Awareness of the possibility of adverse effects is obviously important and a close working relationship with either a clinical pharmacologist or a specialist in the use of antimicrobial agents will help to overcome problems as they arise.

When toxic effects develop or are suspected, the decision has to be made as to whether to stop or change the patient's treatment. The drug may frequently be continued provided the dose is adjusted, either by reducing each individual dose or by prolonging the interval between doses.

Antibiotic assays (Chapter 8) are an important means of determining whether dosage adjustment is necessary, particularly in the case of aminoglycosides, in which the leeway between effective and toxic levels is small. Chloramphenicol should be assayed when used in the newborn child, to prevent excessive accumulation.

Finally, the reporting of adverse drug reactions, whether caused by antimicrobial agents or other drugs, remains the responsibility of all practising doctors. In the UK the Committee on Safety of Medicines operates a voluntary adverse reactions reporting system (see Postscript).

19

Chemoprophylaxis

R. C. B. Slack

Chemoprophylaxis is the prevention of infection by the administration of antimicrobial agents as distinct from prevention by immunization. Individuals who require prophylaxis differ from the normal population in that they are known to be exposed to a particular infectious hazard and/or their ability to respond to infection is impaired.

Prophylaxis should be confined to those periods for which the risk is maximum, so that the problems of disturbance of the normal flora, superinfection with resistant organisms, untoward reactions, and cost will be minimized. If chemoprophylaxis is to have a place in the management of infection it is likely to be most effective when we can identify:

(1)   individuals in whom the risk of infection is high;

(2)   the organisms likely to be responsible;

(3)   the agent likely to be active against those organisms.

Failure to establish and adhere to such guidelines has made unnecessary chemoprophylaxis the commonest form of antibiotic misuse in hospitals.

PATIENTS WITH NORMAL RESISTANCE

A clear example is provided by the need to protect travellers to areas where malaria is common. The chances of acquiring the disease are high, the results can be grave, and the period at risk is well defined: from arrival in the area until 4 weeks after departure—the time taken for any parasites that may have been acquired to be finally eliminated. There are agents which are specifically active against the malaria parasite and suitable for prophylaxis, and there is only one complication: the parasite may be resistant to the chosen prophylactic drug and it is plainly important to ensure that the agent used is active against the local parasite (see Chapter 31).

Not all situations are as clear cut as this, however, and a good example of the sort of uncertainties that arise is provided by the situation in which a child develops meningococcal meningitis. Any of the family, the school and social contacts, and the medical attendants might acquire meningococci from the child and become nasopharyngeal carriers. Some of those carriers could themselves develop meningitis. Should all receive chemoprophylaxis? Epidemiological evidence indicates that children are much more likely than adults to develop the disease and that acquisition requires close contact. The general advice, therefore, is to offer chemoprophylaxis only to close contacts and to medical attendants only if they have been exposed to unusual opportunities for transmission of the organism as, for example, during mouth-to-mouth resuscitation.

Again, the choice of agent is complicated by microbial resistance. Sulphonamides are extremely effective in prophylaxis, but sulphonamide-resistant meningococci are now common. This is particularly unfortunate because other agents such as penicillin, which are equally effective in the treatment of the disease, are much less effective (for reasons which are imperfectly understood) in prophylaxis. In the absence of information as to whether the organism is sulphonamide sensitive, rifampicin should be used. Evidence is accumulating that ciprofloxacin may be equally effective.

Surgical sepsis

The commonest circumstance in which patients with otherwise normal resistance to infection become susceptible is in the course of surgical operations. Here two situations must be distinguished: those in which the tissues involved are infected and those in which they are not.

Uninfected tissues

Here, the patient becomes liable to infection through the breach in the normal protective integument by organisms, almost invariably staphylococci, derived from the patient's own carrier sites or from the surgical team. On the face of it, this might appear to fulfil the criteria for necessary prophylaxis: a known organism (*Staphylococcus aureus*) of known susceptibility (to flucloxacillin) with a risk of infection over a clearly defined period. In fact, there is no justification whatsoever for the use of chemoprophylaxis in this way. The incidence of wound sepsis following operations on uninfected tissues, such as thyroidectomy, should be extremely small and the effect in the otherwise normal patient should in any case be easily controlled. If wound sepsis following such operations is common, something is seriously wrong with the hygienic management of the patients, and the source and mode of spread of infection must be identified and eliminated. The use of antimicrobial agents in this situation diverts attention from the real problem and, by failing to control spread, facilitates infection with resistant strains.

Infected tissues

Under this heading we can conveniently dismiss operations conducted in the presence of infection: for example, incision of an abscess, the removal of infected bone, or prostatectomy in the presence of urinary infection. Antibiotics are commonly given in conjunction with such operations, often with the specific intention of controlling any spread of organisms locally or into the bloodstream as a result of the procedure. In this sense, such therapy can be regarded as prophylaxis, but it is more appropriately regarded as part of the treatment, which will often already have begun prior to surgery when the causative organism and the appropriate agent will ordinarily be known from prior laboratory tests.

Contamination by normal flora

True chemoprophylaxis may be required where operations involve organs which are not infected, but which harbour a normal flora, notably the oropharnyx, the gut, and the vagina. As in the case of the skin, the oropharyngeal flora seldom gives rise to local infection following simple procedures such as tonsillectomy, and systemic chemoprophylaxis is not required. However, if there is much tissue damage or local impairment of the blood supply, such as may be seen in destructive wounds, chemically induced abortion, or elaborate vaginal repairs, implanted organisms may give rise to infection. In such cases infection often involves anaerobic organisms and several different species may act in concert to produce a so-called synergic infection. Such conditions require chemoprophylaxis and, where there is necrotic tissue, surgical debridement.

Upper gut surgery

The normal flora of the gut is uniform neither in its distribution nor in its composition. The mouth contains copious organisms, but the oesophagus, stomach, and small gut normally contain only a few passengers derived from the mouth or the food, many of which are destroyed in the acid of the stomach and the rest hurried by peristalsis to the terminal ileum where the mixed flora typical of the large-bowel contents begins to develop. This is notable for its content of Gram-negative rods, both aerobic and anaerobic, and for the extraordinarily high concentrations of bacteria which develop as the gut contents are progressively dehydrated.

It is to be expected from the scanty flora harboured that operations on the upper gut are seldom complicated by infection and do not call for chemoprophylaxis. Indeed, prophylactic antibiotics given to patients undergoing operations on the upper gut are likely to pave the way for the acquisition of hospital strains of bacteria that are highly resistant to antibiotics. A particular hazard is colonization of the anterior nares by antibiotic-resistant staphylococci and facilitation of their access to the stomach by the passage of pernasal gastric tubes. Protection of such patients by tetracycline or other broad-spectrum agents has, in the past, led to severe and sometimes fatal staphylococcal enterocolitis. Similar arguments might apply to operations on the biliary tract, which is normally sterile; antibiotic administration should be required only in patients with bacterial cholangitis and this is treatment, not prophylaxis. Unfortunately, the presence of bacterial infection can be determined with certainty only at the time of operation and antibiotics are, therefore, usually given routinely to patients undergoing cholecystectomy. Because the majority of infecting organisms are aerobic Gram-negative rods, cephalosporins are commonly used.

Large-bowel surgery

The situation in the large bowel is quite different. No other organ is so laden with bacteria able to infect normal tissues, and post-operative infection rates of 30 or 40 per cent are not uncommon. The problem of controlling microbial spillage from the large bowel in the course of surgery has been approached in the following ways.

Bowel sterilization   The first and original procedure was to remove as far as possible the large-bowel contents by purging and enema. Poorly absorbed agents, such as neomycin and some sulphonamides, were (and in some places still are) widely used in conjunction with mechanical cleansing of the gut to 'sterilize' the bowel before operation. In fact, this failed to render the residual bowel contents sterile because of inactivity against the most numerous bowel inhabitants, the non-sporing Gram-negative anaerobic bacteria. Nevertheless, vigorous pursuit of these procedures sometimes managed to leave the large bowel sufficiently microbially denuded for the patients to become superinfected with antibiotic-resistant hospital strains of staphylococci and to suffer severe and even fatal staphylococcal enterocolitis.

Tissue sterilization   An alternative approach is to attempt to sterilize all the tissues exposed to faecal organisms by irrigation at the end of operation with a potent antiseptic or antibiotic. Considerable reduction in the incidence of post-operative sepsis has been obtained following the use of antibiotics, commonly tetracycline, or non-specific agents such as povidone-iodine or noxytiolin. Unfortunately, absorption of drugs from large raw areas or the peritoneum is at least as rapid as from intramuscular injections and, as a result, the local concentration of agent rapidly falls and the patient is exposed to remote toxic effects of the drug just as if it had been parenterally administered.

Mechanical removal of organisms by irrigation (with saline alone) before closure of the wound is effective in reducing post-operative sepsis.

Systemic chemoprophylaxis Recognition of this problem has led to prophylaxis based on two separate procedures: elimination, as far as possible, of faecal organisms by mechanical means (possibly supplemented by oral antibacterial agents), and systemic administration of drug active against the principal potential pathogens over the period during which implantation and invasion by the organism is likely to occur. In some places, systemic antibiotics have been given for a week or two before operation—a procedure which offends against many of the rules of effective prophylaxis: it contributes nothing beyond the most recent dose to the concentration of drug in the tissues at the time of operation, it exposes patients to the risk of superinfection with resistant organisms and to increased risk of untoward reactions, and it increases the cost.

What is required is concentrations of agent adequate to dispose of any organism likely to establish infection implanted in the tissues in the course of the operative procedure. Plainly, this does not include any period before the operation begins but, in order to secure adequate concentrations at the time of operation, the first dose of agent should be given up to an hour before. If intravenous drugs are used, these are often administered by the anaesthetist at the time of induction of anaesthesia. The question of how long tissue concentrations must be maintained cannot be answered with any certainty, but obviously must cover the time of the operation. No trial has convincingly established the period of risk, but the physiology of wound healing suggests that it is relatively short. Many regimens continue post-operative prophylaxis for 24 or 48 h. For many operations, e.g. uncomplicated appendicectomy, single-dose prophylaxis is usually adequate.

Choice of agent Convincing scientific evidence is also lacking on the optimum agent to be used for this purpose. Success was obtained many years ago with chloramphenicol, though the prophylactic use in large numbers of patients of an agent with so potentially dangerous a side-effect as aplastic anaemia must be deplored. The attraction was that it was active against almost all the organisms likely to be involved in bowel infection, including the predominant anaerobes. Later, cephaloridine was shown to reduce significantly the sepsis rate after large-bowel surgery, although it has no activity against anaerobes. It was generally believed that, by eliminating aerobes which consume oxygen and thereby provide the conditions necessary for anaerobic growth, anaerobic activity was abolished. It later become clear that this cannot be the whole explanation when metronidazole, which is active only against anaerobic bacteria, proved to be a most effective chemoprophylactic agent in both large-bowel and gynaecological surgery.

Despite this success, there was concern that metronidazole has no effect against aerobic bacteria and it was consequently combined with agents such as gentamicin, widely active against Gram-negative rods, and cloxacillin, active against staphylococci. Many believe this clumsy therapy to be unnecessarily comprehensive and the cloxacillin is often omitted, the antistaphylococcal activity of gentamicin being deemed to be sufficient. The arguments against using gentamicin (or any aminoglycoside) are those of toxicity and possible bacterial resistance. The development of many broad-spectrum cephalosporins and combinations of penicillins with β-lactamase inhibitors led to numerous clinical trials of these agents in abdominal surgery; subsequently, an expanded spectrum cephalosporin, such as cefotaxime, was included with metronidazole in most regimens used in Europe and North America, although gentamicin plus metronidazole is as effective. The chief drawback of cephalosporins—antibiotic-associated colitis—may occur with short-course prophylactic regimens, and this adverse effect should be balanced against aminoglycoside toxicity, which is rare after a single dose.

A single agent would be preferred by all if one could be agreed upon, but impeccable comparative trials are hard to do and valid comparisons between series hard to make. Some rely on metronidazole alone, believing that the anaerobic element in synergic post-operative sepsis is so dominant that elimination of that alone will abort the process. Others prefer agents with significant intrinsic activity against both aerobes and anaerobes, and cefoxitin, imipenem, co-amoxiclav (or other combinations of penicillins and β-lactamase inhibitors) have been effectively used for this purpose.

PATIENTS WITH IMPAIRED RESISTANCE

What has been said so far applies to patients in whom there is no reason to suspect any impairment of the natural bacterial clearance mechanisms. There are important differences in patients with impaired resistance. Bacterial infection may be caused by a much greater variety of organisms including 'opportunist' commensal bacteria; the occasions of exposure may be everyday occurrences and, therefore, much less easy to identify, and the role of chemoprophylaxis in eliminating implanted bacteria is more decisive than supportive.

Impaired resistance is of two forms: local and general. Local impairment occurs where, for example, the blood supply to the area is defective or foreign bodies are present, or for some other reason the local defences are not mobilized. Important examples are amputations through the mid-thigh for obliterative arterial disease, implantation of surgical prostheses, and rheumatic endocarditis.

Amputation

Surgery in obliterative arterial disease is associated with a specific serious risk. Even in the most fastidious, the perineum, upper thighs, and lower abdomen can be soiled with gut organisms amongst which clostridia are common. Clostridial spores are highly resistant to antiseptics, and skin preparation before operation cannot be relied upon to destroy them. Implantation of such organisms into the oxygen-deprived tissues of the ischaemic limb at amputation provides precisely the conditions most favourable to their proliferation with the production of tissue necrosis and gas gangrene. Only clostridia are responsible for this condition and all are susceptible to penicillin which, given prior to operation and for 48 h after, can be relied upon to prevent this disastrous complication and must be administered whenever such amputations are contemplated. The risk in through or below-knee amputations is far less and penicillin prophylaxis is not mandatory. However, skin sepsis is common in this group of patients and, since antiseptics remove only the most superficial organisms, peri-operative prophylaxis with agents active against staphylococci and anaerobes is commonly given.

Implantation of surgical prostheses

The deliberate introduction of foreign bodies such as cardiac valves or hip joint prostheses carries a risk of infection, the results of which can be disastrous. Chemoprophylaxis is consequently universally used, but its efficacy is almost impossible to calculate, since the incidence of infection even without chemoprophylaxis is extremely low. A very large study mounted by the Medical Research Council and the Public Health Laboratory Service in the UK has shown a significant reduction in sepsis rates in hip replacement operations when peri-operative antibiotics were used. The study also examined the benefits of 'clean air' theatres and meticulous antisepsis. The combination of such special operative techniques and antimicrobial prophylaxis reduced the infection rate to about 0.1 per cent.

There is no unanimity of opinion as to which antibiotic is most appropriate and little likelihood of settling the question by clinical trial since huge numbers of comparable patients would have to be enrolled to detect differences in the efficacy of different agents. Since *Staph. aureus* is often incriminated in orthopaedic sepsis, the agent chosen should clearly be active against this organism. Many orthopaedic surgeons use cephradine, or cefuroxime, which combine adequate antistaphylococcal activity with useful cover for many Gram-negative organisms.

In cardiac surgery, broad-spectrum cover with an antistaphylococcal penicillin and an aminoglycoside has been advocated, but the common occurrence in some units of strains of staphylococci resistant to these agents has led to the adoption of vancomycin as a prophylactic agent, despite its cost.

Infective endocarditis

Patients with certain congenital cardiovascular abnormalities, prosthetic heart valves, rheumatic carditis, or arteriosclerosis are subject to deposition of vegetations on the endocardium which are liable to become infected with bacteria transiently liberated into the bloodstream. For example, salivary organisms enter the blood when a tooth is extracted, and gut organisms can enter the blood during large-bowel operations. In normal subjects these organisms are quickly cleared by the reticuloendothelial system, but in patients with pre-existing endocardial vegetations they may become trapped and grow in the vegetation to give rise to bacterial endocarditis. A great variety of bacterial species can occasionally infect the valves in this way, but much the most important organisms are viridans streptococci from the mouth and enterococci from the gut or bladder (Chapter 23).

Identification of patients at risk

Despite the availability of many agents active against the infecting organisms, treatment of bacterial endocarditis is still far from satisfactory in terms of prolonged survival. Protection against the risks of such infection is therefore essential. The difficulty is that almost none of the requirements of soundly based chemoprophylaxis can be met in full, and because of the infrequency of infection it is impossible to measure the efficacy of chemoprophylaxis and the relative merits of competing regimens.

The best that can be done is to identify all patients with relevant heart disease undergoing all procedures likely to give rise to relevant bacteraemia, recognizing that this will fail to protect those patients who give no history of heart disease—and increasing numbers of older patients in whom the original nidus is presumably arteriosclerotic fall into this category—and those who give no history of dental or other relevant manipulations. This is an unsatisfactory situation, but the alternative is frequent prophylaxis for a much wider section of the population with all the attendant problems of emergent resistance, side-effects, and cost.

Prophylactic regimens

Thus, the choice of subjects and necessary occasions of chemoprophylaxis are hard to establish. The choice of agents and duration of treatment are scarcely less so. Since bactericidal agents are essential to eliminate the causal bacteria of endocarditis, it follows that they are essential for prophylaxis. Penicillin has long been the drug of choice in chemoprophylaxis for dental procedures where the risk is from oral streptococci which are usually penicillin sensitive.

Dentists object to regimens which require injections and are, thus, unsuited to the dental surgery and likely to add substantially to the difficulties of persuading children (and not a few adults) to undergo necessary dental treatment (itself an important part of prophylaxis against infective endocarditis). This has led to the advocacy of large single doses (3g) of amoxycillin, which has the advantage of being well absorbed when given by mouth when it produces concentrations of drug in the blood bactericidal for the majority population of sensitive streptococci for 24 hours. Where enterococci are likely to be liberated into the blood, supplementation of this treatment with streptomycin or gentamicin is essential. In patients allergic to penicillins, oral erythromycin (or clindamycin) or intravenous vancomycin can be substituted for amoxycillin. Parenteral therapy is recommended only for dental procedures carried out under general anaesthesia.

As in the case of surgical sepsis, it is not established (and probably cannot be established) how long bactericidal concentrations of agents must be maintained, but the episodes of bacteraemia are very short and chemoprophylaxis for more than a few hours is unlikely to be necessary. Again, it is important that the agent should be given an hour or so before operation so that the peak concentration is present in the blood at the time of maximum risk.

LONG-TERM CHEMOPROPHYLAXIS

Rheumatic carditis

This is an unusual form of special susceptibility to infection in that the patients are susceptible not to the infection itself—streptococcal pharyngitis—but to remote immunological sequelae involving the heart. The chemoprophylaxis of the condition rests on unusually secure grounds: only one organism is responsible—the haemolytic streptococcus—and that has remained, to date, steadfastly sensitive to penicillin, which will eradicate the organism from the throat. Penicillin is therefore uniquely indicated. Moreover, the patients at risk are clearly identified by having already suffered an attack of rheumatic endocarditis, it being well established that subsequent attacks of streptococcal pharyngitis lead to further cardiac damage. As a fresh attack of pharyngitis may occur at any time and the risk of further cardiac damage persists at least through adolescence, penicillin prophylaxis must be continuous until puberty.

This requires the oral administration of phenoxymethylpenicillin several times every day or, more conveniently, intramuscular injections of benzathine penicillin, which produce adequate concentrations of penicillin in the blood for a month.

Immunocompromised patients

Prolonged penicillin prophylaxis of rheumatic subjects is successful because only one organism can cause the disease, no resistant strains have emerged, and prolonged penicillin treatment is seldom complicated by side-effects. Had the disease been caused by one of the organisms which has become successively resistant to a great variety of agents, for example the staphylococcus or *Escherichia coli*, frequent changes of therapy would have been required, ending almost certainly with the need to choose between abandoning prophylaxis and contemplating long-term therapy with relatively toxic agents. This kind of dilemma has often to be faced in other situations where the patient's resistance to bacterial infection is reduced for prolonged periods. Examples are in patients suffering from immunodeficiency or diseases associated with impaired defences or treated with immunosuppressive agents. Such patients are subject to invasion from their own microflora and from organisms acquired in the hospital environment, including opportunist organisms such as *Pseudomonas* which can give rise to generalized disease. The management of such patients is an intensified variant of that used for surgical patients. Great care is taken to deny access of hospital organisms to them; they may, for example, be physically isolated from the ward in elaborate mechanical isolators, fed sterile food and given mixtures of poorly absorbed antibiotics such as neomycin, vancomycin, bacitracin, polymyxin, and nystatin, collectively active against all the organisms, including both anaerobes and *Candida*, likely to enter the blood from the gut. A refinement of this blunderbuss approach is to attempt *selective decontamination* with two or three agents that remove most of the organisms from the oropharynx and bowel, but preserve the anaerobic flora. This tactic is intended to discourage overgrowth of resistant organisms in the alimentary tract by a process known as *colonization resistance*. Selective decontamination regimens often combine oral and parenteral drugs, although systemic chemoprophylaxis has been objected to in the past on the grounds that the appropriate agents may be required for therapy if infection occurs despite the elaborate precautions.

The unconscious patient

Normally, the respiratory tract below the larynx is sterile in the sense that there is no resident flora, but organisms stray into the bronchi from the oropharynx and are removed by the mucociliary mechanism. Excess mucus excited by attempts at microbial establishment is removed together with the entrapped microbes by coughing. In the unconscious patient this process is suspended and, if artificial means to maintain bronchial toilet are inadequate, multiplication of oropharyngeal organisms in the depths of the bronchi will give rise to bronchopneumonia. It is tempting to guard against this by chemoprophylaxis directed against the common pathogenic organisms: *Streptococcus pneumoniae* and *Haemophilus influenzae*, for example, with ampicillin. In practice, the effect of such therapy is to facilitate the establishment of resistant Gram-negative rods in the oropharynx, which then promptly follow the same route into the depths of the lung where they establish an infection which is more difficult to treat and may well extend to fatal septicaemia. Several studies have confirmed the expectation that chemoprophylaxis in such circumstances increases rather than decreases the mortality from respiratory infection.

Chronic urinary tract infection

In contrast, the long-term chemoprophylaxis of intractable urinary infection in patients who cannot be controlled by short-term therapy is highly successful. Why should this form of long-term chemoprophylaxis succeed when the evidently analogous situation in the respiratory tract is at best a failure and at worst a disaster? The reasons appear to be twofold. Firstly, the agents most widely used for the purpose, nitrofurantoin and trimethoprim, do not encourage the emergence of resistant strains in the gut—from which the urinary infecting organisms are derived—in the way that resistant organisms are encouraged in the oropharynx. Secondly, the drugs are excreted into the urine in very high concentrations, while agents used in the treatment of respiratory infection achieve concentrations in the bronchial secretions which are often considerably lower than those in the blood. The essential ingredients of success, therefore, are unusually favourable pharmacokinetic properties and unusual failure to facilitate the emergence of resistant strains. Continuing freedom from resistance can never be relied upon and there is already some suggestion that the favourable position of trimethoprim in this regard is threatened.

Urinary tract surgery

Having said that the urinary tract is unusually suited for successful long-term chemoprophylaxis, important exceptions must be noted. Unfortunately, patients are still infected in hospital in the course of instrumentation or surgery. Some of these patients have gross abnormalities of the urinary tract and may have greatly impaired defence mechanisms. Catheterization carries a significant risk of urinary infection and short-term chemoprophylaxis (for example, with nitrofurantoin) to cover the period of risk is highly successful. This success is not, however, maintained if the period of catheterization is prolonged. The defences are then set aside in a way that resembles that of the respiratory tract in the unconscious patient. Prolonged chemoprophylaxis results in superinfection with resistant organisms. This is also true of attempts to reduce infection by instillation of antiseptics into the bladder or by impregnation of catheters with antibacterial compounds. The lesson is always the same: patients in hospital, whose defences are impaired, are continuously at risk and must be continuously protected against the access of hospital organisms by appropriate hygienic measures. Attempts to prevent infection by prolonged chemoprophylaxis while hygiene is neglected can be relied upon to ensure infection with resistant organisms that may be inaccessible to treatment.

Apart from special examples in which unusual features of the organism or the agent can be readily identified, chemoprophylaxis is likely to be successful only over short periods of identifiable exposure to identifiable organisms susceptible to identifiable agents. It is likely to be worthwhile only if the risk to the patient of developing the infection it is desired to prevent clearly outweighs the possible untoward effects and cost of chemoprophylaxis.

Part V

The therapeutic use of antimicrobial agents

20

Respiratory tract infections

A. M. Emmerson

It has been traditional to subdivide the respiratory tract into upper and lower regions, above and below the epiglottis, and to talk of upper respiratory tract infection and lower respiratory tract infection separately. To a large extent this is reasonable; the upper respiratory tract has a rich and varied microbial population at all times, while in most healthy people the lower respiratory tract, protected by ciliated epithelium, mucus, and macrophages, is virtually free from microbes.

Similarly, fairly well-recognized collections of symptoms and signs have been held to define illnesses which can be diagnosed with variable confidence. These include the common cold, pharyngitis, tonsillitis, otitis media, croup, bronchitis, bronchiolitis, and pneumonia, as well as specific infections, such as influenza, diphtheria, and whooping cough.

Some bacteria and viruses can, however, play a part in several of these conditions, and there is considerable overlap between lower and upper tract disease. Fever, excess serous and mucous secretion in the nose and paranasal sinuses, inflammation of the throat and respiratory passages, stimulation of the cough reflex, loss of ciliary activity, shedding of superficial mucosa, spasm of bronchial smooth muscle, and collapse of alveoli can all be found in many respiratory infections. Between them they give rise to the runny noses, headache, earache, cough, sputum production, malaise, and chest pain which, in different combinations, make up the varying clinical pictures of acute respiratory disease.

Respiratory infections are caused by viruses, or bacteria, or both. If the illness is entirely viral in origin, an antibiotic will not help. If there is a bacterial component, antibiotic treatment will probably help, and may be vital. It is often difficult to recognize when bacteria may be involved. Secondary bacterial infection is often, but not always, present in otitis media, sinusitis, and pneumonia, and few would withhold antibiotics for these conditions. Other conditions such as pharyngitis (sore throat) and croup are more controversial.

UPPER RESPIRATORY TRACT INFECTION

Sore throat

This is one of the commonest problems seen in general medical practice and one of the most controversial. The most important causal organism is *Streptococcus pyogenes*, which has been said, in different surveys, to cause less than 20 per cent or more than 50 per cent of all sore throats. All authorities agree that viruses, and particularly the adenoviruses, account for most of the others.

Streptococcal sore throat is important because it may lead to serious complications. It is not possible on clinical findings alone to distinguish between streptococcal and non-streptococcal sore throat, and rapid tests for the detection of β-haemolytic streptococci in throat swabs are not sufficiently reliable for routine use. The question is, therefore, whether to take a throat swab for culture before starting specific treatment or to treat all sore throats as though they were streptococcal, without culture.

The aims of treatment are:

(1) to prevent non-suppurative sequelae (rheumatic fever and acute glomerulonephritis);

(2) to prevent suppurative complications such as sinusitis, periton-sillar abscess, otitis media, cervical adenitis, and pneumonia;

(3) to decrease the spread of infection by removing the source;

(4) to shorten the course of the disease.

Antibiotic treatment of streptococcal sore throat will prevent subsequent rheumatic fever, which may follow in 0.4 to 2.8 per cent of untreated cases, even if treatment is delayed for up to 9 days after onset. Patients who have had an attack of rheumatic fever should be treated with continuous oral penicillin for several years, to prevent a recurrence. There is no convincing evidence that acute nephritis can be prevented by treating a streptococcal sore throat. Suppurative complications are also markedly decreased by prompt treatment, as is spread of infection to contacts. Treatment probably shortens the duration of the sore throat, but not by much. Controlled studies are unconvincing. On balance, since little is lost by delaying the start of treatment by 24 h, where adequate bacteriological facilities are available it is worthwhile treating with antibiotics only those sore throats shown to be streptococcal by culture. In the absence of bacteriological guidance it is reasonable to err on the side of caution and to treat as though all were streptococcal. There is, however, room for discretion and many general practitioners are guided more by the severity of the disease and the social circumstances of their patients than by any consideration of the presumed aetiology.

The antibiotic of choice is either penicillin or, for penicillin-hypersensitive patients, erythromycin, and there is evidence that these should be given for at least 10 days to eradicate the organism. Ampicillin should not be used, as it will cause a rash if the sore throat is the herald of glandular fever. Tetracyclines are also inappropriate because of the high incidence of resistance among streptococci. For those patients with recurrent streptococcal throats, co-amoxiclav or cefaclor appear to eradicate the organism better than oral penicillin.

Diphtheria

At present uncommon in Britain, and indeed everywhere that an effective vaccination policy is practised, diphtheria is nevertheless important in the differential diagnosis of sore throat. Diagnosis must be made on clinical grounds—the severity of the illness, the presence of a diphtheritic membranous exudate—as treatment of the acute illness with antitoxin is life saving and must be started before bacteriological confirmation can be completed. Penicillin and erythromycin are both effective in eradicating the organism, but nose and throat cultures should be repeated 2 or 3 weeks after treatment to detect patients who continue to harbour the organism. Most of these will be cleared by a repeat course of antibiotic.

Croup

Noisy difficult breathing, hoarseness, and stridor are common signs of acute laryngo-tracheo-bronchitis in children in winter. This distressing condition is usually viral in origin; parainfluenza viruses, the respiratory syncytial virus, and adenoviruses being particularly common causes. Treatment is supportive; the condition is usually self limiting and resolves in 2–4 days if uncomplicated. Endotracheal intubation or tracheostomy may be needed to relieve respiratory obstruction.

Acute epiglottitis

This is a much less common, but much more dangerous, cause of croup caused by infection with *Haemophilus influenzae* of capsular type b; it can occur in adults as well as in children. There is systemic illness as well as local respiratory difficulty, and the swollen oedematous epiglottis can cause complete airway obstruction with dramatic suddenness. It is this complication which makes acute epiglottitis such a life-threatening condition. Treatment is as much concerned with maintaining the airway as with controlling the infection, but, as soon as the condition is suspected, treatment should be started with parenteral cefotaxime or, if that is not readily available, intramuscular ampicillin or intravenous chloramphenicol. Some strains of *H. influenzae* are resistant to chloramphenicol or ampicillin (occasionally both) and these cannot be used with full confidence.

Pertussis (whooping cough)

Antibiotics are notoriously ineffective in controlling the distressing cough of pertussis; nevertheless, erythromycin has been shown to eradicate the organism from the respiratory tract and can also be used for the protection of susceptible close contacts. Vaccination is the only reliable way of preventing and controlling this early childhood infectious disease.

Acute otitis media and sinusitis

Mild catarrhal inflammation spreading up the Eustachian tubes and into the paranasal sinuses is a common accompaniment of most viral upper respiratory infections, and often resolves without chemotherapy as the cold subsides. More severe illness, with toothache, facial pain and tenderness, and a purulent nasal discharge, or earache, pain on moving the pinna, and a red bulging eardrum, indicates bacterial infection and demands antibiotic treatment.

Acute sinusitis and acute otitis media are both caused predominantly by *H. influenzae* and *Streptococcus pneumoniae*. Staphylococci, *Str. pyogenes*, and α-haemolytic streptococci are less often involved. The antibiotic of choice is amoxycillin; erythromycin and co-amoxiclav are logical alternatives and may be necessary if β-lactamase-producing *H. influenzae* is involved. The optimal duration of therapy is unknown, but 10 days is conventional. Supportive measures such as elevation of the head of the bed, humidification, analgesics, and decongestants may be helpful. Patients with acute fulminating infection which fails to resolve rapidly should be referred to an ENT surgeon for possible surgical drainage.

Acute bacterial parotitis

As a rule, bacteria reach the parotid gland by retrograde passage from the mouth. The infection is usually unilateral and used to be a common complication of abdominal surgery. Today, good control of post-operative fluid balance, prompt blood replacement, and attention to oral hygiene have made post-operative parotitis a rarity, and the condition is now more often seen in debilitating medical disease, as a result of a dry infected mouth. Occasional cases may follow obstruction of the parotid duct by calculus or a foreign body, or even occur as an embolic complication of septicaemia.

Treatment consists of correction of dehydration, oral toilet, and antibiotics. As the infection is usually due to *Staphylococcus aureus*, the antibiotic of choice is flucloxacillin. Surgical drainage may be necessary if these measures fail to bring prompt relief.

Infection in the mouth

Almost all acute suppurative mouth infections originate in the teeth, and are usually the result of dental caries and periodontal disease. Both of these are caused by the metabolism of sugars by oral bacteria, mainly streptococci. The sugars are converted into dextrans and mucopolysaccharides which accumulate as dental plaque, localizing the bacteria to the tooth surface and gingival margins, and allowing acid production to attack the tooth substance.

Chronic gingivitis

When plaque develops under the gingival margin and the periodontal membrane is broken, particles of food accumulate and become infected. The gums retract and become inflamed, and chronic gingivitis results. Acute infection may punctuate the course of chronic periodontal disease, but is usually well localized as an acute dental abscess.

The bacteria usually involved are streptococci, mainly of the α-haemolytic and non-haemolytic varieties, and when antibiotic treatment is indicated, penicillin and erythromycin are both effective. The mainstay of treatment and prevention is, however, proper mouth hygiene, dental care, and attention to diet. Soft sugary foods cause dental disease; crisp abrasive fibrous foods prevent it.

Vincent's gingivitis

This is an acute ulcerative gingivitis accompanied by, and probably caused by, proliferation of normal mouth microbes, including a spirochaete, *Treponema vincenti*, fusiform bacilli, and other oral anaerobes. The main symptoms are bleeding gums, soreness of the mouth, a bad taste, and offensive breath. The disease always occurs in a mouth already ravaged by preexisting gingivitis and poor oral hygiene. There is extensive gingival ulceration, and contact ulcers may form on the sides of the tongue and the cheek. Occasionally, the infection may spread to cause an acute ulcerative tonsillitis and pharyngitis, a condition known as Vincent's angina.

Vincent's infection responds rapidly to penicillin or metronidazole. When the condition has subsided proper attention should be given to dental care and the correction of underlying mouth disease. Acute ulcerative gingivitis may be an early sign of serious haematological diseases, such as acute leukaemia or agranulocytosis, and these should be excluded.

Thrush

Thrush, infection of the mucous membrane with the yeast *Candida albicans*, is predominantly a neonatal infection. Candida is a common vaginal commensal, especially in pregnancy, and infection is acquired by the infant during passage through the birth canal. It presents in the first few days of life as white curdy patches on cheeks, lips, palate, and tongue. Treatment is with local nystatin.

In adults, oral thrush is more sinister and is almost always indicative of serious underlying disease, among which endocrine disturbances such as diabetes mellitus, severe blood dyscrasias, and disseminated malignancy are prominent; it may herald the onset of AIDS. The condition may complicate treatment with broad-spectrum antibiotics or steroids. A less sinister, but more common manifestation of oral candida infection is the chronic atrophic candidosis which may plague people wearing ill-fitting dentures. In all these conditions one of the oral polyene or azole derivatives may be used to control the candida, but treatment is essentially that appropriate to the underlying condition.

Actinomycosis

This is another condition closely associated with poor oral hygiene, gingivitis, dental decay, and especially tooth extraction, in which a normal mouth organism, *Actinomyces israelii*, gains access to already unhealthy tissues and causes a subacute or chronic suppurative infection.

A. israelii is an anaerobic Gram-positive bacillus which shows true branching. On the rare occasions on which it invades tissues it causes an intense polymorphonuclear neutrophil reaction. The most usual mode of infection is through a tooth socket after extraction. Within 1–6 weeks after extraction, the patient notices a small swelling over the mandible. This enlarges and, if untreated, the infection spreads to form an extensive abscess cavity, with extension to involve overlying skin and the formation of one or more sinuses. The pus characteristically contains 'sulphur granules', which are colonies of the actinomycete, and the diagnosis is confirmed by culture. Usually, medical advice is sought before the abscess points. Incision, drainage, and treatment with penicillin will control the infection, but the antibiotic needs to be given for 2 or 3 months if relapse is to be avoided. Fusidic acid, clindamycin, erythromycin, and tetracycline are also active against actinomyces, but again prolonged treatment is necessary to effect cure.

LOWER RESPIRATORY TRACT INFECTION

Acute bronchitis

Most cases of acute bronchitis in a previously healthy adult are caused by viruses, although some may be caused by *Mycoplasma pneumoniae*. The illness is characterized by chest tightness, wheeze, breathlessness, and cough. Usually mild, it can be severe in the very young, the very old, the debilitated, and in acute exacerbations of chronic bronchitis. If mild, treatment is symptomatic and antibiotics are rarely indicated, especially when the sputum remains mucoid. Purulent sputum or severe illness makes secondary bacterial infection likely, and the most probable offending organisms are *Str. pneumoniae, Moraxella catarrhalis*, and *H. influenzae*, for which cefuroxime and erythromycin are appropriate. The possibility of *M. pneumoniae* infection makes erythromycin or a tetracycline a logical initial choice of antibiotic.

Chronic bronchitis

This term covers a very wide range of diseases, from the irritating, trivial, but persistent cough with some sputum most days in winter and little else, to advanced chronic obstructive airways disease with severe disability and constant respiratory distress. This makes the role of antibiotics in the management of chronic bronchitis particularly difficult to assess. The aim of treatment has been to control acute exacerbations when they occur; long-term prophylaxis has been used for patients with advanced illness and constantly purulent sputum. It now seems clear that those patients who regularly suffer frequent acute exacerbations throughout winter do benefit from long-term antibiotic treatment throughout the winter months, but that for most patients prompt early treatment of acute exacerbations as they occur is just as good. Tetracyclines, ampicillin, amoxycillin, and co-trimoxazole can all be used, and there is little to choose between them. Patient preference and experience of side-effects often decide which is used. A supply of the chosen drug is given at the beginning of winter and the patient instructed to start taking it as soon as symptoms dictate. Patients who do not respond to the chosen antibiotic may benefit from a course of co-amoxiclav or ciprofloxacin.

Pneumonia

Any interference with the defences of the respiratory tract or the normal drainage of the lung may predispose to pneumonia. Such interference may be caused by antecedent upper respiratory infection such as a common cold, and many patients with pneumonia give a history of such an infection. At any time, but usually within a week of the onset of the cold, the patient rapidly becomes more ill, with a rise in temperature, cough, at first dry and painful, but later productive of viscid purulent or blood-stained sputum, pleuritic pain, and rapid respiration. The diagnosis is made by finding clinical or radiological evidence of consolidation.

Most pneumonias are caused by infective agents, although chemical or allergic pneumonias do occur. The consolidation may be confined to part or the whole of one or more lobes of the lungs—lobar pneumonia—or may be patchily distributed in a lobular pattern throughout the lung fields— bronchopneumonia.

Pneumococcal pneumonia

The pneumococcus is by far the commonest cause of lobar pneumonia in previously healthy children and adults, and is also prominent in pneumonias following acute exacerbations of chronic bronchitis, together with *H. influenzae*, and occasionally staphylococci, klebsiellae, and a variety of upper respiratory organisms. Nevertheless, lobar pneumonia is not always pneumococcal; any anatomical type of pneumonia can on occasion be caused by almost any respiratory pathogen. Patients with pneumonia require treatment before the results of bacterial investigation are known, and it is seldom possible to be sure of the cause before starting therapy.

In the previously healthy child or relatively young adult it is reasonable to assume that the infection is pneumococcal and to start treatment with high-dose penicillin by injection; if there is a possibility of infection by penicillin-resistant pneumococci then cefotaxime or ceftriaxone should be given. Alternatively, a combination of ampicillin and erythromycin can be used. This covers not only pneumococci and *H. influenzae*, but also *L. pneumophila* (see below) and *M. pneumoniae*, a fairly common cause of atypical pneumonia which occurs in epidemic waves and often affects young adults in schools, colleges, or army camps.

Nosocomial pneumonia

Pneumonia is the leading cause of mortality resulting from infection acquired in hospital. The incidence of nosocomial pneumonia in intensive care units ranges from 10–65 per cent, with reported case fatalities of 13–55 per cent. It is often associated with mechanical ventilation. The micro-organisms isolated from tracheal aspirates are primarily Gram-negative bacilli, which may be antibiotic resistant. The source of these is primarily exogenous, but secondarily from stomach or oropharyngeal aspirates. Since tracheal aspirates are poor indicators of ventilator-associated pneumonia, protected bronchoscopic techniques are recommended to confirm the diagnosis. The initial use of cefotaxime can be modified following appropriate culture results from the laboratory.

Legionnaire's disease

Legionella pneumophila has proved to be a surprisingly frequent cause of lobar pneumonia, accounting for 10 per cent or more of cases in some series. It can occur in explosive outbreaks, but is more commonly sporadic, and, contrary to popular belief, is far more often relatively mild and self limiting than fulminating and lethal. More than half the cases diagnosed in the UK are found retrospectively by antibody studies on follow-up after recovery from the acute illness. Erythromycin is the antibiotic of choice, and is usually given together with rifampicin in proven cases of severe *Legionella* pneumonia.

Staphylococcal pneumonia

This serious infection is uncommon except during epidemics of influenza. It is an occasional complication of viral pneumonia at any age, but is especially dangerous in infancy. Any patient who becomes rapidly and gravely ill with pneumonia should be treated with high-dose antistaphylococcal therapy. Flucloxacillin and fusidic acid are commonly used in the UK.

Opportunistic infections

Patients developing pneumonia as a complication of some other serious underlying disease are at special risk of infection with unusual organisms. Hospital staphylococci and a variety of Gram-negative organisms, including *Klebsiella* and *Pseudomonas*, are important. Speculative treatment with a combination of an aminoglycoside (e.g. gentamicin) and an expanded-spectrum cephalosporin (e.g. cefotaxime) is indicated while an attempt is made to isolate a significant organism from sputum, blood, pleural fluid, lung puncture, trans-tracheal aspirate, or broncho-alveolar lavage.

Pneumonia developing in association with neutropenia following treatment with cytotoxic drugs, or in patients with immunosuppression, including those suffering from AIDS, may be due to *Pneumocystis carinii*, fungi, or viruses. Appropriate treatment is discussed in Chapters 28 and 29.

It must be stressed that, in the treatment of all severe pneumonias, general medical and nursing care and physiotherapy are as important as antibiotic administration. Close monitoring of blood gases, prompt relief of hypoxia, a readiness to resort to mechanical ventilation early, the correction of dehydration, and the relief of pain are all of great importance in the management of this condition.

Empyema

The commonest cause of empyema (purulent pleural effusion) is extension of infection from the lung, but infection can also result from penetrating chest wounds, as a complication of thoracic surgery or by extension upwards from a sub-phrenic abscess. The commonest infecting organisms are *Staph. aureus, Str. pneumoniae, Str. pyogenes,* anaerobic streptococci, *Bacteroides,* and other anaerobic bacteria. Mixed infections are frequent, and even when bulk pus from the empyema is cultured the causal organism may not be isolated in up to a quarter of cases, usually because of prior antibiotic treatment. Treatment is by drainage of pus and administration of antibiotics. Initial treatment with penicillin and metronidazole can be modified when the results of examination of the aspirated pus become known, but chemotherapy must in any case be continued for several weeks, or until the empyema cavity is satisfactorily obliterated. A similar regimen of high-dose penicillin or flucloxacillin and metronidazole should also be used in the treatment of aspiration pneumonia and lung abscess, in which a similar range of organisms may be involved.

Cystic fibrosis

The susceptibility of patients with cystic fibrosis to pulmonary infection is well recognized and is often the cause of early death. One of the striking features of chest infections in cystic fibrosis is that relatively few pathogens are involved. Early in the disease the organisms implicated are frequently *Staph. aureus* or *H. influenzae,* or both. As patients progress through adolescence to adulthood, these pathogens are replaced by *Pseudomonas aeruginosa.* These are difficult to treat, but clinical improvement, without eradication of the organism, is often achieved with a combination of ceftazidime and gentamicin given in high doses intravenously.

Oral ciprofloxacin may also be useful, and, although resistance may supervene, sensitivity often returns during inter-treatment periods.

Major problems arise when *Ps. aeruginosa* is replaced by *Xanthomonas maltophilia* or *Ps. cepacia;* these organisms are often resistant to many antibiotics and treatment should be guided by laboratory findings.

Tuberculosis

The other major cause of respiratory disease, *Mycobacterium tuberculosis,* is considered in Chapter 26.

21

Urinary infections

R. C. B. Slack

TYPES OF INFECTION

Symptoms of urinary tract infection are usually frequency of micturition and dysuria. Lower abdominal pain, loin pain, and fever are less often seen with acute uncomplicated cystitis—in which infection is confined to the bladder—but are invariably found in acute pyelonephritis, or other upper tract disease involving the kidney. Diagnosis of urinary tract infection requires bacteriological examination of urine.

Bacteriuria

This, the presence of bacteria in a freshly passed mid-stream specimen of urine, is a laboratory finding. When more than 10^5 organisms/ml are cultured from a specimen of urine the term 'significant' bacteriuria is used. This figure correlates well with urinary infection, but should not be taken to imply that lower numbers are necessarily 'insignificant'. The figure of 10^5 has been established as the cut-off point for significance in order to exclude perineal contaminants which may be present in urine in considerable numbers.

Asymptomatic bacteriuria

This is found frequently in surveys of normal populations and the prevalence increases with age. Except at both extremes of life it is found more frequently in females—an indication of the ease of ascent of organisms from the introitus to the bladder. Asymptomatic infection does not need to be treated except where it has been shown to lead to upper tract infection as, for example, in pregnancy.

Acute cystitis

Infection confined to the lower urinary tract is usually self limiting. The hydrodynamic effect of continual urine production and micturition tends to wash organisms out of the bladder. The natural defences of the urinary epithelium, both phagocytic and humoral, also limit the natural history of urinary infection. Unless there are anatomical abnormalities—partial obstruction or an inability to empty the bladder completely—or a focus of infection such as a renal calculus (stone) or abscess, infection of the urinary tract often lasts only a few days, although the duration of symptoms may be shortened by appropriate chemotherapy. Indeed, old remedies such as high fluid intake may be as efficacious as the newest antibiotic!

Recurrent bacteriuria

In some patients recurrent bacteriuria may be shown to be associated with pyelonephritis. This is an indication for treatment and further investigation.

Symptomatic abacteriuria

In general practice about half the patients presenting with frequency and dysuria have sterile urine cultures. This abacteriuric condition is sometimes referred to as the *urethral syndrome*—a common, but largely unexplained condition. Some cases may be due to sexually transmitted organisms, such as chlamydia, and some may represent the early stages of urinary infection.

Post-operative infection

Bacterial infection following surgery or instrumentation of the urinary tract is often seen in hospitalized patients and presents special problems in therapy because of the relatively antibiotic-resistant organisms found in many of these cases. The presence of foreign material such as a urinary catheter, which may act as a focus of infection, also makes treatment more difficult.

Urinary infection in children

This is especially important in the very young whose kidneys are growing, because of the possible sequela of pyelonephritis, an important cause of terminal renal failure. Making an accurate laboratory diagnosis is difficult; collecting an uncontaminated urine from an infant requires patience and skill in catching it. In some cases it is necessary to collect supra-pubic aspirates by direct needle puncture through the abdominal wall. This method is of particular value in babies, where it is relatively easy to perform.

LABORATORY METHODS

The confirmation of urinary tract infection is made in the laboratory by quantitative culture of an uncontaminated specimen. Skin and perineal flora shed into urine in sufficient numbers will multiply in a few hours at room temperature and give false positive results. These can be reduced by refrigeration and rapid processing in the laboratory. Alternatively, the possibility of contaminants growing in the urine during transit can be circumvented by culturing the urine as soon as it is passed. This is achieved by using dip-inoculum methods which consist of agar attached to slides or spoons which are dipped in the urine, drained, and transported in a stoppered bottle to the laboratory where any bacterial cultures are counted after overnight incubation at 37 °C. A rough quantification is possible by this method or by other simple methods of direct plating of a fixed volume of urine on appropriate culture media. Simple identification of the resulting significant isolates is made and antimicrobial susceptibility tests performed as described in Chapter 7. The common bacterial causes of urinary infection and their usual antibiotic sensitivity patterns are listed in Table 21.1. Many of the bacteria listed may be present as truly infecting organisms or as contaminants. This is a particular problem in urine collected from women, which is commonly contaminated with perineal or vaginal organisms. Mixtures of bacteria usually indicate

Table 21.1. Frequency of isolation and usual antibiotic susceptibility of organisms causing urinary tract infection

Organism	Percentage isolates		Sulphonamides	Trimethoprim	Ampicillin	Nitrofurantoin	Nalidixic acid	Gentamicin	Fluoroquinolones
	Hospital	General practice							
Escherichia coli	50	75	(S)	S	(S)	S	S	S	S
Proteus mirabilis	14	8	S	(S)	S	R	S	S	S
Klebsiella aerogenes	12	5	(S)	(S)	R	S	S	S	S
Other coliforms	4	1	R	(S)	(S)	S	S	S	S
Staphylococci	6	7	S	S	R	R	R	S	S
Enterococcus faecalis	10	3	R	(S)	S	R	R	R	S
Pseudomonas aeruginosa	3	<1	R	R	R	R	R	S	S
Candida albicans	<1	0	—— Use antifungal agents ——						
Mycobacterium tuberculosis	<<1	<<1	—— See Chapter 26 ——						

S = usually sensitive; R = usually resistant; (S) = resistance common (> 25 per cent of strains).

contamination, although mixed infections do occur in catheterized patients.

THERAPY

Choice of agent

In a condition with such a high spontaneous cure rate it may not be always possible to judge comparative efficacy of different regimens. Urinary infections have been the subject of numerous trials and for most antibiotics a cure rate of over 80 per cent is expected. In acute, uncomplicated cystitis seen in general practice, over 90 per cent of patients would be expected to be asymptomatic after a few days' antibiotic and remain free from bacteriuria for some weeks following. It is an advantage to know the susceptibility of the infecting strain before starting treatment, but delay is justified only in asymptomatic and chronic recurrent cases. The vast majority of acute urinary infections present with painful symptoms and treatment should start before sensitivity results are available. A 'best guess' antibiotic should be selected based on past history, knowledge of likely pathogens, and local resistance patterns. In domiciliary practice *Escherichia coli* predominates and the majority will be fully sensitive to all the commonly used antimicrobials listed in Table 21.1. However, in some communities, sulphonamide and ampicillin-resistant coliforms are sufficiently common for these drugs to be abandoned in favour of trimethoprim or one of the other urinary antimicrobials. The use of co-trimoxazole is not recommended in the treatment of a urinary infection, since the sulphonamide component plays an insignificant role and one might as well use the less toxic trimethoprim alone, unless the infecting organism is known to be resistant.

Two agents, nitrofurantoin and nalidixic acid, achieve adequate concentrations only in urine and are exclusively of use in urinary tract infection. Nitrofurantoin is cheap, but it often causes nausea; the macrocrystalline formulation is better in this respect. It is only effective in an acidic urine; thus in *Proteus* infections, where the ammonia-producing bacteria raise the pH to over 8, it is ineffective. Nalidixic acid and its early congeners (including cinoxacin, oxolinic acid, flumequine, and pipemidic acid) are inactive against staphylococci and streptococci, and may also exhibit some unpleasant side-effects. Fluoroquinolones, such as ciprofloxacin, norfloxacin, and ofloxacin, combine much improved intrinsic activity with an expanded spectrum which covers not only Gram-positive cocci, but also problem bacteria such as *Pseudomonas aeruginosa*.

Alternative agents to the drugs so far mentioned are often less effective. Most oral cephalosporins and mecillinam fail to produce better results than the traditional drugs. Tetracyclines are effective against many urinary pathogens, but resistance is common and they have sufficient side-effects not to be widely used in practice. The combination of amoxycillin and clavulanic acid, co-amoxiclav, is useful in the therapy of resistant strains.

In countries in which it is available, fosfomycin has proved useful in the treatment of cystitis. The spectrum of activity of this antibiotic embraces most urinary tract pathogens, but the calcium salt commonly used for oral administration is erratically absorbed, and resistance may supervene if insufficient concentrations are achieved in urine. The trometamol salt of fosfomycin has much better bioavailability and is potentially advantageous for the oral treatment of bacterial cystitis.

Therapeutic regimens

Conventional treatment of urinary infection has been extrapolated from general principles of therapy of tissue infections, often without due regard to the special circumstances obtaining in the infected urinary tract. Thus, it has been advocated for many drugs that they be taken several times a day for 7—10 days. In fact, many antibacterial drugs are preferentially excreted into the urine and attain very high concentrations there, sometimes for long periods. Moreover, in the treatment of bacterial cystitis (in contrast to pyelonephritis or infections complicating urinary tract abnormalities) antibacterial drugs are generally needed only to tip the balance in favour of normal clearance mechanisms. Several studies have shown that much-curtailed regimens, lasting for 1—3 days, are as successful as prolonged therapy in curing bacterial cystitis. Indeed, longer courses are wasteful of resources especially since many patients, wiser than their doctors, abandon treatment once the symptoms abate.

Short-course treatment has an additional potential benefit in serving to identify those few patients (the ones who fail short-course therapy) who are likely to require more extensive urological investigation. Many of the commonly used antibacterial agents are suitable for this type of approach, although those such as trimethoprim, the newer fluroquinolones, or trometamol fosfomycin which are slowly excreted into urine over a long period have an advantage over rapidly excreted compounds (β-lactam agents and nitrofurantoin) which achieve high, but transient, concentrations in bladder urine. The practice of giving one or two massive doses of amoxycillin, which is sometimes advocated, would seem to have little to recommend it, since the enormous urinary levels produced are no more bactericidal than are those achieved by conventional doses.

Symptomatic abacteriuria (urethral syndrome)

The 'urethral syndrome' is usually seen in young women and, although the patients are generally given antibiotics, the symptoms are probably self limiting. Some patients get intractable symptoms and seek relief from non-medical practitioners; as there may be a psychological element to the urethral syndrome this is reasonable practice. It is, however, important to exclude any known microbial cause. A proportion of women suffering from the urethral syndrome do display intermittent bacteriuria, and sexually transmitted diseases may mimic the frequency and dysuria syndrome. Anticholinergic preparations are commonly used in the management of cystitis and may be beneficial—an example is emepronium (Cetiprin).

Sexual and emotional difficulties may aggravate symptoms, and counselling is important. Frequency and dysuria are sometimes related to vaginal hygiene and deodorants or to sexual technique. It is probably worth investigating such patients and monitoring their response to antibiotics if symptoms persist after excluding other organic causes. Those with no bacteria or pus cells in any urine sample require 'talking therapy', whereas a positive laboratory test should alert the physician to a condition amenable to 'swallowing therapy'.

The chronic sufferer from frequency and dysuria is a persistent visitor to the surgery and may consume more antibiotics than most patients, hoping for relief from this distressing condition.

Difficult infections

In a small minority of patients, symptoms persist or rapidly recur after short-course therapy. Inappropriate choice of agent accounts for a few of these, but many of them will be shown to have abnormalities on intravenous urogram. Radiological or ultrasonic assessment of patients failing therapy or presenting with recurrent urinary infection is important and must be considered mandatory in children and young adult males. Urograms and micturating cystograms often show an anatomical abnormality such as vesico-ureteric reflux or a contracted kidney indicative of pyelonephritis. Bacteriuria in such patients is an indication for antibiotics even in the absence of symptoms. If repeated conventional courses of treatment fail to prevent relapse and bacteriuria relatively soon after stopping the drug there is a case for long-term antibiotics to suppress the infection. There is some debate about how long this prophylaxis should continue and which patients should receive it. In adults the decision should not be taken lightly and it should be reviewed every 6 months. It is common practice to maintain children with vesico-ureteric reflux and evidence of kidney damage on suppressive antibiotics until they reach puberty. Co-trimoxazole and, more recently, trimethoprim alone are the most widely used agents for this purpose. There is very little evidence for the emergence of trimethoprim-resistant strains on this regimen. Drugs which rapidly select resistant mutants during a course of treatment, such as nalidixic acid, are not suitable, but nitrofurantoin may be useful, if tolerated, in patients who develop infection with trimethoprim-resistant organisms. Adverse reactions and superinfection limit the choice of antimicrobial when used long term and it may be necessary to ring the changes after a few years.

Calculi

Stones in the collecting system are a common cause of urinary tract obstruction and this may predispose to urinary infection. Some calculi, especially those containing hydroxyapatite, may harbour the infecting organism within the substance of the stone. Urease-positive bacteria such as *Proteus* species are commonly incriminated because the alkaline conditions produced by the production of ammonia by the bacterial enzyme favour stone formation. Large infected calculi cannot be treated by chemotherapy, and surgery or lithotripsy is necessary. Infection often relapses after lithotomy and there may be small stones left in the kidneys which can act as a further source of bacteriuria. Long-term drug suppression is indicated for these patients. Trimethoprim is the most favoured drug for this indication as nitrofurantoin is ineffective against *Proteus* infections.

Catheters

Urinary catheterization is an essential and commonly performed procedure, but it is not without complications to the patient, the commonest of which is infection. Organisms may be introduced into the bladder on insertion of the catheter or may ascend between the catheter and urethra or up the lumen of the tube. Ascending infection results first in bladder colonization with no symptoms except a 'cloudy' urine, followed by cystitis which may lead to bladder calculi. In some cases with long-term indwelling catheters, infection may reach the kidneys to result in pyelonephritis. Instrumentation or catheter removal from an infected urine may give rise to bacteraemia, which may present as a mild 'catheter fever' or a life-threatening Gram-negative septicaemia.

Prevention of bacterial colonization is obviously a desirable goal, but, even with careful aseptic technique and the use of closed drainage systems, bacteriuria is a frequent finding in patients after the catheter has been in position for a few days. The decision to use an indwelling urinary catheter should be tempered by awareness of this complication. In the management of the young chronically sick with neurogenic

bladders, many authorities advocate intermittent self-catheterization
to overcome the inherent problems of a foreign body in the bladder. Attempts at chemoprophylaxis with antibiotics inevitably lead to
colonization with resistant organisms including, eventually, *Candida*.
Hexamine (methenamine), the oldest antibacterial drug used in urinary
infection, may have some benefit when used prophylactically since
the active component, formaldehyde, which is released in the acid
conditions of the urine, is active against all bacteria and yeasts. In
the face of established infection, however, hexamine is ineffective.
Prophylactic bladder irrigation with antiseptics, such as chlorhexidine
and noxytiolin, is sometimes advocated, but this has the disadvantage
of breaking the closed drainage system which offers the best means of
keeping infection at bay, and infection rates are not improved. Again,
in the face of long-term bacteriuria the procedure is of limited value and
may provoke bacteraemia.

Treatment of catheter-associated urinary infection with antibiotics
is only of short-term value. However, in the symptomatic febrile
patient Gram-negative septicaemia may supervene and it is important
to abort this complication. The chances of treatment being successful
are considerably improved if the catheter can be removed. Symptomless
infection present at the time of removal of a catheter can be treated as an
ordinary urinary infection. In patients with indwelling urinary catheters
and minimal symptoms there is little to be gained by chemotherapy as
candiduria will inevitably follow.

Choice of antimicrobial to treat infection in a catheterized patient may
be severely limited as the organisms responsible are often antibiotic-
resistant nosocomial strains and infections are frequently due to mixed
organisms.

22

Gastrointestinal infections

R. G. Finch

Gastrointestinal infections are among the commonest infections suffered by mankind. World-wide it has been estimated that on any one day 200 million people are suffering from acute infective gastroenteritis. In developing countries, diarrhoeal disease superimposed on severe protein-calorie malnutrition is responsible for much mortality. Even in Britain the morbidity produced is profound and the economic impact significant. For example, approximately 4.3 million working days per annum are lost as a result of acute diarrhoea, much of which is infective in origin. Death may occur from electrolyte and fluid loss, particularly in the very young, elderly, or malnourished who can ill withstand such severe metabolic disturbances that sometimes accompany acute infectious diarrhoea.

Gastrointestinal pathogens are transmitted directly from person to person or indirectly through faecal contamination of the environment, food, or water supply. Hence the high frequency of such infections in underdeveloped countries where the absence of a clean water supply and safe sewage disposal compound the problems of poverty. Some pathogens, most notably salmonellae, are common to both humans and farm animals.

Food may be contaminated by various gut pathogens or their toxins. When illness occurs as a sudden outbreak which can be traced to a common meal, the term *food poisoning* is applied. Non-microbial food poisoning occasionally results from the ingestion of chemicals, fungi, and other toxins such as scombrotoxin and ciguatoxin.

CLINICAL MANIFESTATIONS

The incubation period of gastrointestinal infections varies according to the ingested dose, the site of infection in the gut, and the pathogenic mechanism of diarrhoea. The shortest incubation periods are seen with *Staphylococcus aureus* food poisoning where a pre-formed toxin produces symptoms within $1/2$–8 hours of ingestion. Longer incubation periods are associated with salmonellosis and shigellosis, in which microbial replication within the bowel may take a day or so before disease is produced.

Symptoms of nausea and vomiting are more frequently associated with small-bowel infection. Large-bowel involvement is often associated with tenderness over the colon. In dysentery, diarrhoea is accompanied by a profuse, bloody exudate. Regardless of the major site of action, colicky pain is the commonest symptom associated with gastrointestinal infection. The severity of illness is essentially dictated by the degree of fluid loss. Losses of less than 3 per cent body weight are usually undetectable. Once fluid loss exceeds 10 per cent body weight oliguria, cyanosis, and cardiovascular collapse develop and may be fatal unless rapidly corrected.

Systemic symptoms of fever, headache, and rigors are seen in shigellosis and salmonellosis where the intestinal mucosa is involved. Bacteraemia may complicate a severe attack of gastrointestinal salmonellosis and occasionally result in metastatic infection.

GENERAL MANAGEMENT

Fluid replacement

The management of acute gastroenteritis is largely dictated by the severity of the illness. Most attacks are self limiting and adequate oral fluid replacement is usually possible. Admission to hospital may be required when vomiting persists or clinically detectable dehydration has developed. In most instances, oral fluid replacements are successful. In infants oral treatment with glucose–electrolyte solution is usually given and milk feeding temporarily stopped since lactose deficiency frequently complicates gastroenteritis in early childhood. Therefore, unhydrolysed lactose remaining in the bowel is broken down by gut organisms to lactic and acetic acid, which produce diarrhoea through the effects of an osmotic load. Older children and adults can usually replace fluid losses by drinking water, fruit juices, or soft drinks. Few patients require intravenous fluid replacement. However, under such circumstances normal saline and bicarbonate are usually rapidly effective in the severely dehydrated.

The glucose–salts solution recommended for oral rehydration by the World Health Organization and the United Nations Children's Fund is shown in Table 22.1. Over-the-counter preparations available in the UK generally contain less sodium chloride and more glucose. They are not as effective as the WHO formulation in severe dehydration.

Use of antibiotics in gastrointestinal infections

Since most episodes of acute gastroenteritis are self limiting, antibiotics are not generally indicated. Furthermore, the use of antibiotics carries

Table 22.1. Formula for oral rehydration fluid recommended by the World Health Organization

Substance	Weight (g)
Sodium chloride	3.5
Potassium chloride	1.5
Sodium citrate*	2.9
Glucose (anhydrous)	20.0

To be dissolved in 1 litre of clean drinking water.
* Sodium bicarbonate 2.5 g may be used, but this is less stable and should be freshly prepared.

the risk of directly irritating an inflamed bowel mucosa, or of producing diarrhoea from superinfection. In addition, their use may encourage transferable drug resistance among such pathogens as *Salmonella*.

None the less, there are specific circumstances where antibiotics are appropriate for gastrointestinal infections and associated with clear benefits. Table 22.2 summarizes the chief indications for antimicrobial therapy.

Bowel sedatives and adsorbents

Various agents are available for the symptomatic control of gastrointestinal symptoms. They are frequently prescribed yet little definite evidence exists for their efficacy. They act either by slowing gastrointestinal motility or by fluid adsorption. Diphenoxylate with atropine, loperamide, and codeine slow gastrointestinal motility, and may have an additional mild analgesic effect. Adsorbants include kaolin, chalk, aluminium hydroxide, and cellulose, which tend to increase the stool bulk. Their use should not minimize the importance of adequate fluid and electrolyte replacement. This is especially important in infancy and early childhood where bowel sedatives may induce an ileus and mask fluid loss. Moreover, excessive dosing with diphenoxylate may induce respiratory depression in the young child. Bowel sedatives should also be used cautiously in those with fever or bloody diarrhoea since it is possible to potentiate invasive bacterial disease.

Table 22.2. Major gastrointestinal infections and their antimicrobial therapy

Organism	Major site of infection	Disease produced	Antimicrobial therapy	Comments
Bacillus cereus	SB	Food poisoning (nausea and vomiting)	None	Reheated rice often incriminated
Campylobacter jejuni	SB	Enteritis	(None)	Erythromycin in severe cases
Clostridium botulinum	CNS	Botulism (neural paralysis)	Penicillin	Neurotoxin: antitoxin more important than antibiotics
Clostridium difficile	LB	Pseudomembranous colitis	Vancomycin or metronidazole	Antibiotic-associated
Clostridium perfringens	SB	Food poisoning (diarrhoea)	None	Due to toxin production
Entamoeba histolytica	LB*	Amoebic dysentery	Metronidazole	See Chapter 31
Escherichia coli	SB	(i)Infantile diarrhoea		Rare above age of two. Fluid replacement more important than antibiotics
		(ii) Traveller's diarrhoea	Ciprofloxacin or norfloxacin†	Due to cholera-like toxins; usefulness of antibiotics unproven; self limiting
Giardia lamblia	SB	Giardiasis	Metronidazole	See Chapter 31
Rotavirus	SB*	Diarrhoea	None	Hospital and community outbreaks occur
Salmonella typhi (and *S. paratyphi*)	Extraintestinal	Enteric fever	Co-trimoxazole, chloramphenicol or ciprofloxacin	Antibiotic treatment mandatory; resistant strains occur

Table 22.2. cont.

Organism	Major site of infection	Disease produced	Antimicrobial therapy	Comments
Other salmonellae	SB*	Diarrhoea	None, unless complicated by systemic infection (ciprofloxacin)	Antibiotics prolong excretion
Shigella sonnei	LB*	Sonnei dysentery	None	Usually self limiting
Sh. dysenteriae Sh. flexneri Sh. boydii	LB*	Bacillary dysentery	Co-trimoxazole or ciprofloxacin	Antibiotics only in severe cases
Staphylococcus aureus	SB	(i)Food poisoning (nausea and vomiting)	None	Due to toxin; usually self limiting
		(ii)Enterocolitis	Flucloxacillin +fusidic acid	Antibiotic-associated
Vibrio cholerae	SB	Cholera	Tetracycline	Fluid replacement essential, but antibiotics reduce disease severity
Yersinia enterocolitica	SB	Mesenteric adenitis/ diarrhoea/ileitis	(Co-trimoxazole, tetracycline)	Antibiotics only in severe cases

* Mucosal invasion.
† Prophylactic use in selected persons.
LB=large bowel; SB=small bowel; CNS=central nervous system.

SPECIFIC INFECTIONS

Virus infections

Viral infections of the bowel are common and produce both sporadic and epidemic disease. Many viruses may cause infection; however, numerically the most important is *rotavirus*, which causes both community- and hospital-acquired gastroenteritis. The virus can be demonstrated by electron microscopy. Several other viruses may be associated with acute gastroenteritis; these include adenoviruses, Norwalk agent, caliciviruses, and astroviruses. The infections are usually self limiting and antimicrobial chemotherapy is not indicated.

Cholera

Cholera is an important world-wide cause of serious gastrointestinal infection. It is prevalent throughout the Indian subcontinent and South East Asia from where it has spread to many parts of Africa and to Central and South America. The infection is spread by faecal contamination of water supplies. The cholera vibrio is present in large numbers in the stools of infected patients. The present pandemic is caused by the El Tor biotype.

The onset of cholera is sudden with the development of profuse, pale, watery diarrhoea which may reach several litres a day; the so-called rice water stools which are isotonic with plasma. The patient rapidly becomes dehydrated and, unless fluid and electrolytes are replaced, becomes apathetic with subsequent hypotension and death. Mortality is highest in the elderly, the very young, and the malnourished.

Recognition of the pathophysiological role of cholera toxin in the production of the disease by activating cyclic AMP, which in turn stimulates water and electrolyte secretion by the intestinal epithelial cells, has justified the empirical benefit of a glucose–electrolyte oral replacement regimen. The addition of glucose considerably reduces the total volume of replacement fluid required by enhancing the absorption of sodium and water from the small bowel.

Cholera is one of the few gastrointestinal diseases for which there is little argument concerning the merits of antibiotic treatment as an adjunct to fluid replacement therapy. It has been shown that the duration of cholera is abbreviated by 60 per cent by the use of an oral tetracycline such as doxycycline, prescribed for 4 days. The vibrio is eliminated from the bowel and toxin production ceases rapidly. The carrier state does not occur. Resistance to tetracycline is, unfortunately, increasing and may limit the usefulness of antibiotic therapy in the future.

Campylobacter infection

Campylobacter jejuni is now recognized as one of the commonest world-wide causes of acute gastrointestinal infection which may be sporadic or epidemic. The organism produces infection in all age groups, but most frequently in young adults and pre-school children. Epidemics have occurred involving several thousand people following the ingestion of contaminated milk or water supplies. The organism itself is widespread in nature, producing infection in both domestic and farm animals, including poultry, and hence there are many opportunities for spread to humans.

Campylobacter gastroenteritis generally lasts for a few days, but may occasionally be more protracted with marked abdominal symptoms of colicky pain and tenderness as well as profuse diarrhoea. Acute appendicitis may be mimicked. Attacks are self limiting and managed by increasing the oral fluid intake. More severe attacks sometimes require hospitalization, and under these circumstances oral antibiotic treatment with erythromycin or a quinolone such as ciprofloxacin is indicated, although the latter is contraindicated in childhood.

There is little information to suggest that any of the different salts or esters of erythromycin has any advantage over erythromycin base, although the former are more readily absorbed from the bowel. The drugs are well tolerated, but occasional gastrointestinal intolerance may aggravate the patient's condition. Campylobacter infection is common, but fatalities are rare. Excretion ceases soon after clinical recovery.

Helicobacter infection

Helicobacter pylori is a recently described spiral organism linked with chronic gastritis and peptic ulceration. Treatment with amoxycillin and metronidozole in combination with bismuth salts clears the infection, but relapse may occur. Alternative regimens include omeprazole plus amoxycillin or clarithromycin. Other macrolides and quinolones seem to be ineffective.

Salmonellosis

Gastrointestinal salmonellosis is second only to campylobacter as a cause of gastrointestinal infection in the UK where several thousand cases are reported annually. There are more than 1700 different serotypes of salmonella but relatively few produce human disease with any regularity. Some common strains are *Salmonella typhimurium, S. enteritidis, S. hadar* and *S. virchow.* Frozen poultry and eggs are a common source of human infection by *S. enteritidis* phage type 4 and are linked to the ease of transmission among battery raised hens and contamination of the carcasses during evisceration.

Illness is commonly associated with systemic features of fever and malaise, in addition to the gastrointestinal symptoms. Bloodstream invasion may also occur following mucosal penetration. This occurs more frequently in the very young, the elderly, and those with underlying diseases such as alcoholism, cirrhosis, and AIDS. Achlorhydria from pernicious anaemia, atrophic gastritis, gastrectomy or H_2 receptor antagonists enhances the risk of salmonellosis by eliminating the protection afforded by the normal gastric acid.

Treatment of acute gastrointestinal salmonellosis is essentially directed at the replacement of any lost fluid or electrolytes, either by mouth or intravenously. Until recently antibiotics were considered to be contraindicated in the management of gastrointestinal salmonellosis, unless there is secondary bloodstream invasion, since they do not reduce the duration of illness and may prolong the period of excretion. However, for severe or invasive infections fluoroquinolones have gained increasing use, although they remain of equivocal efficacy in less severe disease. Apart from the fluoroquinolones, co-trimoxazole or a cephalosporin, such as ceftriaxone, provide alternative choices.

Enteric fever

This is caused by *Salmonella typhi* or *S. paratyphi* A, B, or C. The illness is usually designated typhoid or paratyphoid fever when the aetiological agent is known. Enteric fever is primarily a septicaemic illness acquired by ingestion. The gastrointestinal mucosa is readily penetrated, and the pathogen gains access to the lymphatics and blood from where it infects the liver and other parts of the reticuloendothelial system. The bowel is also involved since the lymphoid tissue in Peyer's patches is inflamed and often ulcerates. Constipation is more common than diarrhoea. Perforation and peritonitis are not uncommon in the untreated disease.

Enteric fever is potentially fatal and, unlike gastrointestinal salmonellosis, should always be treated with antibiotics. The bacteria are frequently located intracellularly and not all drugs shown to be active *in vitro* evoke satisfactory clinical response. The drug of choice is chloramphenicol, which produces the most rapid resolution of fever and best cure rates. Treatment must be continued for 2 weeks and, even so, relapse may occur. Alternative agents include ciprofloxacin, co-trimoxazole, and high-dose amoxycillin; all are effective, although the time taken for resolution of the fever may not be as rapid as with chloramphenicol and relapses also occur. Relapses should be treated with a further 2 weeks' treatment.

Following clinical recovery, salmonella may be excreted in the stool for several weeks. Should this continue for a period in excess of 3 months it is likely that the patient will become a persistent carrier.

In general the chronic carrier state is harmless to the individual.

However, there is a potential threat to his household and the community should lapses in personal hygiene produce contamination of food or water supplies. For this reason chronic excretion precludes employment requiring the handling of food. Prolonged high-dose ampicillin therapy is occasionally curative although ciprofloxacin is now preferred.

Shigellosis

In its severe form shigellosis produces classic bacillary dysentery characterized by profuse diarrhoea with blood and pus. Infection is world-wide but is more common in underdeveloped countries where sanitation and levels of hygiene are low. In Britain outbreaks occur, particularly among young children in low socioeconomic circumstances and also in long-stay institutions such as prisons and hospitals for the mentally ill. The spectrum of illness ranges from mild diarrhoea to a fulminating attack of dysentery. The more severe forms of disease are in general associated with *Shigella dysenteriae*, whilst more mild attacks are associated with *Sh. sonnei. Sh. flexneri* and *Sh. boydii* tend to produce disease of intermediate severity, although there is considerable individual variation. *Sh. sonnei* is the most frequent isolate in Britain.

Shigella spp. are amongst the most virulent gastrointestinal pathogens, requiring only a few bacteria to produce disease. The organism multiplies in the small bowel with subsequent invasion of the mucosa of the terminal ileum and colon. The intense inflammatory response produces a hyperaemic bowel which readily bleeds. Despite the severity of the infection, bloodstream invasion is uncommon in shigellosis. Some strains, notably *Sh. dysenteriae*, also produce an enterotoxin which stimulates fluid secretion within the small bowel so that watery diarrhoea may precede frank dysenteric symptoms.

Treatment of shigellosis is dependent upon the severity of the diarrhoea and blood loss. Mild attacks may be managed with fluid and electrolyte replacement by mouth, whereas more severe cases may require hospitalization and intravenous fluids. In shigellosis there is a definite place for antibiotic therapy for the severe attack, and to curtail the milder attacks associated with epidemic disease. Unfortunately, resistance among *Shigella* is increasing, and laboratory testing of antibiotic susceptibility is important.

Ampicillin, co-trimoxazole, or tetracycline have been widely used and may be administered orally provided they are shown to be active *in vitro*. Increasing problems with antibiotic resistance have led to an increased use of oral quinolones, notably ciprofloxacin. Antibiotic therapy shortens the illness, controls symptoms, and speeds elimination of the organism from the bowel. For most mild attacks of *Sh. sonnei*, antibiotics are unnecessary.

Yersiniosis

Infection with *Yersinia enterocolitica* may produce mesenteric adenitis, terminal ileitis, and also acute diarrhoea. For obscure reasons it is more common in Scandinavia, but its occurrence is worldwide. Erythema nodosum and a reactive arthritis may complicate such infections. The illness is usually self limiting and, unless complicated by extragastrointestinal symptoms, is infrequently suspected. Co-trimoxazole or tetracycline are effective if an antibiotic appears justified. For invasive disease gentamicin is appropriate.

Food poisoning

Food may be contaminated at source, in the abattoir, subsequent to marketing, or during preparation. Storing at ambient temperatures encourages microbial growth, hence the importance of adequate refrigeration. Foods frequently associated with outbreaks of disease include poultry, meats, shellfish, and those containing dairy products, notably cream. Foodhandlers may excrete salmonellae and contaminate food by lapses in personal hygiene, whilst staphylococcal food poisoning is often the result of contamination of food from infected skin lesions.

Clostridium perfringens produces powerful exotoxins which may contaminate meats, gravies, and sauces that are either inadequately refrigerated or partially reheated. True mucosal invasion is uncommon with *Cl. perfringens* food poisoning, although a severe invasive infection, enteritis necroticans, may rarely occur. This has been described from New Guinea where pork feasts produce disease known locally as 'pig bel'.

Occasional outbreaks of gastroenteritis are caused by *Bacillus cereus*, most frequently in association with the reheating of rice in restaurants. The organism is ubiquitous and produces disease by elaborating an enterotoxin. The disease is self limiting.

Botulism is fortunately a rare disease which develops after ingesting inadequately sterilized canned products. Spores of *Cl. botulinum* produce a powerful neurotoxin that is readily absorbed from the gut and produces neural paralysis which in particular affects the respiratory musculature. Treatment is aimed at supporting the patient whilst the fixed neurotoxin undergoes degradation. Prompt treatment with antitoxin is essential to prevent more severe disease.

In most forms of food poisoning specific antimicrobial chemotherapy is contra-indicated. Treatment is essentially supportive with the notable exception of the use of specific antitoxin for botulism. The exception is symptomatic bloodstream invasion complicating gastrointestinal salmonellosis or severe shigellosis and campylobacteriosis, as discussed above.

Escherichia coli

Acute gastroenteritis is common among travellers to tropical and subtropical regions where it has been known to generations of travellers as 'Delhi belly', 'Gyppy tummy', or 'Montezuma's revenge'. In many instances disease is caused by toxin-producing strains of *Esch. coli*. The toxins have many similarities to the cholera toxin and the pathophysiology of the illness is similar. *Enterotoxigenic* strains differ from the *enteropathogenic Esch. coli* responsible for infantile gastroenteritis which is associated with a few clearly defined serotypes. The latter illness, once a scourge of obstetric units, is now uncommon, at least in the UK, although it may still produce severe dehydration, requiring intravenous fluids. Two other kinds of pathogenic *Esch. coli* are recognized: *enteroinvasive* strains that can produce severe invasive infection of the bowel, but are fortunately uncommon; and *enterohaemorrhagic* strains that produce a toxin detectable by a cytotoxic effect on Vero tissue culture cells (Vero toxin), and have been associated with haemorrhagic colitis and the haemolytic uraemic syndrome.

Antimicrobial therapy is generally unnecessary in the management of traveller's diarrhoea or infantile gastroenteritis caused by *Esch. coli*. However, for severe infection or if the patient is immunocompromised, has inflammatory bowel disease, or has experienced previous severe traveller's diarrhoea, treatment with an oral quinolone, such as norfloxacin or ciprofloxacin, can be considered. These agents are still unlicensed for use in children. Attempts at chemoprophylaxis against traveller's diarrhoea with oral doxycycline, co-trimoxazole or a quinolone have been reasonably successful, but their widespread use for this indication is not recommended except in the higher risk groups mentioned. Drug resistance among *Esch. coli* strains is an increasing problem in developing and tropical countries where enterotoxigenic strains are endemic; resistance would inevitably increase further with widespread prophylactic use.

Antibiotic-associated diarrhoea

Paradoxically, the use of antimicrobial agents is occasionally complicated by diarrhoea. This is usually due to a direct irritating effect on the bowel mucosa. However, alteration of the bowel flora may rarely be followed by frank infection with *Candida* spp. or *Staph. aureus*.

A more serious consequence of antibiotics is disease caused by toxin producing strains of *Clostridium difficile*. In severe cases bloody diarrhoea and a frank colitis develop. The bowel appearances are characteristic and aptly described by the term 'pseudomembranous colitis'. Use of clindamycin or β-lactam antibiotics are most frequently complicated by this disease which occurs in sporadic or epidemic form in hospital practice. The condition is potentially fatal and should be treated with oral vancomycin or metronidazole.

Intestinal parasites

Symptoms ranging from mild diarrhoea to severe dysentery may be caused by some protozoa and helminths. These are considered in Chapters 5 and 31.

23

Bacteraemia and endocarditis

P. Ispahani

BACTERAEMIA

Bacteraemia refers to the presence of viable bacteria in the blood detected in the laboratory by blood culture. The clinical manifestations associated with bacteraemia range from the patient being completely asymptomatic to the presence of fever, rigors, tachycardia, shock, multi-organ failure, and death. When bacteraemia is associated with clinical signs and symptoms it is referred to as *septicaemia*. Thus bacteraemia is a laboratory finding, whereas septicaemia is a clinical term.

In recent years, however, the widespread use of haemodynamic monitoring in intensive care units has shown that not all patients with septicaemia are bacteraemic and the terms *sepsis* and *sepsis syndrome* have become popular. This takes into account that the sepsis syndrome results from the release of cytokines (inflammatory mediators such as tumour necrosis factor, interleukin-1, etc: 'host poisons') stimulated by microbial substances (structural components of organisms, e.g. lipopolysaccharide, teichoic acid, or exotoxins: 'bacterial poisons'). On the other hand, the term sepsis has been used loosely by some to mean any infection with or without blood involvement. In this chapter the term septicaemia will be used to indicate the presence of signs and symptoms in infections involving the bloodstream.

Any traumatic procedure that facilitates entry of organisms from an infected cutaneous lesion or bacteria-laden mucosal surface may cause bacteraemia (Table 23.1). In addition, invasive infections such as pneumococcal pneumonia, meningitis, or osteomyelitis may be associated with bacteraemia.

In the last 50 years, changes have taken place in the type of organism most frequently encountered. In the pre-antibiotic era *Streptococcus pyogenes* and *Str. pneumoniae* accounted for the majority of positive blood cultures and fatalities, but by 1960 *Staphylococcus aureus* had become dominant. Today, staphylococci and pneumococci are still important, but are outnumbered by Gram-negative bacilli as causes of septicaemia and death (Table 23.2). Anaerobes such as *Bacteroides fragilis* are also encountered more frequently, perhaps because of improved anaerobic techniques.

The increase in bacteraemic infections due to Gram-negative bacilli

Table 23.1. Procedures that may produce transient bacteraemia

Predominant organism	Procedure
Viridans streptococci	Dental extraction
	Periodontal surgery
	Surgery or instrumentation of the upper respiratory tract
Enterococci	Surgery or instrumentation of:
	urinary tract
	gastrointestinal tract
	bilary tract
	Obstetric or gynaecological surgery
Staphylococcus aureus	Manipulation or drainage of a septic focus

Table 23.2. Distribution of organisms in 3740 episodes of bacteraemia (1980–1991) at University Hospital, Nottingham

Gram-negative	%	Gram-positive	%
Escherichia coli	25.4	*Staph. aureus*	13.0
Klebsiella spp.	5.2	*Staph. epidermidis*	3.5
Proteus spp.	4.1	*Str. pneumoniae*	10.8
Salmonella spp.	2.1	Haemolytic streptococci	5.2
Other Enterobacteriaceae	2.3	(Groups A, B, C and G)	
Pseudomonas spp.	3.6	Other streptococci	3.5
Haemophilus influenzae	4.7	Enterococci	1.9
Neisseria meningitidis	2.1	Fungi	0.6
'Others'	0.7	'Others'	0.6
Anaerobes	2.5	Anaerobes	0.6
Total	52.7	Total	39.7

——————————————— Polymicrobial 7.6% ———————————————

follows the success of antibiotics in controlling many Gram-positive infections, but advances in medical and surgical expertise have also played an important part: Gram-negative septicaemia is common in patients undergoing extensive surgery, aggressive immunosuppressive therapy, and invasive procedures at the extremes of age, in the very ill, or in patients whose normal defence mechanisms are already compromised by the underlying disease. These infections are mostly hospital acquired, the widespread use of antibiotics having promoted the selection of Gram-negative organisms (which may be resistant to many antibiotics) in the hospital environment.

The use of vascular catheters has become an indispensable feature of medical management and this has resulted in an increase in bacteraemia caused by Gram-positive cocci, notably *Staph. aureus, Staph. epidermidis*, and enterococci. Polymicrobial bacteraemia and recurrent bacteraemia have also become more common in recent years.

The duration of bacteraemia may be transient (lasting for several minutes) intermittent, or continuous (lasting for several hours to days). The danger of transient bacteraemia depends on the host and the organism. Thus, transient bacteraemia due to viridans streptococci after dental extraction is of no consequence in an otherwise healthy individual, but in those patients with abnormal heart valves it may produce endocarditis (see below). *Staph. aureus* may localize in the metaphyses of long bones in children or the vertebrae in adults and lead to osteomyelitis. Transient bacteraemia with Gram-negative bacilli following instrumentation of an infected urinary tract may produce rigor and fever.

Continuous bacteraemia is the hallmark of intravascular infection and also occurs in infections in patients with neutropenia, overwhelming septicaemia, acute haematogenous osteomyelitis, and infections with intracellular organisms such as *Salmonella typhi* and *Brucella* spp., during the early stage of the illness.

Most other bacteraemias are intermittent and are characteristic of abscesses and certain types of chronic infection such as meningococcal or gonococcal septicaemia or brucellosis.

Laboratory investigation and antibiotic therapy

If death is to be prevented and shock avoided, the clinician must react promptly and aggressively to the early signs of septicaemia with appropriate 'best-guess' parenteral therapy. Mortality in patients who are shocked is still over 50 per cent.

There are no specific clinical findings that are diagnostic of bacteraemia or fungaemia or, for that matter, that differentiate between Gram-negative and Gram-positive septicaemia. Hence the importance of blood cultures so that the pathogen is identified and specific therapy is instituted as early as possible.

Most bacteraemias are intermittent, hence the importance of more than one set of blood cultures prior to starting antibiotics. Ideally, at least two sets from two separate venepunctures at intervals of a few minutes to a few hours (depending upon the clinical urgency) should be taken. Since bacteraemias are usually low grade, the volume of blood drawn at each venepuncture is important; in adults at least 10 ml should be taken; in infants and young children 1–3 ml. Other appropriate specimens from likely foci of infection must also be sent to the laboratory; these may include urine, sputum, CSF, pus, pleural or joint fluids, etc. Often a Gram-stained smear of a specimen from the presumed site of infection gives the vital clue on which the choice of best-guess therapy can be based.

Secondary bacteraemia

When bacteraemia is secondary to a focus of infection which is readily apparent or clinically suspected, it is usually possible to predict the most likely organisms from the clinical presentation. The selection of antibiotics is guided not only by the suspicion of the focus of infection but also whether the infection was community or hospital acquired. The most appropriate antibiotic or combination can then be chosen in the light of local knowledge of resistance patterns and changed later, if necessary, on the basis of bacteriological findings.

Primary bacteraemia

Certain groups of patients give no clue as to the primary focus of infection or its likely source. Such 'primary' bacteraemia of unknown source may occur in neonates, immunocompromised patients, and, rarely, normal individuals.

The neonate. The newborn baby is comparatively more susceptible to bacterial invasion of the bloodstream, but the recognition and localization of infection may be difficult because the manifestations are frequently non-specific. However, it is imperative that the diagnosis is made early and antibiotic treatment started at once, (after specimens have been taken for microscopy and culture, but before the results are known) to avoid complications like meningitis and death.

The initial blind choice in a neonate with 'early-onset' ($\leqslant 7$ days) sepsis is most often a combination of benzylpenicillin and gentamicin, which covers the two most common organisms, *Escherichia coli* and group B haemolytic streptococci, as well as other streptococci, many other Gram-negative bacteria, and *Listeria monocytogenes*. If however, there is an obvious staphylococcal skin infection, flucloxacillin should be substituted for benzylpenicillin.

Empiric treatment for 'late-onset' (>7 days) sepsis varies according to the clinical setting. The combination of cefotaxime and gentamicin should be considered in neonates who are ventilated, known to be colonized with enterobacteria, or have had previous exposure to antibiotics. Since *Staph. epidermidis* is the commonest isolate in patients with long-lines *in situ* and vancomycin is the only reliable agent against these organisms, a combination of vancomycin with gentamicin or cefotaxime would be a reasonable choice in neonates in whom catheter-associated sepsis is strongly suspected.

Immunocompromised patients. Bacteraemia frequently develops without previous surgery or instrumentation in immunocompromised patients, especially those with haematological disease, whose underlying condition or therapy increases susceptibility to infection. Among the major predisposing factors are profound neutropenia, mucosal ulcerations, and administration of corticosteroid, cytotoxic, and immunosuppressive drugs. Neutropenic patients are unable to localize an infection at the point of entry due to their inability to mount an inflammatory response; bloodstream invasion occurs frequently without any clinical evidence of the source of bacteraemia. Despite the fact that blood cultures from immunocompromised patients yield Gram-positive organisms more frequently than Gram-negative organisms, it is the Gram-negatives, in particular *Pseudomonas aeruginosa*, which are feared, for if left untreated most patients will die within 48 h. Therefore, it has been customary to provide a broad-spectrum synergistic bactericidal combination of antibiotics as initial blind therapy in febrile neutropenic patients. Precise choice of the empiric regimen will depend on local experience and knowledge of resistance patterns. Most successful and widely used regimens have included an aminoglycoside (e.g. gentamicin) together with either an antipseudomonal penicillin (e.g. azlocillin) or an expanded-spectrum cephalosporin with antipseudomonal activity (e.g. ceftazidime). Concern about aminoglycoside toxicity has led some to advocate monotherapy with ceftazidime, the imipenem/cilastatin combination or ciprofloxacin. If blood cultures are positive, relevant modifications in the antibiotic regimen are made. However, it is advisable not to narrow the spectrum of antibiotic cover in febrile neutropenic patients for there is a risk of breakthrough bacteraemia.

If fever persists for more than 72 h despite broad-spectrum antibiotics and blood cultures remain negative, the patient should be reassessed and, after appropriate samples for culture including targeted blood cultures have been taken, vancomycin or teicoplanin may be added to the regimen of those who have vascular catheters *in situ*. Empiric antifungal therapy with amphotericin B should be considered in selected patients who remain febrile and neutropenic for 7 days despite broad-spectrum antibiotics.

Normal individuals. Primary bacteraemia in normal individuals is rare. The most common type seen the UK is that due to *Neisseria meningitidis*. In infants, children or young adults it can produce a fulminating septicaemia with petechial rash progressing to shock and death in a matter of hours. Mortality in this type of presentation can be as high as 30 per cent. General practitioners and hospital doctors suspecting this condition should give benzylpenicillin immediately. Since it is unlikely that subsequent blood or CSF cultures from these patients would be positive, a throat or pernasal swab must always be obtained and a special request made for the isolation of *N. meningitidis*.

Str. pneumoniae and *Haemophilus influenzae* occasionally cause bacteraemia in an otherwise healthy, but febrile child. Those aged 6 months to 2 years are most at risk. Although such bacteraemias may resolve spontaneously, a small minority of patients remain ill and a few develop severe disease, including meningitis. Antibiotic therapy with amoxycillin is warranted.

Other important causes of primary bacteraemia include *Salmonella typhi* and *S. paratyphi* (see Chapter 22), *Brucella abortus*, and *Br. melitensis*. In the UK brucellosis in humans is usually caused by *Br. abortus*, acquired by direct contact with animals, or from consumption of unpasteurized milk and its products. It is difficult to culture *Br. abortus* from blood, even in the acute stages. The diagnosis may rest on clinical presentation with a history of occupational exposure or of drinking raw milk. Serological tests are also helpful. Doxycycline (100 mg twice daily) given in combination with rifampicin (900 mg daily) for at least 6 weeks is the treatment of choice. Co-trimoxazole has also been used, but seems to be associated with a high relapse rate.

Management of septicaemic shock

Septicaemic shock results in profound and complex effects on the cardio-vascular system (hypotension, decreased systemic vascular resistance, myocardial depression, maldistribution of blood flow, and multi-organ system failure). The management of septicaemia is based on two basic principles:

(1) to eradicate the source of infection with appropriate antibiotics and drainage or debridement of the septic focus, whenever possible;

(2) to stabilize the haemodynamic status with the administration of intravenous fluids, oxygen, inotropic agents, and vasopressors.

However, even when such patients are managed aggressively in intensive care units, the mortality in those who have reached the organ failure stage is depressingly high (approximately 50 per cent).

Since the manifestations of septicaemia are associated with an exaggerated release of cytokines by macrophages stimulated by microbial products, there has been much interest in the possibility that interference with bacterial or host mediators might be beneficial and serve as an adjunct to antimicrobial therapy in septicaemia.

Monoclonal antibodies against lipid A of Gram-negative organisms and against tumour necrosis factor have been subjected to therapeutic trial, but neither have lived up to their early promise. The routine use of such a strategy in patients with septicaemia still seems some way off.

INFECTIVE ENDOCARDITIS

Endocarditis is an inflammation of the endocardial surface of the heart. An infection of the endocardium with micro-organisms is known as 'infective' endocarditis, which is preferable to the old term 'bacterial' endocarditis, since fungi, rickettsiae, or chlamydia may be involved. Although the infection may be located anywhere in the heart chamber, the lesion is usually on the heart valves. The words *acute* and *subacute* are still used to describe endocarditis, though the terms originated in the pre-antibiotic era when all patients with endocarditis died. Those who died in less than 6 weeks following a fulminant course due to infection of normal valves by virulent organisms such as *Staph. aureus, Str. pneumoniae* or *Neisseria gonorrhoeae* were said to have acute bacterial endocarditis, whereas those who suffered a more indolent course due to infection of abnormal valves by relatively avirulent organisms (e.g. viridans streptococci), and died much later, sometimes after a year of illness, were said to have subacute bacterial endocarditis.

Nowadays, most patients are cured provided the diagnosis is made, and treatment with appropriate antibiotics is begun, sufficiently early. Therefore, it is more useful not only to classify endocarditis according to the infecting organism but also to refer to the underlying anatomy which, besides giving an idea of the probable course of the disease, has therapeutic implications suggesting the antibiotic regimen to be used.

Epidemiology

Infective edocarditis, although not common (approximately 2000 cases per year in England and Wales), is still a dangerous condition with a mortality of 15–30 per cent. In recent years the spectrum of recognized underlying cardiac lesions in infective endocarditis in adults has been changing as a result of a decline in rheumatic heart disease (in the developed world) and improvement in cardiac diagnostic imaging techniques (echocardiography). The following trends have been noted:

1. The median age of the patient has increased. Whereas in the past the mean age of the patients was less than 40 years, today more than half of the patients are over 50 for the following reasons:

   (a) people with congenital heart disease or rheumatic heart disease survive longer because of advances in medical and surgical expertise to correct valve dysfunction;

(b) a longer average life span of the general population is associated with an increased incidence of degenerative valve disease; almost 30 per cent of elderly patients who develop endocarditis do not have a pre-existing cardiac condition, but may have minor degenerative valvular lesions which serve as a nidus for the initiation of infection;

(c) genitourinary tract infections and manipulations, gastrointestinal malignancies, and hospital-acquired bacteraemias are more common in the elderly.

2. The proportion of acute cases has risen, partly because of the preponderance of *Staph. aureus* endocarditis in intravenous drug-abusers, which occurs predominantly in young adults.

3. The 'classic' physical signs of subacute bacterial endocarditis are seen in fewer patients.

4. Mitral valve prolapse with regurgitation is recognized more frequently as an underlying cardiac condition.

5. Prosthetic valve endocarditis (PVE) is more common.

Pathogenesis

Infective endocarditis is most likely to result from the interaction of several events (Fig. 23.1):

(1) structural alteration of the endothelial surface of the valve (e.g. turbulence of blood flow from an incompetent valve can denude the endothelium);

(2) deposition of platelets and fibrin on the edges of the valve, resulting in the formation of a non-bacterial thrombotic vegetation (NBTV);

(3) colonization of NBTV by micro-organisms transiently circulating in the blood.

After certain procedures, transient bacteraemia is a common event (Table 23.1). Furthermore, a wide variety of trivial events such as chewing and tooth brushing induce streptococcal bacteraemia. Indeed, 85 per cent of cases of streptococcal endocarditis cannot be related to any iatrogenic procedure. To cause endocarditis organisms must not only enter the circulation, but must also be able to survive complement-mediated serum bactericidal activity and adhere to NBTV. Certain streptococci capable of producing extracelluar dextran tend to stick to fibrin–platelet vegetations and are known to cause endocarditis more frequently than do non-dextran-producing strains. However, organisms such as enterococci and *Staph. aureus* that do not produce dextran are important causes of endocarditis. In these cases adherence may be mediated by host proteins such as fibronectin and fibrinogen.

Pathogenesis of Infective Endocarditis

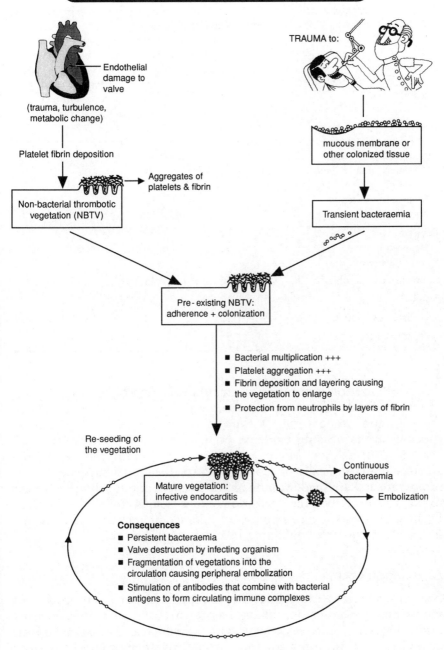

Fig. 23.1. Pathogenesis of infective endocarditis.

Table 23.3 Aetiological agents in infective endocarditis and their approximate frequency

| Organism | Native valve % | Prosthetic valve/cardiac surgery | | Intravenous drug-abuser % |
		Early-onset < 2 months %	Late-onset >2 months %	
Streptococci (all)	65	5	35	15
Viridans, (alpha haemolytic)	35	<5	25	5
Str. bovis	15	<5	<5	<5
Enterococcus faecalis	10	<5	<5	8
Other streptococci	<5	<5	<5	<5
Staphylococci (all)	25	50	30	50
Staph. aureus	23	20	10	50
Staph. epidermidis	2	30	20	<5
Gram-negative aerobic bacilli	<5	20	15	15
Fungi	<5	10	5	5
Miscellaneous bacteria	<5	10	10	10
Culture negative	5–10	5	<5	<5

Once colonization occurs there is rapid deposition of additional layers of platelets and fibrin over and around the growing colonies, causing the vegetation to enlarge. Within 24–48 h marked proliferation of bacteria occurs, leading to dense populations of organisms (10^9–10^{10} bacteria/g of tissue). Micro-organisms deep within the vegetations are often metabolically inactive, whereas the more superficial ones proliferate and are shed into the bloodstream continuously; they return to the heart to reseed the vegetation, and a vicious circle is established. Fresh vegetations are composed of colonies of micro-organisms in a fibrin-platelet matrix containing relatively few leucocytes.

Aetiological agents

Any organism can cause infective endocarditis, but streptococci and staphylococci account for more than 90 per cent of culture-positive cases. However, the frequency with which various organisms are involved differs not only for the type of valve that is infected (native or prosthetic) but also with the causative event (e.g. dental manipulation, intravenous drug abuse, or a hospital-acquired infection) (Table 23.3).

Native valve endocarditis

Streptococci. Streptococci account for about 65 per cent of all cases of native valve endocarditis. Most common of all are the 'viridans streptococci', a heterogenous group including *Streptococcus mitis, Str. sanguis, Str. mutans, Str. milleri* group, and *Str. salivarius,* normally present as commensals in the mouth; most are highly sensitive to penicillin and cause infections primarily on abnormal heart valves. A few cases are caused by 'nutritionally variant streptococci', which are not only difficult to isolate from blood but seem to be harder to eradicate with antibiotic treatment; relapses are more frequent than with the other viridans streptococci.

Str. bovis is an important cause of endocarditis in the elderly, and is frequently associated with colonic polyps and carcinoma. Recovery of this organism should prompt an early investigation for colonic disease. It is sensitive to penicillin.

Enterococci are related to streptococci, but are classified as a separate genus. They are gut commensals and cause 10 per cent of all streptococcal cases. Enterococci commonly cause urinary tract, wound, and intravenous line infections; they often give rise to hospital-acquired bacteraemias, commonly in association with other organisms, but endocarditis is rare (<5 per cent). However, persistent enterococcal bacteraemia in an elderly male with a recent history of genitourinary manipulation, trauma or disease requires investigation for infective endocarditis.

Haemolytic streptococci of Lancefield Groups B and G are occasionally incriminated in endocarditis. Diabetic patients are particularly at risk for Group B infections. Group A haemolytic streptococci which were an important cause of acute endocarditis in the pre-penicillin period are rarely reported now.

Staphylococci. Staphylococci account for 25 per cent of cases of native valve endocarditis; over 90 per cent is due to *Staph. aureus,* which is the leading cause of of acute endocarditis. The course is frequently fulminant with widespread metastatic abscesses, and results in death in approximately 40 per cent of cases. The organism can attack either normal or damaged valves and cause rapid destruction of the affected valves. Surgery is often required. *Staph. epidermidis,* in contrast, causes an indolent infection on previously damaged valves.

Other bacteria. Almost all species of bacteria have occasionally been reported as causes of native valve endocarditis. Most commonly encountered are the fastidious, slow-growing Gram-negative bacilli of the 'HACEK' group (*Haemophilus* spp., *Actinobacillus actinomycetemcomitans, Cardiobacterium hominis, Eikenella corrodens,* and *Kingella* spp.). *Erysipelothrix rhusiopathiae*, *Listeria monocytogenes*, *Rothia dentocariosa*, *N. gonorrhoeae* and *Str. pneumoniae* are also occasionally involved.

Gram-negative enteric bacteria rarely cause endocarditis, except in intravenous drug abusers and patients with prosthetic valves. However, *Salmonella* spp. have an affinity for abnormal cardiac valves and for aneurysms of major vessels.

Fungi. These organisms seldom cause native valve endocarditis. Risk factors include: major underlying illnesses, prolonged courses of broad-spectrum antibiotics, corticosteroids or cytotoxic agents, and a central venous line that has been in place for a considerable length of time. The course is indolent but grave. Large vegetations frequently embolize, occluding major vessels in the lower extremities. When this occurs culture of the material obtained at embolectomy may yield the offending organism, when blood cultures are negative. Fungal endocarditis is more often seen in intravenous drug abusers or after reconstructive cardiovascular surgery. *Candida*, *Torulopsis*, and *Aspergillus* species are usually implicated.

Prosthetic valve endocarditis

Endocarditis involving a prosthetic valve is termed 'early onset' when symptoms appear within 60 days of insertion and 'late onset' when symptoms occur after that time. Early-onset disease usually reflects contamination arising in the peri-operative period. Despite prophylactic antibiotics, staphylococci account for 50 per cent of all cases, and *Staph. epidermidis* is more common than *Staph. aureus*. Early-onset infection is often associated with valve dehiscence, a fulminant course, and a high mortality. Late-onset prosthetic valve endocarditis occurs after the valve has become endothelialized. The source of infection (as in native valve endocarditis) is seeding of the valves following transient bacteraemia from dental, genito-urinary or gastrointestinal manipulation, and viridans streptococci again become the commonest organism. Late-onset disease caused by *Staph. epidermidis*, diphtheroids or other organisms of the early-onset type may simply reflect a delayed manifestation of the infection acquired in the peri-operative period.

Infective endocarditis in intravenous drug abusers

The skin, rather than the contaminated drug or its associated paraphernalia, is the commonest source of micro-organisms responsible for infective endocarditis in intravenous drug abusers. *Staph. aureus* is the predominant cause, but other organisms, including *Pseudomonas* spp., Group A haemolytic streptococci, other streptococci, and fungi, etc., are also important. In this group of patients, endocarditis often involves the tricuspid valve especially when *Staph. aureus* is the causative agent.

Laboratory diagnosis

Blood cultures must be obtained from all patients with fever and heart murmur, irrespective of the initial diagnosis, before contemplating antibiotic therapy.

Bacteraemia is usually low-grade, but continuous, so it does not really matter when blood cultures are obtained. In the absence of previous antimicrobial therapy, blood cultures are positive in more than 95 per cent of cases.

Blood for culture should be collected aseptically as a separate procedure from other investigations such as blood count or erythrocyte sedimentation rate (ESR) to minimize the chances of 'pseudobacteraemia'. At least three sets of blood cultures are obtained, irrespective of temperature, from three separate venepunctures over a period of time. *Staph. epidermidis* and diphtheroids are important causes of endocarditis as well as common blood culture contaminants from the skin, and isolation of the same relatively 'avirulent' organism repeatedly in the absence of an intravascular catheter is highly suggestive of infective endocarditis. At each venepuncture at least 10 ml of blood should be withdrawn and inoculated in equal amounts aseptically into two bottles (one set). The practice of obtaining a large volume of blood at one venepuncture, distributing it into 4–6 bottles, and passing it off as 2–3 sets, does not answer the basic question of continuous bacteraemia, and may result in dangerous diagnostic confusion.

It is immensely important to pay strict attention to skin preparation and to aseptic techniques while performing the venepuncture and inoculating the culture bottles. Casual stroking of the skin with a 'medi-swab' followed by the use of the ungloved finger to palpate the vein is a sure way to cause contamination of the cultures. Similarly, blood should not be drawn through an indwelling catheter, since peri-catheter contaminants may be picked up.

The interval between each venepuncture depends upon the clinical urgency. In acute cases, when antimicrobial therapy should be commenced within 2–3 h, three sets from separate venepunctures should be taken at intervals of at least 30 min apart before the start of therapy; if there is no urgency then the three sets are taken over a 24 h period with intervals of 6–8 h between each set. All blood culture bottles must be taken to the laboratory promptly and incubated for up to 3 weeks to cater for fastidious organisms.

It may be difficult to isolate bacteria from patients who have received antibiotics in the preceding 2 weeks. If the clinical situation permits, repeated blood cultures spread over several days may be necessary in such patients, for occasionally, negative blood culture during the first week is followed by continuous bacteraemia thereafter.

Blood culture may remain persistently negative in a small number of patients with suspected endocarditis. Likely explanations are:

(1) prior administration of antibiotics (the most common cause);

(2) infection with fastidious organisms including those of the 'HACEK' group, *Coxiella burnetii*, *Chlamydia psittaci* or *Brucella* spp.;

(3) infection with *Candida*, in which only 50 per cent of blood cultures may be positive;

(4) infection of the right side of the heart, which is occasionally accompanied by negative blood cultures;

(5) disease other than infective endocarditis (e.g. left atrial myxoma).

When blood cultures are negative, paired samples of sera (one taken on admission and another 10–14 days later) should be examined for antibodies against other infective agents of endocarditis.

Echocardiography has assumed an increasingly important role in the diagnosis, assessment, and management of patients with suspected infective endocarditis, but negative results do not exclude the diagnosis especially in those with prosthetic valves.

General principles of therapy

The chief aims of management are to sterilize the vegetation and to ensure that relapse will not occur.

Bactericidal antibiotics

For most other infections bacteriostatic agents are capable of eradicating the offending microbe in support of host defence mechanisms. However, in endocarditis, organisms reach extremely high densities within the depths of the vegetation encased in layers of fibrin, where the bacteria are free to divide without interference from phagocytic cells or humoral defences. Hence, bactericidal antibiotics are necessary, which must sterilize the vegetation on their own without any help. Bacteriostatic agents such as tetracycline or chloramphenicol may produce a symptomatic response, but, once discontinued, relapse is common and they should not be used. The most commonly used bactericidal agents are the penicillins, in particular benzylpenicillin. In penicillin-hypersensitive patients, vancomycin or a cephalosporin offer suitable alternatives.

Parenteral route

The administration of antimicrobial agents by the parenteral route is the only reliable way of ensuring that high doses of antibiotics can be given and that sufficient antibiotic is present in the serum to guarantee its penetration into the depths of relatively avascular vegetations. Oral treatment can be recommended only in selected cases of native valve endocarditis during the last 2 weeks of treatment, provided facilities exist for frequent monitoring of serum bactericidal activity and patient compliance is assured.

Prolonged therapy

Organisms buried deep in the infected vegetations exist in a state of reduced metabolic activity and cell division. Bactericidal antibiotics that have a cell wall site of action (e.g. penicillin) are relatively inactive in this situation so that the antibiotic must be administered for a prolonged period. Short-term therapy is associated with relapse. Most patients with endocarditis are cured by 4 weeks of treatment; some may require treatment up to 6 weeks or more, whilst a selected group may be cured in only 2 weeks.

Synergistic combination therapy

Aminoglycosides, though generally bactericidal, have little activity against streptococci and cannot be used alone. But the combination of gentamicin with penicillin produces a more rapid and complete bactericidal effect than that obtained with penicillin alone. It has therefore become a common practice to recommend combination therapy in the initial stages of management of infective endocarditis.

Laboratory control of antibiotic therapy

Determination of MIC and MBC

Ordinary disc diffusion or break-point sensitivities are not recommended in the laboratory management of endocarditis. Instead, the MIC and MBC of the antibiotics to be used, for the organism isolated, should be precisely determined (see Chapter 7). In difficult cases, tests for antibiotic synergy may also be required for optimal combination therapy.

Serum bactericidal levels

As an additional control of adequate therapy, testing of the bactericidal activity of the patient's serum for the patient's own organism just before, and 1 h after, administering a dose, has been widely advocated. However, because of the inherent technical variability of this test, together with varying interpretations, serum bactericidal levels correlate poorly with clinical outcome. However, a trough titre >1/32 and a peak of >1/64 is said to predict bacteriological cure.

In endocarditis caused by sensitive viridans streptococci or *Staph. aureus*, appropriate high-dose parenteral antibiotics reliably produce titres of 128 or 1024, and this test is most likely to be helpful when treating difficult or unusual organisms, or when using unusual antibiotics or the oral route.

Aminoglycoside assays

When aminoglycosides (usually gentamicin) are being used for synergistic activity with penicillins in patients with endocarditis, a serum concentration of gentamicin lower than that considered therapeutic for Gram-negative infections should be adequate, thus lessening the potential for toxicity. It seems reasonable therefore that adults or elderly patients with normal renal function should receive a loading dose of 120–160 mg of gentamicin (depending upon the age and body weight) followed by a maintenance dose of 1.5 mg/kg twice daily for adults, and once daily for the elderly. The concentration of antibiotic in the serum should be periodically monitored and the dose adjusted accordingly (a pre-dose concentration ≤1.0 mg/l; post-dose of 4–5 mg/l should be adequate).

Blood culture organism

This must be fully identified and saved in case future tests are needed; e.g. serum bactericidal levels, further antimicrobial sensitivities, synergy tests or comparisons with a strain causing relapse, should this occur.

Specific antimicrobial regimens

Streptococci

Isolates highly sensitive to penicillin (MIC ≤0.1 mg/l) e.g. viridans streptococci, Str. bovis, other streptococci. Approximately 80 per cent of viridans streptococci are highly sensitive to penicillin, and such cases have been successfully treated with penicillin for 6 weeks. Addition of an aminoglycoside, such as gentamicin, produces synergistic killing and sterilizes the cardiac vegetations more rapidly. Thus it became a common practice to recommend combination therapy for the first 2 weeks followed by a further 2 weeks of benzylpenicillin alone on the grounds that the duration of treatment may be shortened from 6 to 4 weeks and the few relapses that occurred with penicillin alone prevented completely. However, by using a much higher dose of penicillin, a 99 per cent cure rate can be achieved with a 4-week regimen of benzylpenicillin alone. Such a regimen is recommended in elderly patients or those with impaired renal function in whom aminoglycosides are best avoided, when treating uncomplicated native valve endocarditis. In selected cases, just 2 weeks of combination therapy may be adequate. For uncomplicated native valve endocarditis it is common practice in the UK to give an initial 2 weeks of combination therapy and then to consider oral amoxycillin for the last 2 weeks, provided patient compliance can be guaranteed and facilities for monitoring serum bactericidal activity are available. Patients with prosthetic value endocarditis should be treated more aggressively and for a longer duration to ensure cure.

Isolates relatively resistant to penicillin (MIC >0.1 mg/l but <0.5 µg/ml) e.g. viridans streptococci or nutritionally variant streptococci (NVS). Viridans streptococci that are relatively resistant to penicillin are increasingly encountered. The relapse rate in endocarditis caused by NVS is high, even when 2 weeks of combination therapy is followed by a further 2 weeks of benzylpenicillin. Endocarditis caused by such strains, or other streptococci which are relatively resistant to penicillin, is best treated with high-dose benzylpenicillin and a more prolonged combination therapy, with appropriate monitoring of serum gentamicin levels.

Isolates resistant to penicillin (MIC ≥0.5 mg/l) e.g. Enterococcus faecalis, Ent. faecium, and other streptococci. Enterococcal endocarditis is the third most common type of endocarditis and is among the most difficult to treat. Mortality is around 20 per cent and relapses are not uncommon. Although penicillin, ampicillin, and vancomycin inhibit the growth of enterococci they are not bactericidal for most strains, and therapy with these agents alone results in a high relapse rate. For a bactericidal effect, it is usually necessary to add an aminoglycoside to penicillin, ampicillin or vancomycin (which is appropriate for patients who are allergic to penicillin); this results in marked enhancement of killing. A combination of penicillin or ampicillin with an aminoglycoside is the treatment of choice for enterococcal endocarditis. In the past, streptomycin was used, but about 40 per cent of enterococcal strains are highly resistant to streptomycin (MIC >2000 mg/l), and in such strains synergy cannot be demonstrated. For this reason gentamicin is now the preferred aminoglycoside. High-level resistance to gentamicin also occurs in enterococci and is becoming more common. Thus *in vitro* testing (using a disc containing 100 µg of gentamicin) should be a routine procedure in all isolates of enterococci.

High-level gentamicin-resistant strains may retain sensitivity to other aminoglycosides; if such a strain is encountered then all available aminoglycosides should be tested. The optimal therapy of endocarditis due to these high-level gentamicin or multiply aminoglycoside resistant enterococci has not been established. High-dose ampicillin for 2–3 months or valve replacement may be necessary for cure.

Ent. faecium strains are generally more resistant to β-lactam antibiotics than are *Ent. faecalis* strains, and β-lactamase-producing *Ent. faecalis* strains have also been reported. Such patients are best treated with vancomycin and gentamicin, unless the isolate is resistant to glycopeptide antibiotics. Enterococci are uniformly resistant to all cephalosporins. Patients with enterococcal endocarditis should receive at least 4–6 weeks of combination therapy.

Staphylococci

Staph. aureus.   In approximately one-third of all patients with *Staph. aureus* endocarditis the underlying heart valves are normal. The infection results in rapid and severe valvular destruction and the mortality, even with appropriate treatment, is about 40 per cent.

The mortality in hospital-acquired (secondary to infected intravascular devices) *Staph. aureus* endocarditis in those over 50 years of age is more than 50 per cent. Most patients with prosthetic valves need further surgery to replace the infected valve, because of valve dysfunction, dehiscence, and myocardial abscesses. But the outcome of *Staph. aureus* endocarditis involving the tricuspid valve in intravenous drug abusers is not so grim. It is much easier to cure than the left-sided *Staph. aureus* endocarditis and the mortality is less than 10 per cent.

Since the vast majority of *Staph. aureus* strains produce a β-lactamase which destroys penicillin, the initial choice is a penicillinase-stable penicillin such as flucloxacillin. However, the choice and the duration of treatment with a synergistic agent (e.g. gentamicin) are controversial. A clinical trial of flucloxacillin plus gentamicin versus flucloxacillin alone failed to show an improved outcome with combined therapy, and gentamicin is now recommended only for the first 3–5 days of treatment of complicated cases of native valve endocarditis and for 2 weeks when a prosthetic valve is involved. However, the clinical trial did demonstrate that combination therapy was associated with a more rapid clearance of bacteraemia. In the UK, low-dose gentamicin is still widely used with flucloxacillin for both native valve and prosthetic valve endocarditis, at least for the first 2 weeks of therapy. Some prefer to use oral fusidic acid instead of gentamicin.

In selected patients, such as an intravenous drug abuser with a right-sided endocarditis, in whom venous access is a problem, or a patient with uncomplicated native valve endocarditis, who has responded dramatically to 2 weeks of combination therapy, oral flucloxacillin (1.5 g/6 hourly) may be considered for the remaining 2 weeks of therapy. The remaining patients should receive high-dose flucloxacillin intravenously for at least 4 weeks or longer in complicated cases.

If the patient is allergic to penicillin or the *Staph. aureus* is multiply resistant, then vancomycin should be used. Rifampicin, a very potent antistaphylococcal agent (which, however, must never be used alone, owing to the emergence of resistance) should be added in difficult cases.

If laboratory tests reveal that the *Staph. aureus* is penicillinase negative and the MIC for penicillin is 0.1 mg/l or less, then penicillin may be used, and the regimen is the same as that used for endocarditis due to highly sensitive viridans streptococci.

Staph. epidermidis. This organism rarely infects a native valve but is a common cause of both early-and late-onset prosthetic valve endocarditis. It is difficult to cure with antibiotics alone and surgery is almost always required in patients with early-onset endocarditis. Isolates are frequently resistant to flucloxacillin, therefore flucloxacillin must not be used unless carefully performed sensitivities (which might take several days) confirm that the strain is sensitive. Therapy must therefore be started with vancomycin and rifampicin. Gentamicin may also be added for the first 2–3 weeks if the strain is sensitive. Frequent monitoring of drug levels in the blood is mandatory to minimize the chances of toxicity. If the organism is indeed sensitive to flucloxacillin then vancomycin is dropped and flucloxacillin and rifampicin is continued. All strains of *Staph. epidermidis* should be carefully tested for vancomycin sensitivity, since resistance among coagulase-negative staphylococci has been documented.

Recommended antibiotic regimens for streptococcal and staphylococcal endocarditis are shown in Table 23.4. Recommended antibiotic regimens for other organisms or clinical settings are shown in Table 23.5.

Surgical management

Emergency valve replacement in patients with infective endocarditis has now become an important adjunct to medical therapy. In selected patients, it is a life-saving procedure at any stage of the disease. The major indications for surgical intervention include:

(1) refractory heart failure related to structural valvular damage;
(2) myocardial or perivalvular abscess;
(3) untreatable or uncontrolled infection (e.g. fungal or Gram-negative bacillary infection of the prosthetic valve);
(4) repeated relapses with a difficult organism (e.g. *E. faecium*),
(5) multiple embolic episodes.

Prognosis

Infective endocarditis remains a life-threatening infection. The prognosis varies according to the infecting micro-organism, the type of cardiac valve (native versus prosthetic and aortic versus mitral versus tricuspid), the age of the patient, and the presence or absence of complications. Mortality is lowest (<10 per cent) in viridans streptococcal endocarditis of the native valve and highest (40–80 per cent) in early-onset prosthetic valve endocarditis.

Table 23.4. Recommended antibiotic treatment regimens for streptococcal and staphylococcal endocarditis

Organism	Treatment of choice (1st week / 2nd week / 3rd week / 4th week)	Suggested adult dosage/interval/route	Comments
Streptococci (a) Highly sensitive to penicillin (MIC ≤0.1 mg/l) Viridans streptococci Str. bovis Other streptococci	Benzylpenicillin Gentamicin	1.8 g/4 h/IV	**Native valve endocarditis (NVE):** Benzylpenicillin alone for 4 wks may be considered for the elderly or those at risk of renal problems Consider changing to oral amoxycillin (1 g/6 h) after 2 wks of combination therapy In selected uncomplicated infections combination therapy for 2 wks may be adequate **Prosthetic valve endocarditis (PVE):** Gentamicin should always be included for at least the first 2 wks followed by benzylpenicillin for a further 4 wks or oral amoxycillin 1 g/6 h for the last 2 wks is a reasonable alternative after 4 wks of parenteral benzylpenicillin. (Cephalosporins/vancomycin)*
(b) Relatively resistant to penicillin (MIC >0.1 mg/l but <0.5 mg/l) NVS† Viridans streptococci	Benzylpenicillin Gentamicin	2.4 g/4 h/IV	The relapse rate with these organisms is high Combination therapy may be prolonged for 4 weeks High doses of benzylpenicillin should be used
(c) Resistant to penicillin (MIC ≥0.5 mg/l) Enterococci Viridans streptococci	Ampicillin Gentamicin	2 g/4 h/IV	Ampicillin is twice as active as benzylpenicillin for enterococci To avoid relapse, combination therapy should be prolonged for at least 6 wks if: (1) PVE; (2) The duration of symptoms is more than 3 months; (3) The mitral valve is involved; (4) It is a relapse of enterococcal endocarditis. (Vancomycin)*

Table 23.4. cont.

Organism	Treatment of choice 1st week	2nd week	3rd week	4th week	Suggested adult dosage/interval/ route	Comments
Staph. aureus	Flucloxacillin				2 g/4 h/IV	In selected patients, e.g. right-sided endocarditis in IV drug abuser or a patient with NVE who has responded dramatically to treatment; consider oral flucloxacillin after 2 wks of combination therapy
	Gentamicin					Parenteral flucloxacillin may be prolonged for 6 wks in complicated and/or PVE
						Consider adding rifampicin (300 mg bd oral) in complicated and/or PVE
						Use vancomycin 1 g/12 h/IV for methicillin-resistant strains, or if the patient is allergic to penicillin
						Surgery is often required
Staph. epidermidis	Vancomycin				1 g/12 h/IV	Most common aetiological agent in PVE (early-onset)
	Rifampicin				300 mg/12 h/ oral	Use vancomycin as most strains are resistant to flucloxacillin
	Gentamicin					Use rifampicin if the strain is sensitive
						Consider using gentamicin as well (if the strain is sensitive)
						Combination treatment using vancomycin and rifampicin should be prolonged for 6–8 wks
						Surgery is often required

*Alternative drugs if the patient is allergic to penicillin.

† Nutritionally variant streptococci.

Table 23.5. Recommended antibiotic treatment regimens for endocarditis other than that caused by streptococci and staphylococci (adult with normal renal and hepatic function)

Organism/serology result/clinical setting	Antibiotic	Suggested dose/ interval/route	Duration (weeks)	Comments
'HACEK' group* Other unusual bacteria	Ampicillin+ gentamicin	2 g/4 h/IV Synergistic dose	4	Sensitivity tests are difficult to perform or interpret Attempt bactericidal levels, if possible
Enterobacteriaceae	Cefotaxime+ gentamicin	2 g/4 h/IV Full dose	4–6	Choice depends upon antibiotic sensitivity results. For *Salmonella* spp. consider ceftriaxone 2 g/12 h/IV instead of cefotaxime Gentamicin must be used in full doses and throughout the course, or resistant strains may emerge Mortality is high. Surgery is often required
Ps. aeruginosa	Ceftazidime+ gentamicin or tobramycin	3 g/8 h/IV Full dose	6	Left-sided endocarditis requires immediate surgery Right-sided may be treated medically first
N. gonorrhoeae *N. meningitidis* *Str. pneumoniae* Group A haemolytic streptococci	Benzylpenicillin	2.4 g/4 h/IV	3–4	Rare causes of IE nowadays All are highly sensitive to penicillin Use cefotaxime if the patient is allergic to penicillin or the strain (e.g. *Str. pneumoniae*) shows reduced sensitivity to penicillin
Fungi	Amphotericin B +flucytosine	1 mg/kg/24 h/IV 37.5 mg/kg/6h/oral	6–8	Outlook is grim Medical treatment alone is unlikely to succeed Early surgical excision plus medical treatment may be successful

Table 23.5. cont.

Organism/serology result/clinical setting	Antibiotic	Suggested dose/ interval/route	Duration (weeks)	Comments
Culture-negative, serology positive: *Coxiella burnetii*	Doxycycline + co-trimoxazole or rifampicin	100 mg/12 h/oral	Months & years	*Cox. burnetii*: rare cause of IE; phase 1 antibody >200 is considered virtually diagnostic of IE; valve replacement is often needed for cure; mortality with medical treatment alone is high. *Chlamydia psittaci*: experience limited
Clinically suspected acute bacterial endocarditis (awaiting blood culture results)	Benzylpenicillin + flucloxacillin + gentamicin	2.4 g/4 h/IV 2 g/4 h/IV Synergistic dose	Not applic- able	Regimen is modified, once the organism has been identified When empirical therapy of SBE is required as a therapeutic trial for a genuine culture-negative case, the choice of regimen depends upon the clinical setting. The following regimen is recommended for 4 weeks, if clinical response is demonstrated after 2 weeks: NVE: Use enterococcal regimen PVE: Use *Staph. epidermidis* regimen (vancomycin + gentamicin)

* See text for meaning of this acronym. IE = infective endocarditis; NVE = native valve endocarditis; PVE = prosthetic valve endocarditis; SBE = subacute bacterial endocarditis.

24

Skin and soft-tissue infections

P. J. Wilkinson

GENERAL CONSIDERATIONS

At birth the skin of the baby rapidly becomes colonized with bacteria from the mother, other handlers, and the environment. Only a limited number of species, for example *Staphylococcus epidermidis*, micrococci, *Propionibacterium acnes*, and coryneform bacteria, all of which are essentially non-pathogenic, finally become resident flora of the normal skin. In intact skin, these micro-organisms usually prevent potential pathogens such as *Staphylococcus aureus* and *Streptococcus pyogenes* (haemolytic streptococci of Lancefield group A) from becoming established. However, if the skin is broken by accidental or surgical trauma, burns, a foreign body, or a primary skin disease (psoriasis, atopic dermatitis), these pathogens may not only become established as resident organisms; they may also give rise to infection of the skin and subcutaneous tissue.

Other bacteria from, for example, faeces or the environment, can briefly colonize the skin as transient flora; they are readily removed by washing, whereas resident organisms will persist in moderate numbers despite even the most thorough skin disinfection. If introduced through, for example, a dirty wound or compound fracture, transient micro-organisms can also give rise to skin and soft-tissue infection. Such infections often involve several different bacterial species.

The general condition of the patient, including factors such as underlying immunodeficiency, diabetes mellitus or systemic or topical treatment with corticosteroids, can also predispose to skin infection. Treatment with broad-spectrum antibiotics, which disrupts the resident flora, can give rise to cutaneous candidiasis. However, in one of the commonest skin infections, namely a boil or furuncle, there is usually no evident breach in the skin nor any other predisposing factor.

Many different micro-organisms, including bacteria, fungi, and some viruses, may be involved in skin and soft-tissue infections. The commonest bacterial causes are *Staph. aureus, Str. pyogenes, Clostridium perfringens, and Bacteroides* species. Thrush is usually caused by the yeast *Candida albicans*, and cold sores by the virus *Herpes simplex*.

STAPHYLOCOCCAL INFECTIONS

Staph. aureus is the commonest cause of infection of traumatic wounds (accidental or surgical), burns, and skin diseases. The adult intact skin does not readily accept *Staph. aureus* except as transient flora, whereas the skin of the newborn is readily colonized. However, approximately one in four people, and more in a hospital environment, carry the organism in their nostrils. Other sites of skin carriage of this species are the perineum and axilla.

Skin infection with *Staph. aureus* may involve the hair follicles or the surface, and the lesions produced may be pustular or exfoliative.

Pustular lesions

Such lesions of the skin are by far the commonest bacterial infection in man and include:

1. *Folliculitis* (pimples), in which the infection is confined to the hair follicle and does not involve the surrounding skin or subcutaneous tissue. Such infections are usually mild, self limiting, and do not need medical attention.
2. *Furuncle* (boil), in which the folliculitis has spread deeper and is surrounded by an area of cellulitis.
3. *Carbuncle*, in which several furuncles have coalesced to form a large, indurated, painful lesion that contains loculated pus with multiple drainage points.

Exfoliative lesions

These involve the superficial layers of the skin and are characterized by stripping of the epidermis as a result of the action of an exfoliative toxin produced by certain phage types of *Staph. aureus*. When such lesions are localized and limited the condition is known as *impetigo*, but this form may also be caused by *Str. pyogenes* (see below). Not infrequently, both organisms can be isolated from the lesions. In the newborn the more pronounced lesions may give rise to large flaccid blisters, or *bullous impetigo*, which occasionally may spread in an epidemic form in baby nurseries or neonatal units.

Rarely, in the very young or the immunosuppressed adult, extensive, continuous lesions affect large areas of the body. The patient is generally ill with fever and skin tenderness, and the epidermis may separate in sheets in response to gentle stroking (*Nikolsky's sign*). Various names have been given to this generalized form of the disease, such as *scalded skin syndrome, toxic epidermal necrolysis, Ritter's disease,* and *pemphigus neonatorum. Staph. aureus* may not be found in the skin lesions and the infection may be at a remote site (e.g. the conjunctiva) from where the toxin causing the generalized skin lesions is absorbed.

Toxic shock syndrome

Certain phage types of *Staph. aureus* produce toxins which cause a multi-system disease characterized by the sudden onset of fever, myalgia, vomiting, diarrhoea, hypotension, and an erythematous rash: the *toxic shock syndrome*. Originally thought to affect only menstruating women who used a particular type of tampon, it is now known to be a rare sequel of any type of staphylococcal infection.

MANAGEMENT OF STAPHYLOCOCCAL INFECTIONS

Pustular lesions

Minor, well-localized staphylococcal skin lesions usually resolve without medical attention. Larger boils, carbuncles, and infected wounds, however, need not only surgical drainage but also systemic antimicrobial therapy, which may have little effect on the local lesion but prevents local extension or metastatic infection. This is particularly important when lesions are on the face and the consequences of retrograde spread along the emissary veins to the cavernous sinus are severe, so that antibiotic treatment of even small lesions around the nose and lips is justified.

Most isolates of *Staph. aureus* now produce penicillinase and therefore require treatment with a penicillinase-stable penicillin such as flucloxacillin. Erythromycin or clindamycin are suitable alternatives for patients who are allergic to penicillin. Topical antimicrobials applied in ointments, powders or sprays diffuse unevenly to the site of all but the most superficial skin infections, and are therefore not recommended for their treatment (see Chapter 32).

To prevent haematogenous dissemination of infection, antibiotic treatment should be started before any drainage procedure, and in high-risk situations should be given parenterally at first. Treatment should continue until the acute inflammation has subsided. It is always good practice to send a sample of pus for bacterial culture and determination of the antibiotic sensitivities of the causal bacteria, which may be found to have multiple antibiotic resistances (e.g. a multi-resistant strain of *Staph. aureus*) or to be an organism other than *Staph. aureus*.

The management of patients with *recurrent boils* poses a special problem. Although any one episode is treated in the standard way, to prevent further episodes the site of staphylococcal carriage (which may involve another person, partner or family member) should be determined and steps taken to eradicate the source of infection (see Chapter 32).

The minor pustular lesions of *acne* and *rosacea* are not bacterial in origin, although commensal bacteria may contribute to their persistence and tetracyclines may help to keep the lesions under control. Topical clindamycin is also useful in acne, and topical metronidazole gel in rosacea.

Exfoliative lesions

Very superficial lesions such as impetigo may be controlled by topical agents only (see Chapter 32), but if *Str. pyogenes* is involved then systemic penicillin should be given for at least 10 days to eradicate the organisms from skin lesions and thereby avoid the possible risk of post-streptococcal glomerulonephritis. Erythromycin is suitable for patients who are allergic to penicillin.

Extensive impetigenous or bullous lesions, as well as staphylococcal scalded-skin syndrome and toxic shock syndrome, are potentially life threatening and require urgent medical attention. They should be treated with a parenteral antistaphylococcal agent such as flucloxacillin or erythromycin.

STREPTOCOCCAL SKIN INFECTIONS

Str. pyogenes does not form part of the normal skin flora, and primary streptococcal skin infections are now far less common than those due to *Staph. aureus* in communities in which poor hygiene is practised. Streptococci probably enter the skin through minor cuts, scratches or puncture wounds, or become superimposed on some pre-existing skin disease. Lapses in personal hygiene favour initiation of the infective process.

Impetigo

Streptococcal impetigo is very similar to the non-bullous form of staphylococcal impetigo, except that regional lymphadenopathy is commoner with the streptococcal variety. Characteristically, a pre-school child develops lesions around the mouth and nostrils, or on the extremities. Systemic antibiotics were not generally used until reports of outbreaks of impetigo in which the causative streptococcal strains were nephritogenic; in certain parts of the world, impetigo is now the commonest form of streptococcal infection to precede acute glomerulonephritis. It is therefore now advisable to treat all cases with systemic antibiotics, preferably a penicillin, and to limit topical antimicrobials to patients with small numbers of lesions or as supplemental therapy. Antibiotic treatment is also justified as a public health measure to decrease the reservoir of pyogenic streptococci in a population and to limit the spread of potentially nephritogenic strains.

Cellulitis

Cellulitis in its broadest sense is an acute infection of the subcutaneous tissues and is usually streptococcal in origin, though it can be staphylococcal or polymicrobial, particularly after operations on the intestinal or female genital tracts, when spreading infections with mixed aerobic and anaerobic bacteria of gut or genital origin can occur. *Erysipelas*, a more superficial form of cellulitis which usually affects the face or lower limbs, is almost always caused by haemolytic streptococci of Lancefield group A. In the neonate, erysipelas may develop from an infection of the umbilical stump.

Previous accidental or surgical trauma or a pre-existent skin lesion are the usual predisposing factors in cellulitis. Rarely, however, blood-borne bacteria may localize in subcutaneous tissue, or an underlying osteomyelitis may present as cellulitis.

If material for bacteriological examination is difficult to obtain because there is no exudate or superficial skin lesion, clinical appearances may help to differentiate staphylococcal from streptococcal cellulitis. In a typical streptococcal case the involved lymphatic ducts show up as a red streak that extends towards the regional lymph nodes, which are enlarged and tender. Bacteraemia is common.

Although various kinds of haemolytic streptococci other than *Str. pyogenes* may be involved, benzylpenicillin remains the treatment of choice. Staphylococcal cellulitis requires flucloxacillin or erythromycin, which will provide cover for both organisms if the bacterial aetiology is in doubt.

NON-STREPTOCOCCAL CELLULITIC INFECTION

Haemophilus infection

Haemophilus influenzae (serotype b) is an important cause of cellulitis in infants under the age of 3 years, although its incidence has been reduced in countries in which immunization has been introduced in childhood. Facial swelling, often of the cheek or periorbital region, is a common presenting feature and blood cultures are usually positive. In such cases, a parenteral, broad-spectrum cephalosporin such as cefotaxime or ceftriaxone should be given initially, followed by oral therapy where necessary with cefixime, cefuroxime axetil, co-amoxiclav or (if sensitive) amoxycillin. Chloramphenicol, although effective, has now been superseded on account of its toxicity. Benzylpenicillin is not effective against *H. influenzae* and should not be used in such cases.

Anthrax

This is an animal disease that occasionally spreads to workers who handle animal hides, wool, or animal products contaminated with the spores of *Bacillus anthracis*; it may present as an oedematous cellulitis. Characteristically, a large, painless necrotic lesion (*malignant pustule*) develops on the face, neck or arm over 2–3 days and can lead to septicaemia which is sometimes fatal. The characteristic lesion and the patient's occupation should alert the doctor to this rare condition. Parenteral penicillin is the treatment of choice, or a tetracycline for those allergic to penicillin.

Necrotizing infections

The classification of necrotizing, subcutaneous infections is confusing and controversial. *Necrotizing fasciitis* (streptococcal gangrene) is a rapidly spreading and life-threatening form of cellulitis that involves skin, subcutaneous tissue, and fascia. Most cases are caused by *Str. pyogenes* either alone or in combination with other bacteria, including *Staph. aureus*, coliform bacilli, and anaerobes. The initial cellulitis advances aggressively and the patient becomes toxic. Blood cultures are often positive and streptococci can also be isolated from the bullous lesions.

Progressive synergistic bacterial gangrene usually complicates surgical abdominal wounds. It starts as an ulcer near the wound and can spread to much of the anterior abdominal wall. Micro-aerophilic streptococci, together with *Staph. aureus* and, occasionally, coliform bacilli, have typically been isolated from such lesions.

The management of these rare conditions is primarily surgical, with radical debridement of all necrotic tissue, intensive life-support therapy, and the treatment of shock. Antibiotics are initially of only secondary importance, but should nevertheless be given as indicated by bacteriological results. Suitable initial combinations include ampicillin with gentamicin and metronidazole, and imipenem.

CLOSTRIDIAL INFECTION

Gas gangrene (clostridial myositis) is a life-threatening, invasive infection that can be caused by several species of *Clostridium*, principally *C. perfringens*. These bacteria are part of the normal intestinal flora of humans and animals, and clostridial spores are common in soil. Gas gangrene develops only when impaired blood supply, tissue necrosis, or the presence of foreign bodies produces a low oxygen tension in the tissues and thus creates conditions in which the spores can germinate. Extensive soft-tissue injury contaminated with soil or dirt, for example a compound fracture in a road accident, or a bullet or shrapnel wound, all carry an increased risk of gas gangrene. Gas gangrene may rarely complicate surgical wounds, particularly after intestinal or biliary surgery, or be a complication of septic abortion. Clostridial anaerobic cellulitis occurs under similar circumstances, but exploration of the wound usually reveals that the muscle is spared.

Prevention of gas gangrene

Patients undergoing above-knee amputation for peripheral vascular disease are at risk of developing gas gangrene from faecal clostridia that contaminate the buttocks, and should be given penicillin prophylaxis (see Chapter 19).

Management of gas gangrene

A clinical diagnosis of gas gangrene is made on the basis of palpable (crepitus) or radiological signs of a spreading, gas-producing infection in a toxic patient with the above risk factors. Immediate and extensive surgical excision of all involved tissues and the removal of any foreign body are essential, and may mean hysterectomy (after septic abortion), excision of subcutaneous tissue and muscle of the abdominal wall, or amputation of a limb. Parenteral benzylpenicillin should also be given promptly in high dosage. For patients allergic to penicillin, metronidazole may be used. Some authorities also advocate local irrigation with penicillin and hydrogen peroxide, or the use of hyperbaric oxygen.

Despite these desperate and mutilating measures, the mortality in gas gangrene remains high. Antitoxin therapy has no place in the management of gas gangrene, whereas in tetanus and botulism, the other important clostridial diseases caused by *C. tetani* and *C. botulinum* respectively, antitoxin is much more important than antibiotic therapy.

ANAEROBES OTHER THAN CLOSTRIDIA

Bacteroides fragilis and other non-sporing, Gram-negative anaerobes form a major part of the normal bacterial flora of the upper respiratory, gastrointestinal, and female genital tracts. These organisms and anaerobic streptococci are often found with coliform bacilli in mixed infections in intra-abdominal sepsis following appendicectomy, abdominal, ano-rectal, and gynaecological surgery.

In the elderly, diabetic or obese patient, post-operative infection or infected pressure sores may give rise to a rapidly spreading infection that involves deeper tissues, including muscle, to produce *synergistic necrotizing cellulitis*, a variant of necrotizing fasciitis. *Fournier's gangrene*, another form of necrotizing fasciitis that involves the perineum, scrotum or penis, is also associated with mixed organisms including anaerobes. Infection may spread to the anterior abdominal wall. The incidence of post-operative infection following certain types of abdominal operation is high, but is very substantially reduced by antimicrobial prophylaxis (see Chapter 19).

For established infection, surgical intervention is the most important treatment and antimicrobial therapy plays a supportive role. The antibiotics given must cover coliform bacilli and anaerobes, and combinations of a broad-spectrum cephalosporin (e.g. cefotaxime, ceftazidime), or ampicillin plus an aminoglycoside (e.g. gentamicin), with metronidazole, are all reasonable choices. Alternatively, imipenem may be used as a single agent.

MISCELLANEOUS INFECTIONS

A wide variety of organisms, alone or in combination, may occasionally give rise to infection of, for example, human or animal bites, or gangrenous lesions in diabetics. Wounds close to bones or joints may extend to involve these structures. A definitive bacteriological diagnosis should be sought and appropriate treatment given on the basis of laboratory results.

Viral infections of the skin, such as herpes simplex and varicella zoster, are discussed in Chapter 28. Superficial fungal infections usually respond to topical therapy (see Chapter 32) although dermatophyte infections of finger- or toenails may require oral treatment with terbinafine for up to 3 months, or with griseofulvin for a year or more. These agents are deposited in newly formed keratin and the prolonged treatment is needed to allow healthy nail to replace the diseased tissue. Even so, treatment of chronic infections of toenails may be unsuccessful, although terbinafine is more reliable in this respect than griseofulvin.

25

Bone and joint infections

P. J. Wilkinson

SEPTIC ARTHRITIS

Septic or pyogenic arthritis can be defined as the invasion of the synovial membrane by micro-organisms, usually with extension into the joint to produce an infection in a closed space. In most cases, bacteria reach the joint through the bloodstream from a distant focus of infection such as a septic skin lesion, otitis media, pneumonia, meningitis, gonorrhoea or an infection of the urinary tract. Some infections may spread to joints while the primary focus remains undetected. Rarely, bacteria may be introduced directly into the synovial space following a penetrating wound, an operation on the joint or an intra-articular injection. Alternatively, the joint may become infected by direct spread from an adjacent area of osteomyelitis or cellulitis. Once established, septic arthritis can give rise to secondary bacteraemia.

Aetiology

Staphylococcus aureus accounts for 60–90 per cent of all proven joint infections. Other bacteria are important in specific age groups: *Escherichia coli* and streptococci of Lancefield group B in neonates; pneumococci, *Streptococcus pyogenes*, and coliform bacilli in the elderly. *Haemophilus influenzae* of serotype b may be responsible in children under the age of 6 years, although childhood immunization has already markedly reduced the incidence of this. *Neisseria gonorrhoeae* occasionally causes septic arthritis in young adults, and patients with meningococcal infection may develop septic arthritis during the course of their illness. Other rare causes of septic arthritis include *Mycobacterium tuberculosis*, opportunist mycobacteria, *Brucella* spp., fungi, and *Borrelia burgdorferi*, the spirochaete that causes Lyme disease.

Clinical and diagnostic considerations

In nine cases out of ten, a single joint is involved, most commonly the knee, followed by the hip. Typically, the patient is a child with a high temperature and a red, hot, swollen joint with restricted movement. However, septic arthritis is not uncommon in the elderly and the debilitated, who may have non-specific symptoms. Patients with rheumatoid arthritis have an increased incidence of septic arthritis, but the clinical diagnosis may be delayed or overlooked—a fact which could contribute to the poor prognosis.

A presumptive diagnosis of septic arthritis rests on the immediate examination of the joint fluid, because of the difficulty on clinical grounds in distinguishing other conditions with similar features, such as an exacerbation of rheumatoid arthritis, gout, acute rheumatic fever, or trauma to the joint. Typically, the fluid is cloudy or purulent with a marked excess of neutrophils. The Gram-film is of immediate help not only in confirming the diagnosis but also in the choice of the most appropriate antimicrobial therapy. In patients who have not had antibiotics prior to arthrocentesis and whose infection is with Gram-positive organisms, the bacteria should be evident microscopically in most cases. Gram-negative bacteria are less obvious, but Gram-negative cocci are typically seen clustered in the cytoplasm of pus cells. Despite the microscopic evidence of bacterial infection, culture of synovial fluid may sometimes fail to yield the pathogen, and blood cultures must always be taken at the same time since the organism is sometimes isolated only by this means. In suspected gonococcal arthritis, cervical, urethral, rectal, and throat swabs must also be taken for culture before starting antimicrobial therapy.

Guidelines to antibiotic therapy and management

It is very important that a diagnosis is made rapidly and appropriate therapy started immediately because permanent damage to the joint may occur and lead to long-term residual abnormalities. Most patients who are treated promptly recover completely. Infection of the hip joint is more difficult to treat since, in addition to antibiotics, open surgical drainage is needed because of the technical difficulty of needle aspiration. The key to success in managing a patient with septic arthritis is a combination of antibiotics and drainage. In most cases this is achieved by needle aspiration, which should be repeated daily, if indicated, in an attempt to 'drain the joint dry'.

The choice of initial antibiotic therapy depends on the age of the patient and the findings in the Gram-film. If organisms can be identified with reasonable confidence before culture (see Table 25.1), the appropriate antibiotic for that particular organism is the automatic choice irrespective of the age. If bacteria are not seen at this stage, however, the initial choice is influenced by the age of the patient and/or the underlying disease. Antibiotics are chosen to cover

Table 25.1. Initial antimicrobial therapy in septic arthritis when bacteria are seen in the Gram-film of the joint aspirate

Description of the Gram-film	Probable organism	Initial choice of antibiotic	Comments
Gram-positive cocci in clusters	Staphylococci	Flucloxacillin	Fusidic acid may be added
Gram-positive cocci in chains or pairs	Streptococci	Benzylpenicillin	
Gram-negative coccobacilli	*H. influenzae*	Cefotaxime or ceftriaxone	Chloramphenicol effective but toxic May change to ampicillin if sensitive
Gram-negative large rods	Coliform bacilli or *Pseudomonas*	Cefotaxime + gentamicin	Change cefotaxime to ceftazidime if *Ps. aeruginosa*
Gram-negative diplococci	*Neisseria* spp.	Benzylpenicillin	

the most likely bacterial causes of the infection (Table 25.2) and can be modified subsequently if a pathogen is isolated.

Most antimicrobial agents given parenterally achieve therapeutic levels in the infected joint, so the intra-articular injection of antibiotics is not recommended, particularly as it may induce chemical synovitis. There is no consensus of opinion about the type of surgical intervention that is appropriate in septic arthritis and haematogenous osteomyelitis, nor about the choice of antibiotics, route of administration, and duration of treatment. A sequential intravenous–oral regimen, carefully monitored at the time of oral therapy, is widely used in children. In all cases, the initial treatment must be with parenteral antibiotics until the condition of the patient has stabilized (usually 7–10 days) and the joint is reasonably dry. In selected patients, high-dose oral therapy may be used in the last 2–3 weeks of treatment, provided the patient can be relied upon to comply and serum bactericidal concentrations are satisfactory (see Chapter 8). The duration of treatment depends on the organism and the age of the patient. Neonates and young infants, in whom there may be concurrent osteomyelitis, should receive intravenous therapy for at least 3–4 weeks. Ten to fourteen days of therapy may be adequate for septic arthritis caused by *Str. pyogenes*, pneumococci or *Neisseria* spp., whereas *Pseudomonas aeruginosa* may require as long as 6–8 weeks. Most cases of septic

Table 25.2. Initial antimicrobial therapy in septic arthritis when no organisms are seen in the Gram-film of joint aspirate

Type of patient	Most common organisms	Less common organisms	Initial choice of antibiotic
Neonate (0–2 m)	*Staph. aureus* Group B streptococci Gram-negative bacilli		Flucoxacillin + gentamicin
Infant (2 m–6 y)	*Staph. aureus*	*Str. pyogenes* *Str. pneumoniae* *H. influenzae*	Flucloxacillin + cefotaxime
Child (7–14 y)	*Staph. aureus*		Flucloxacillin
Adult (>15 y)	*Staph. aureus*	*N. gonorrhoeae*	Flucloxacillin
Elderly or debilitated	*Staph. aureus*	*Str. pyogenes* *Str. pneumoniae* Gram-negative bacilli	Flucloxacillin + gentamicin

arthritis caused by *Staph. aureus* or *H. influenzae* are treated for at least 3–4 weeks.

OSTEOMYELITIS

Osteomyelitis is infection of bone and is usually caused by bacteria. In the days before antibiotics, osteomyelitis was a dreaded disease not only because it was frequently fatal, but also because those who survived were often left seriously disabled with chronic discharging sinuses from the affected bone. This complication may still occur when acute osteomyelitis has not been treated promptly and adequately. Unlike soft tissues, bone is a rigid structure and cannot swell so that, as infection proceeds and pus forms, there is a marked rise of pressure in the affected part of the bone which, if unchecked or unrelieved, may impair the blood supply to a wide area and result in areas of infected dead bone. Once this chronic phase of osteomyelitis is established, necrotic bone (sequestrum) must be removed surgically in addition to the use of antibiotics if the infection is to be eradicated.

Pathogenesis and aetiology

Osteomyelitis may be haematogenous (infected through the blood-stream) or non-haematogenous (infected directly through a wound).

Haematogenous osteomyelitis

This type of infection is most commonly caused by staphylococci that reach the site from a boil or other focus of infection through the bloodstream. The primary focus of infection is often not apparent. Acute haematogenous osteomyelitis is primarily a disease of children under 16 years, in whom more than 85 per cent of cases occur. The usual sites are the long bones (femur, tibia, humerus) near the metaphysis, where the blood supply to the bone is most dense. However, when the disease occurs in adults the vertebrae are commonly affected.

Staph. aureus accounts for about half of all cases and for more than 90 per cent of cases in otherwise normal children. In the elderly with underlying malignancies and other diseases, and in drug addicts, Gram-negative bacilli (coliform bacilli and *Ps. aeruginosa*) are being reported with increasing frequency. Coliforms are also commonly involved in vertebral osteomyelitis. In neonates, the diagnosis of osteomyelitis is often difficult and many bones are involved as well as their adjacent joints. In addition to *Staph. aureus*, *Esch. coli* and group B haemolytic streptococci are the main bacterial causes. Group B streptococci seem to have a predilection for the humerus in neonates. As in septic arthritis, *H. influenzae*, *Str. pyogenes*, and *Str. pneumoniae* may occur (Table 25.2), but they are even less common in osteomyelitis. Rare causes of haematogenous osteomyelitis include *M. tuberculosis*, *Brucella abortus* and, particularly in parts of the world where sickle cell anaemia is prevalent, salmonellae.

Non-haematogenous osteomyelitis

When bones are infected by the introduction of organisms through traumatic or post-operative wounds, *Staph. aureus* is still the commonest cause, but Gram-negative bacteria are also found. *Ps. aeruginosa* may occasionally produce osteomyelitis of the metatarsals or calcaneum following a puncture wound of the sole of the foot, and *Pasteurella multocida* infection may follow animal bites. Patients with infected pressure sores over a bone, or those with peripheral vascular disease or diabetes mellitus, may develop osteomyelitis with mixed aerobic and anaerobic organisms (coliforms and *Bacteroides* species), although *Staph. aureus* is an important cause of osteomyelitis by this route also.

Clinical and diagnostic considerations

The typical manifestations of acute, haematogenous osteomyelitis include the abrupt onset of high fever and systemic toxicity, with marked redness, pain, and swelling over the bone involved. In adults, the presentation may not be so dramatic as in children. The most important physical sign is bony tenderness at the metaphysis; this is particularly helpful in older children and adults in whom the features of infection are not so pronounced. In vertebral osteomyelitis there may be general malaise, with or without low-grade fever and low back pain. If the infection is not controlled it may spread to produce a spinal epidural abscess with consequent neurological symptoms.

The diagnosis of osteomyelitis is confirmed by bone aspiration, which will also reveal any abscess that requires surgical drainage, and the isolation of the causative organism from material from the lesion. A bone scan may help to localize the site and extent of the infection. At least two sets of blood cultures must be taken; this will confirm the diagnosis in about half the cases and remove the need for bone biopsy. In patients with chronic osteomyelitis it may be misleading to base antibiotic treatment on the results of cultures of pus obtained from a draining sinus, which will often yield organisms from the exterior that are secondarily colonizing the sinus. For precise bacteriological diagnosis, material must be obtained during the surgical removal of dead bone and tissue, or by deep needle aspiration of exudate.

Guidelines for antibiotic therapy and management

It is generally agreed that acute haematogenous osteomyelitis can be cured without surgical intervention provided that antibiotics are given while the bone retains its blood supply and before extensive necrosis has occurred, in practice within the first 72 h of the development of symptoms. Antibiotic therapy must, therefore, start immediately after a bone aspirate and blood cultures have been obtained. Results from a Gram-film of aspirated material may help in the initial choice of antibiotic. If no organisms are seen, *Staph. aureus* is the prime suspect in any age group, and an antistaphylococcal agent that penetrates well into bone and pus should be used. Penicillins and fusidic acid fulfil this criterion; however, since *Staph. aureus* is usually resistant to benzylpenicillin and resistance to fusidic acid arises easily when that drug is used alone, a combination of flucloxacillin and fusidic acid is recommended. If the patient is a child under the age of 6 years, flucloxacillin and cefotaxime should be used to cover the rare possibility of *H. influenzae*. In the neonate, where group B streptococci are possible, benzylpenicillin may be used instead of cefotaxime. Alternative antistaphylococcal agents include clindamycin, vancomycin, teicoplanin, and rifampicin.

To ensure adequate concentration at the site of infection, high doses of antibiotics should be given parenterally. If an abscess has already formed when the patient is first seen, or there is no significant clinical improvement within 24 h of starting parenteral therapy, then surgical drainage of the abscess is essential.

The duration of antimicrobial therapy of acute staphylococcal osteomyelitis should be not less than 4 weeks and may need to be much longer. This is a long period for a patient, particularly a young child, to receive intravenous therapy. If the initial clinical response is good, the patient can be relied upon to comply, and the serum antibiotic activity can be monitored, parenteral therapy may be changed to high-dose oral therapy for the remaining 3–4 weeks. Flucloxacillin and fusidic acid are both suitable for oral therapy. The recommended duration of treatment of osteomyelitis caused by *Str. pneumoniae* or *Str. pyogenes* is 10–14 days, but this may need to be prolonged in individual cases.

The management of osteomyelitis caused by enteric Gram-negative bacilli is difficult. Appropriate surgical intervention should be accompanied by prolonged intravenous therapy with an aminoglycoside such as gentamicin, in combination with an extended-spectrum cephalosporin such as cefotaxime (enterobacteria) or ceftazidime (*Ps. aeruginosa*). Until recently, there has been a lack of a suitable oral agent that is both active against this group of bacteria and also achieves good penetration into bone. The fluoroquinolones, such as ofloxacin and ciprofloxacin, meet these criteria and may be given both orally and parenterally. They are particularly useful in osteomyelitis caused by *Brucella* spp., *Ps. aeruginosa, Esch. coli, Proteus* spp., and *Salmonella* spp. The development of resistance has been reported when fluoroquinolones have been used as single agents, however, and combination with another effective antimicrobial is recommended.

In chronic osteomyelitis where surgical drainage and excision of dead bone and tissue are essential, high-dose oral antibiotics have to be continued post-operatively for several months if the infection is to be eradicated. Improvements in techniques for venous access now make long-term intravenous therapy with antibiotics such as ceftriaxone or gentamicin possible for outpatients, who can visit a clinic daily or on alternate days. This approach is particularly useful where there is no suitable oral agent for the causative organism, and also offers the opportunity for regular monitoring of aminoglycoside concentrations and serum antimicrobial activity without the need for expensive, inconvenient, hospital inpatient care.

26

Mycobacterial disease

A. M. Emmerson

TUBERCULOSIS

Tuberculosis is one of the most widespread infections known to man; an estimated 1.7 billion people, or a third of the world's population, harbour the pathogen *Mycobacterium tuberculosis*, and every year 8 million individuals develop new clinical disease. The pulmonary form was described by Hippocrates, and characteristic lesions of tuberculosis of the spine have been demonstrated in the mummies of ancient Egypt. It attacks both humans and animals (e.g. badgers, cattle), affects all ages and every organ in the body, and ranges from latent to hyperacute (the 'galloping consumption' of Victorian times), killing young and old alike, the famous and the unknown. This reservoir of infected persons results in 3.6 million people with infectious pulmonary tuberculosis (sputum-smear positive) with an overall annual mortality of 2.9 million. Infection with human immunodeficiency virus (HIV) is the most potent risk factor for development of tuberculosis (TB) and, at the time of writing, 3.1 million people are co-infected with HIV and TB according to World Health Organization figures.

In 1882, Robert Koch published his epoch-making study of the tubercle bacillus and its causative role in the disease tuberculosis. This was almost 100 years after the death of Dr Samuel Johnson who during his lifetime suffered from scrofula—superficial tuberculous lymphadenitis which usually affects the lymph nodes of the neck. Johnson, like many people, was touched by his sovereign, Queen Anne, for the 'king's evil'. As an alternative the ill were often bled directly or indirectly with leeches and liberally treated both topically and systemically, with rum, madeira, cayenne pepper, tartar emetic ointment, and the juice of liquorice!

However, the last 40 years have seen enormous progress in the understanding of the epidemiology, prevention, and treatment of TB and, although far from eradicated, this age-old killer of man has become a preventable and curable disease. Disturbing new problems have arisen with the treatment of co-existing infection of HIV and TB.

This chapter will deal principally with the treatment of pulmonary TB because it remains the commonest form of the disease (65 per cent of cases) and practically the only form responsible for human transmission.

Landmarks in the treatment of tuberculosis

Before the advent of chemotherapy during the 1940s, the treatment of tuberculosis was largely restricted to attempts to increase the patient's resistance to the disease. Prolonged rest in hospital and sanatoria, special diets, and avoidance of physical activity were all thought to be important. Attempts were made to immobilize affected lung tissue by artificial pneumothorax, removal of ribs, or, more radically, removal of affected lung tissue itself. Amputation of affected limbs was common, as was surgical resection of other diseased tissues. Today, most of these methods have become almost forgotten history, as the action of drugs on the tubercle bacillus itself has assumed overwhelming importance.

The main landmarks in this story are summarized in Table 26.1. The first was the discovery, in 1940, of the bacteriostatic effect of sulphonamides in guinea-pigs infected with tubercle bacilli. The most effective were diamino-sulphones such as dapsone, and the discovery was less than earth-shattering because these agents were found to have little if any activity against tuberculosis in humans. They were, however, effective in the treatment of leprosy and remain so today.

The next major advance was the introduction in 1944 of streptomycin, the first drug shown to be effective in the treatment of human tuberculosis. Its use was, however, limited by the ready emergence of streptomycin-resistant tubercle bacilli during treatment, and also by adverse reactions to the drug. In 1949, it was discovered that combined therapy with *p*-aminosalicylic acid (PAS) and streptomycin prevented the emergence of strains resistant to either, and since then the administration of two or more drugs in combination has been considered essential for adequate treatment of tuberculosis.

The third of the classical antituberculous drugs, isoniazid (INH), was introduced in 1952 and, for the first time, uniformly successful primary chemotherapy of tuberculosis became possible. Initial treatment with streptomycin alone, in courses lasting from 6 weeks to 3 months, had

Table 26.1. Landmarks in the treatment of tuberculosis

Year	Treatment
1944	Streptomycin
1949	Combination chemotherapy: streptomycin and PAS
1952	Isoniazid
1956	Ambulatory outpatient treatment
1964	Intermittent regimens, fully supervised
1967	Rifampicin
1972	Short-course chemotherapy

a very high relapse rate after cessation of treatment, while prolonged treatment led to a high incidence of toxicity from the drug, and emergence of drug resistance was common. The addition of PAS almost eliminated the emergence of resistant strains, and allowed treatment to be prolonged to 12 months or longer. Relapses after treatment were still common, but longer periods of treatment with streptomycin, which could only be given by daily injection, were increasingly unacceptable to patients and it needed the introduction of INH, another oral agent, for really long-course treatment to be possible. Eventually, a classical regimen evolved in which streptomycin, PAS, and INH were given for 2–3 months, followed by PAS and INH for a further 18 months to 2 years. Until the late 1950s, patients were usually confined to hospital for most of this time. This was a very successful regimen (more than 90 per cent of patients completing the course were cured), but it was also a very exacting ordeal in itself, and patients commonly absconded from treatment. Among absconders, relapse was common.

Between 1955 and 1960 a controlled clinical trial was carried out in Madras to compare the effect of 12 months of chemotherapy in two groups of patients: one group treated under good conditions in a sanatorium, the other under poor conditions at home. The results were startling. Despite good accommodation, nursing, rich diet, and prolonged bed rest the sanatorium patients did no better than similar patients treated in overcrowded homes, who had a poor diet, much less rest, and who often worked long hours under poor conditions. The risk to close family contacts was studied for over 5 years, and showed that there was no difference in the incidence of disease between the contacts of patients treated at home and those of sanatorium patients. The major risk to contacts lay in exposure to the index case before diagnosis was made and treatment initiated. Once effective treatment had been started there was little further risk to contacts. Also, the study showed that treatment in a sanatorium is no safeguard against irregularity of drug taking unless the patient is actually seen to swallow every dose or receive every injection. It was this study which caused the dramatic change from institutional to ambulatory outpatient treatment as a general policy. TB sanatoriums were closed as public health authorities recognized that patients receiving combination chemotherapy did not constitute a contagious risk.

During the 1960s several new antituberculous drugs were brought into use, of which three—rifampicin, pyrazinamide, and ethambutol—have emerged as of particular importance. Exploitation of these drugs has allowed investigation of intermittent chemotherapy regimens, in which individual drug doses are given at intervals of more than a day (in some cases only once or twice a week)—of particular importance in developing countries where fully supervised daily medication is difficult to deliver—and also, more recently, the development of much shorter regimens, several being curative in less than 12 months.

Factors involved in the response to chemotherapy

Tubercle bacilli: number, site, and activity

In human pulmonary tuberculosis, most of the tubercle bacilli are found on the walls of cavities in the lungs open to the bronchi. Here the pH is relatively high, at least on the alkaline side of neutrality. The oxygen tension is also high and the bacilli are actively multiplying. However, there is another smaller population of bacilli, dormant in closed cavities, or in caseating tissue, or inside macrophages, where the pH and oxygen tension are both low, and bacterial multiplication is slow.

Antituberculous drugs and their mode of action

The drugs available for the treatment of tuberculosis differ in their activity against tubercle bacilli under different conditions. For example, streptomycin and INH are bactericidal against actively multiplying bacteria under alkaline conditions, while pyrazinamide acts largely on intracellular organisms in an acid medium. Rifampicin is active against both extracellular and intracellular organisms, and also on those dormant in caseous nodules. Bactericidal activity against actively mult- iplying bacteria largely determines the acute response of the sick patient to chemotherapy, but sterilizing activity against the dormant 'persisters' in the bacterial population is most important when considering the incidence of relapse after cessation of treatment.

Effects of the body's defences and immune response: species variation

Host factors and defence mechanisms have, in recent years, been shown to be of much less importance in determining the outcome of tuberculous infection than is the effective use of antituberculous drugs. However, species differences in the response to tuberculosis are of considerable interest and have been the source of some confusion. In the mouse, unlike the human, tubercle bacilli multiply readily inside macrophages, while there is much less multiplication in cavities and tissue spaces. In the guinea-pig, multiplication of bacilli more nearly resembles that in humans, but the human immune response, based on the bacteristatic effect of low pH and low oxygen tension in caseous tissue, is nearer that of the mouse than the guinea-pig. The effect of these differences on the experimental investigation of the drug treatment of tuberculosis has been to complicate an already difficult picture. For example, streptomycin has high bactericidal activity in humans and moderate activity against actively multiplying bacilli in the guinea-pig, but is virtually inactive in the mouse. Pyrazinamide, bactericidal in the mouse, is without effect on tuberculosis in the guinea-pig. The practical implication is that the development of effective antituberculous regimens in humans has depended almost entirely on the use of large-scale controlled trials of different regimens in appropriate human populations. There is still no suitable *in vitro* or animal model from which information can be transferred to humans without reservation.

Immunity in TB is cell mediated; the key to restriction of intracellular growth of the bacillus is co-operation between macrophages and sensitized lymphocytes. Humoral reactions are thought to play little part. The generation of clones of antigen-specific T cells initiates the immune response, which is depressed in HIV-positive patients. T cell clones may facilitate elimination of the pathogen by macrophage activation and granuloma formation or by cytotoxic action; or they may interact with B cells to produce specific antibodies which, in conjunction with phagocytic cells or complement, also act as an effector arm. The mechanism by which mycobacteria survive inside activated macrophages is unknown and may be oxygen dependent or oxygen independent. The role of iron in persistence of infection has not been elucidated. Future research is required to establish the interaction between antimycobacterial agents and the immune system, if one exists.

The antituberculous drugs

Streptomycin

This was the first effective drug against tuberculosis in humans. Like all aminoglycosides it is not absorbed when given orally, and must be administered as an intramuscular injection. It is more actively bactericidal in the proliferative than in the resting phase of bacterial growth. Adequate concentrations are attained in lung, muscle, uterus, intestinal mucosa, adrenals, and lymph nodes. Diffusion into bone, brain, and aqueous humour is poor. Little normally enters the CSF, although penetration increases when the meninges are inflamed. Vestibular damage occurs in about 30 per cent of cases and 24 h CSF levels may need to be monitored to keep the trough level below 3 mg/l. The plasma half-life, which is normally 2–3 h, is considerably extended in the newborn, in the elderly, and in patients with severe renal impairment. Serum levels need to be monitored in patients over 40 years of age. Hypersensitivity reactions in the form of fever and skin rashes may develop.

The injections are painful and must be administered by deep intramuscular injection; 1 per day is sufficient but barely tolerable. Duration of treatment is 1–2 months.

p-Aminosalicylic acid (PAS)

This was formerly used in combination regimens to prevent the emergence of drug-resistant organisms. Up to 10–12 g a day was given orally, in two or three doses. The drug tastes most unpleasant, and gastrointestinal intolerance was common. PAS is no longer used and is included for historical reasons only.

Isoniazid (isonicotinic acid hydrazine; INH)

This is active only against the tubercle bacillus, not against other microbes, but against this organism it is potent and bactericidal. It penetrates rapidly into all tissues and lesions, its activity is not affected by the pH of the environment, it is well tolerated, and is cheap. It is not surprising, therefore, that it is the drug most widely used in the treatment of tuberculosis. The drug is given in a single daily oral dose as it is more important to achieve a high peak concentration than to maintain a continuously inhibitory level. In intermittent regimens, large doses can be used and very high peak levels attained. Isoniazid is metabolized mainly by acetylation, at a rate which varies from one individual to another. Patients can be divided into two groups—*rapid* and *slow inactivators*. This is of little clinical importance in patients treated daily, or even twice weekly, but with intermittent regimens in which the drug is given only once a week, rapid inactivators (within 1 h) fare less well than slow inactivators (within 3 h), and there is some practical value in determining, by relatively simple tests, to which group a patient belongs when an intermittent regimen is contemplated.

Adverse reactions are uncommon. Isoniazid tends to raise plasma concentrations of phenytoin and carbamazepine by inhibiting their metabolism in the liver. Overdosage may give rise to vomiting, dizziness, blurred vision, and slurring of speech within 30 min to 3 h.

Hepatitis is an uncommon (0.1 per cent) but potentially serious reaction that can be easily averted by prompt withdrawal of treatment. A sharp rise in serum transaminases at the outset of treatment, which may be enhanced by the concomitant use of rifampicin, is of little significance. Isoniazid interferes competitively with pyridoxine metabolism by inhibiting the formation of the active form of the vitamin and hence often results in peripheral neuropathy, which can be prevented by co-administration of pyridoxine.

Following oral absorption, plasma concentrations are good and CSF penetration is about 50–80 per cent of the serum levels. Urinary concentrations are high. Primary resistance in *M. tuberculosis* in the UK is rare (1–4 per cent) but resistance develops quickly with single-drug therapy.

Pyrazinamide

This has a special sterilizing effect on intracellular tubercle bacilli in acid conditions and has therefore found an important place in short-course chemotherapy, in which the important factor is the incidence of relapse after cessation of treatment. It is given orally, produces high serum levels, and penetrates freely into CSF. Adverse reactions are rare, but hepatic toxicity has been a problem; hypersensitivity reactions and photosensitivity of the skin also occur.

Treatment for longer than 2 months is not recommended. Drug interactions occur with allopurinol, causing hyperuricaemia with attacks of gout, and with oral antidiabetic agents, causing a further fall in blood sugar. The dose should be reduced in renal impairment and avoided in patients with severe liver damage and gout.

Rifampicin

One of the most exciting and potentially valuable of the antituberculous drugs is rifampicin. Active also against a wide range of other bacteria, it has proved a most potent drug against human tuberculosis, both for primary treatment and in treatment of relapses, given daily or intermittently. However, rifampicin has not yet become a universally used standard drug in developing countries because it is expensive, and it has troublesome side-effects requiring special supervision and care. Curiously, several of these are far more common on intermittent regimens than when the drug is taken daily, and typically begin 2–3 h after the single morning dose. Once-weekly regimens give more toxicity than twice-weekly, and with daily regimens side-effects are uncommon and trivial. The side-effects are usually mild, and can usually be controlled by reducing either the dose size or the interval between doses. The exception is that the occurrence of purpura is an indication to stop the drug and not give it again.

Primary resistance in tubercle bacilli is rare (less than 1 per cent). Although rifampicin is sometimes used in the treatment of life-threatening staphylococcal infections and in the prophylaxis of meningococcal and *Haemophilus influenzae* meningitis, there is no evidence that this extended use has jeopardized the value of rifampicin in the treatment of TB.

Ethambutol

Ethambutol is now accepted as a replacement for PAS. In combination with other antituberculous drugs it is active against *M. tuberculosis* and many of the atypical mycobacteria. Resistance develops slowly during therapy, but primary resistance occurs in less than 4 per cent of strains of *M. tuberculosis*. It has a primarily bacteristatic action on proliferating bacteria. It is rapidly absorbed after oral administration and high serum levels are found after 2 h, with even higher levels inside erythrocytes. Adequate levels are found in the CSF. Ethambutol is excreted in the urine both unchanged and as inactive metabolites.

Dose-dependent optic (retrobulbar) neuritis can result in impairment of visual acuity and colour vision. Early changes are usually reversible, but blindness can occur if treatment is not discontinued promptly.

Thiacetazone

Thiacetazone is one of the oldest antituberculous drugs, being known since before 1950. It has about the same rate of toxicity as PAS, with rashes, jaundice, bone marrow depression, and gastrointestinal upsets prominent. It is more convenient to the patient than PAS (one tablet instead of several cachets a day), is much cheaper, and is stable in tropical climates, where PAS tends to deteriorate.

Thiacetazone is bacteristatic against *M. tuberculosis* and is often used in combination with isoniazid to inhibit the emergence of resistance to isoniazid, particularly on the continuation phase of the long-term regimens. It is well absorbed from the gastrointestinal tract and plasma levels are sustained for long periods of time. Side-effects include nausea, vomiting, diarrhoea, and skin rashes. Rare cases of fatal exfoliative dermatitis and acute hepatitis failure have been reported.

Ethionamide and prothionamide

Because of its gastrointestinal side-effects—anorexia, salivation, nausea, abdominal pain, and diarrhoea—ethionamide is one of the most unpleasant of all antituberculous drugs to take. Prothionamide is closely related in structure, but is better tolerated. The role of these drugs is almost entirely as second-line treatment of patients with tuberculosis or leprosy whose bacilli are resistant to first-choice drugs.

Both compounds are absorbed quickly when given by mouth with good tissue and CSF levels. Both are bacteriostatic at therapeutic concentrations but bactericidal at higher concentrations. Complete cross-resistance occurs between both, but not with isoniazid, to which these drugs are related.

Contraindications include pregnancy, severe liver damage, and gastric complaints; care should be exercised in epilepsy and in psychotic patients. Combinations with isoniazid, cycloserine or alcohol should be avoided.

Cycloserine, viomycin, kanamycin, capreomycin

These are four rather weak antituberculous drugs used only in three-drug regimens as reserves for the treatment of tuberculosis resistant to the major antituberculous drugs.

Capreomycin, viomycin, and kanamycin all need to be given by injection. Primary resistance is rare but resistance develops rapidly.

Promising developments

Several new antituberculous compounds are being evaluated, notably the fluoroquinolones, ciprofloxacin, ofloxacin, and sparfloxacin, but clinical experience is presently sparse.

Short-course and intermittent therapy

The discovery that both pyrazinamide and rifampicin are active against dormant as well as actively dividing tubercle bacilli prompted the investigation, mainly in East Africa and Hong Kong, of shorter periods of treatment with a variety of combinations of antituberculous drugs. In the first East African trial streptomycin and isoniazid were used alone and with either pyrazinamide, thiacetazone, or rifampicin. This trial clearly showed that all four regimens were effective in controlling the acute stage of the disease, but that, in addition, the regimens containing rifampicin or pyrazinamide would cure more than 90 per cent of patients in 6 months.

Further trials explored different combinations and also the effect of intermittent treatment. It soon became apparent that all regimens containing two of the three drugs, isoniazid, pyrazinamide, and rifampicin would cure more than 90 per cent of patients in 6 months and virtually all in 9 months. The limitations of treatment became those of cost and of patient compliance in the face of unpleasant side-effects of the drugs. In the developing world the aim was to find acceptable fully supervised mass treatment at a cost the communities could afford.

Affluent countries have different aims. These countries need very effective unsupervised regimens for use where patient motivation is high and good compliance can be assumed. Studies in these countries have shown that rifampicin plus isoniazid daily for 9 months, with streptomycin or ethambutol for the first 2 months, will cure virtually all patients with pulmonary tuberculosis, and these regimens have become standard treatment in Europe. More recently, it has been shown that the total length of treatment can be reduced from 9 to 6 months if pyrazinamide is added for the first 2 months. The British Thoracic Society now recommends a 6-month course of treatment in which rifampicin, isoniazid, and pyrazinamide are given together with either ethambutol or streptomycin for 2 months, then treatment continued for a further 4 months with the two drugs rifampicin and isoniazid (Table 26.2). There is increasing evidence that the fourth drug (ethambutol or streptomycin) can be omitted from this regimen without detriment. Almost all regimens contain an initial intensive phase with three or four drugs as it is important to bring the acute illness under control as rapidly as possible.

Effective chemotherapy rapidly reduces the population of viable bacilli (sputum smears may be positive but cultures remain negative) and consequently reduces the risk of transmission, often within 2 weeks. Institutional care is necessary where supervised therapy can be given to patients who fail to respond to treatment and for those who are severely ill (e.g. massive haemoptysis or pyopneumothorax) or who are bedridden with severe paraparesis. Most patients can be treated

Table 26.2. Recommended treatment regimens for tuberculosis in adults

Drug	Initial (2 months) phase		Continuation (4 months) phase		Major side-effects
Standard regimen					
Rifampicin	10 mg/kg/d (450–600 mg/d)		10 mg/kg/d (450–600 mg/d)		Hepatitis; gastrointestinal upsets
Isoniazid	5 mg/kg/d (200–300 mg/d)		5 mg/kg/d (200–300 mg/d)		Peripheral neuropathy; hepatitis
Pyrazinamide	30 mg/kg/d (1.5gm–2gm/d)				Gastrointestinal upsets; gout
Ethambutol*	15–25 mg/kg/d				Retrobulbar neuritis
Intermittent regimen					
Rifampicin	10 mg/kg	3 times weekly	10 mg/kg	3 times weekly	As above
Isoniazid	15 mg/kg		15 mg/kg		
Pyrazinamide	50 mg/kg		50 mg/kg		

* Or streptomycin (15 mg/kg/d or 0.75–1 g/d for 2 months).

satisfactorily provided that they can be relied upon to take their drugs regularly or are carefully supervised.

Steroids have no place in the routine management of tuberculosis, but in hospital short courses are of value in treating patients with pericarditis, pleural effusion, tuberculous meningitis, and acute miliary tuberculosis with dyspnoea.

Surgical resection is rarely necessary except in severe post-tuberculosis bronchiectasis, particularly when this is a cause of repeated haemoptysis. However, this may change if multidrug-resistant tuberculosis becomes widespread, particularly in immunosuppressed patients.

Monitoring the therapeutic response

Inadequate compliance is by far the most important cause of therapeutic failure. Most cases of chronic or relapsing tuberculosis are the result of irregular, inadequate administration of prescribed drugs or the use of less potent regimens. Response to treatment is most readily evaluated from the clinical response of the patient and particularly by monitoring weight changes, fever, and cough. Where resources permit, cultures and smears should be examined for acid fast bacilli.

Drugs used in pregnancy

Treatment should never be interrupted or postponed during pregnancy or at any time when immunological resistance to the disease is reduced. Because of the risk of ototoxicity to the fetus, aminoglycosides such as streptomycin should be avoided.

Tuberculosis and HIV infection

Because of immunosuppression, patients with HIV infection are at high risk of developing clinical tuberculosis and this may antedate the manifestation of AIDS by months. The disease is frequently caused by atypical mycobacteria; it may present atypically and is often extrapulmonary. Longer courses (>9 months) of treatment are often needed.

Chemoprophylaxis against tuberculosis

Isoniazid is commonly used alone in antituberculosis chemoprophylaxis because it is effective, cheap, acceptable, and has few side-effects. Fears that isoniazid-resistant organisms would emerge have proved unfounded.

Drug-resistant tuberculosis

There is wide variation between different parts of the world in the number of patients found to be infected with tubercle bacilli resistant to one or more antituberculous drugs at the time the disease is diagnosed. High rates of resistance, particularly to isoniazid, have been reported in some places, but short-course chemotherapy may be successful even in the presence of resistance to both isoniazid and streptomycin providing the regimen includes rifampicin and pyrazinamide in the first 2 months, and rifampicin in the continuation phase. This is because initial resistance to rifampicin and pyrazinamide is low everywhere at present, and is another important justification for the use of the complex four-drug regimens already suggested. Drug sensitivity testing (see Chapter 7), is performed in recognized centres as part of national surveillance. Individual patient susceptibility testing should occur if the patient continues to produce culture-positive sputum after 3 months. Where adequate facilities exist for determining drug sensitivities, regimens can be devised for individual patients taking account of both initial resistances and resistances emerging during treatment.

Modern drug regimens are designed to prevent the emergence of drug resistance, but control of tuberculosis is threatened by the widespread emergence of drug resistance in *M. tuberculosis* in certain populations.

The incidence of tuberculosis has increased in the USA and parts of Africa, largely in association with the epidemic of HIV infection. Outbreaks, sometimes caused by bacilli with multiple drug resistance, have occurred in hospitals, centres for the care of patients with AIDS, and in prisons, posing considerable clinical and public health problems. In the UK, resistance to isoniazid alone is presently less than 4 per cent and resistance to isoniazid and rifampicin (with or without resistance to other drugs) is less than 0.6 per cent. However, with the emergence of multiple drug resistance in other parts of the world, enhanced surveillance is required.

Modern molecular methods which allow the rapid detection of resistant strains should help to speed up any necessary change of therapy and prompt patient isolation.

Nosocomial transmission of multidrug-resistant *M. tuberculosis*

Multidrug-resistant tuberculosis is often characterized by a rapid progression from diagnosis to death and a strikingly high case fatality (>80 per cent). Patients are often severely immunocompromised and the clinical diagnosis of tuberculosis may be difficult to recognize. As a result there is often delay in initiating isolation of the patients and in the recognition of drug resistance. Health care workers are at great risk from multidrug-resistant tuberculosis, since these highly infectious patients remain untreated.

Infection control measures require the rapid identification of patients with multidrug-resistant tuberculosis and the immediate isolation of smear positive *M. tuberculosis* patients in isolation rooms. Negative air pressures should be maintained in these rooms and patients should be nursed under 'source control'. To prevent nosocomial transmission, HEPA (high-efficiency particulate air) filters may have to be fitted if there is difficulty in exhausting TB-contaminated air from buildings. Provision of personal respirators to health care workers may be a thing of the near future.

Extrapulmonary tuberculosis

Tuberculous meningitis

This form of tuberculous infection is invariably fatal if untreated, and appropriate chemotherapy is vital. It is a frequent complication of untreated miliary tuberculosis, and may vary from an abrupt and severe illness resembling other acute bacterial meningitis to a subtle and chronic disease extending over several months. Treatment should always include isoniazid and rifampicin. The isoniazid should initially be given in larger than usual dose, with a pyridoxine supplement. During the first intensive phase, these drugs should be accompanied by pyrazinamide and ethambutol. After about 2 months, these can be discontinued, but the isoniazid and rifampicin should be continued for at least a further 8 months. Intrathecal antibiotics are unnecessary, but additional treatment with corticosteroids should be used in severe cases.

Other forms of tuberculosis

Tuberculosis can affect any system in the body including, in decreasing order of frequency, superficial lymph nodes, bone and joints, the genito-urinary tract, the abdomen, the breast, and skin. Patients with non-respiratory tuberculosis can be regarded as non-infectious. Generally, the principles described for the treatment of pulmonary tuberculosis are also appropriate for the treatment of other forms, although few regimens have been given controlled clinical trials. Surgical intervention is sometimes necessary to establish the diagnosis, or to drain large abscesses, relieve pressure from tuberculous masses or repair damage from tuberculous scar tissue, but is no longer the mainstay of antituberculous treatment.

ATYPICAL MYCOBACTERIA

The so-called 'atypical' species of mycobacteria that can cause disease in humans include *M. kansasii*, *M. marinum*, *M. avium*, *M. intracellulare*,

M. fortuitum, and several others. The isolation of pathogenic atypical mycobacteria does not prove that disease is present; colonization with these organisms is not uncommon. Nevertheless, disease caused by these organisms may be indistinguishable from true tuberculosis.

Atypical mycobacteria are usually more resistant to the standard antituberculous agents than is *M. tuberculosis*. However, standard antituberculous chemotherapy is usually effective, although it may have to be prolonged and more often need to be accompanied by surgical resection of affected tissue.

Atypical mycobacteria of the *avium-intracellulare* group have come into prominence since the appearance of AIDS. Patients with defective cell-mediated immunity such as occurs in AIDS seem particularly prone to develop infection with these mycobacteria and the disease may be associated with a severe 'wasting syndrome'. Mycobacteria of the *avium-intracellulare* group are usually highly resistant to the common antituberculous drugs and infected patients respond poorly to antimicrobial therapy (see Chapter 29).

LEPROSY

This is a chronic communicable tropical disease caused by infection with *M. leprae*, and characterized by skin lesions and involvement of peripheral nerves causing anaesthesia, muscle weakness, paralysis, and consequent injury and deformity. Two major types are described: *lepromatous* and *tuberculoid*. In lepromatous leprosy there is diffuse involvement of skin and mucous membranes, with ulceration, iritis, and keratitis; scrapings of skin or mucous membranes contain numerous acid-fast bacilli. The tuberculoid form is more localized, but nerve involvement occurs early; only scanty bacilli are present. In both forms, progress of the disease is slow. The tuberculoid form may heal spontaneously in a few years. Death is usually due to other causes.

The mainstay of treatment of leprosy has been oral dapsone (diaminodiphenylsulphone; DDS) given for 1 or 2 years in tuberculoid disease, but for up to 10 years in lepromatous leprosy. However, resistance to dapsone has become common and leprologists now recommend triple therapy, whenever possible, with rifampicin, clofazimine, and dapsone. Rifampicin is more rapidly bactericidal than dapsone, but resistance may arise if it is used alone. It is also expensive, which is a considerable constraint to its use in countries where it is most needed. Clofazimine is effective, but the compound is pigmented and some patients find the discoloration of the skin that it produces unacceptable. Ethionamide or prothionamide are useful, but more toxic alternatives.

In multibacillary, lepromatous leprosy, triple therapy with monthly rifampicin and daily clofazimine (or alternatives) and dapsone should be given for at least 2 years, or until bacilli can no longer be seen microscopically; in paucibacillary disease, 6 months' therapy with rifampicin and dapsone may be adequate. With such long and complicated regimens, patient compliance is naturally a problem, particularly in areas of the world where leprosy is most prevalent. There are preliminary indications that the fluoroquinolones, notably ofloxacin, and the newer macrolides may have a role in the treatment of lepromatous leprosy. It should be remembered that patients with leprosy may also have tuberculosis; the triple therapy regimen used for the treatment of leprosy is inadequate for the treatment of tuberculosis.

27

Meningitis and brain abscess

P. Ispahani

MENINGITIS

Meningitis is an infection within the subarachnoid space resulting in inflammation of the membranes (arachnoid and piamater) covering the brain and the spinal cord and the intervening cerebrospinal fluid (CSF). Infection may be due to bacteria or viruses. The inflammatory process in bacterial meningitis extends throughout the subarachnoid space and regularly involves the ventricles, but the brain itself is generally not affected by the infecting organism or the inflammatory exudate.

Viral meningitis is usually self limiting. Despite advanced medical intensive care technology and the availability of potent bactericidal antibiotics, bacterial meningitis remains a relatively common and devastating disease with a mortality of 10–30 per cent. The outcome is dependent upon the organism, the age of the patient, the state of consciousness and clinical presentation on admission, and the rapidity of diagnosis and treatment. Furthermore, the long-term neurological sequelae in the survivors is high, especially in neonates, very young infants, and in those with *Streptococcus pneumoniae* meningitis.

If death is to be averted, and neurological complications minimized, the clinician must suspect meningitis early, diagnose it accurately, and initiate appropriate antimicrobial therapy aggressively.

Epidemiology

Until recently in the UK about 2500 cases of bacterial meningitis occurred annually, and some 75 per cent of these were due to infection by one of the three organisms: *Neisseria meningitidis*, *Haemophilus influenzae* (type b), and *Str. pneumoniae*. The remaining 25 per cent of cases had a varied aetiology with Group B haemolytic streptococci and *Escherichia coli* dominant in the neonatal period. However, since the introduction of a conjugate vaccine against *H. influenzae* (type b) in 1992, a dramatic fall in the incidence of invasive infection has been observed. In Finland and the USA where this vaccine was introduced a few years earlier, invasive disease with *H. influenzae* (type b) has been virtually eliminated.

In the UK, *N. meningitidis* is the commonest cause of acute bacterial meningitis and is likely to remain so until a suitable vaccine becomes available for strains of serogroup B, which account for over 60 per cent of all cases of meningococcal disease in the UK.

Age and organisms

The frequency with which various bacterial species are encountered in meningitis is strikingly age related (Table 27.1). In the past, *Esch. coli* and other enterobacteria dominated as agents of neonatal meningitis, but Group B haemolytic streptococci are now the leading cause. Meningitis due to these two classic neonatal pathogens, which account for approximately 75 per cent of cases, can occasionally occur in an infant beyond 28 weeks of age. Less common causes are *Listeria monocytogenes*, other enterobacteria and *Candida albicans*. *Str. pneumoniae* is a rare cause of neonatal meningitis, but it appears to have become more common. From the age of 3 months, 95 per cent of all cases of meningitis in children is due to the three major pathogens of bacterial meningitis. *H. influenzae* (type b) is rare after the age of 6 years and, indeed, 75 per cent of cases occur before the age of 2 years.

After the age of 40 years, meningitis is most commonly due to *Str. pneumoniae*. *L. monocytogenes* (especially in those with underlying diseases), *Esch. coli*, *Staph. aureus* (usually post-neurosurgery), and *Mycobacterium tuberculosis* are some of the other agents producing meningitis in adults.

Pathogenesis and clinical features

Bacterial meningitis most commonly follows haematogenous spread of micro-organisms from the nasopharynx in the case of the three major meningeal pathogens, which are also found as normal commensals in a small proportion of the population. The main sequence of events in the development of meningitis by these three organisms is believed to be: initial mucosal colonization, transgression of the mucosal epithelium, bacteraemia, penetration of the blood–brain barrier, and multiplication within the subarachnoid space. The choroid plexus of the lateral ventricles is probably the initial site of entry of blood-borne bacteria into the CSF. Occasionally, haematogenous spread may follow from a focus of infection in the middle ear, lung, heart valves, skin, gastrointestinal or genito-urinary tracts. Rarely, bacteria may reach the CSF by direct extension from neighbouring suppurative tissues or a ruptured intracranial abscess, or be directly implanted into the subarachnoid space from the nasopharynx through dural defects of congenital or traumatic origin. Once a pathogen is introduced into the subarachnoid

Table 27.1. Bacterial meningitis in Nottingham 1980–1991: distribution of organisms in different age groups in 617 cases

	Neonates	Children		Adults
Organism (number of cases)	≤ 28 weeks (*n* = 60)	5–11 weeks (*n* = 33)	3 mths–14 yrs (*n* = 309)	≥ 15 years (*n* = 215)
Neisseria meningitidis (225)	3.3	27.3	43.7	36.7
Haemophilus influenzae (type b) (126)	1.7	21.2	37.5	0.9
Streptococcus pneumoniae (120)	5.0	15.1	13.0	33.5
Group B haemolytic streptococci (30)	36.7	18.2	0.3	0.5
Other streptococci (8)	1.7	–	0.3	2.8
Escherichia coli (27)	26.7	12.2	0.3	2.8
Other enterobacteria (7)	6.7	3.0	0.6	–
Listeria monocytogenes (26)	8.3	–	0.3	9.3
Pseudomonas aeruginosa (6)	3.3	–	–	1.9
Staphylococcus aureus (13)	1.7	–	1.0	4.2
H. influenzae (non capsulate) (6)	–	–	1.0	1.4
Miscellaneous bacteria (7)	1.6	–	1.0	1.4
Mycobacterium tuberculosis (11)	–	–	1.0	3.7
Fungi (5)	3.3	3.0	–	0.9

Percentage of isolates in:

space, bacteria multiply rapidly because of inadequate local defences. Then an intense inflammatory process is set up with marked congestion, oedema, and outpouring of exudate. Blood vessels and nerves coursing through this space may be involved in the inflammatory process leading to arteritis, infective thrombophlebitis, and cranial nerve palsies, or the thick exudate may interfere with free CSF circulation and absorption, leading to blockage and hydrocephalus.

The clinical picture consists of signs and symptoms of systemic illness (e.g. general malaise, fever, toxicity, poor feeding, and leucocytosis) increased intracranial pressure (e.g. headache, vomiting, irritability, disturbance of consciousness, and seizure), and meningeal irritation (e.g. photophobia, neck pain, and positive Kernig's sign). In neonates, infants, and the aged the signs and symptoms may be non-specific and subtle.

The presence of a petechial or purpuric rash, predominantly on the extremities, in a patient with meningeal signs almost always indicates meningococcal disease and requires immediate antibiotic therapy.

Laboratory diagnosis

CSF examination

Lumbar puncture should be performed with the utmost urgency, and CSF obtained should be sent to the Department of Microbiology within minutes of its collection. Delay in examining the CSF jeopardizes the institution of appropriate therapy. In an adult at least 4–5 ml of CSF is obtained into two or three sterile bottles, which are then labelled sequentially. A sample for the estimation of CSF glucose is collected into a special tube containing fluoride, and a corresponding blood glucose is sent separately to the clinical chemistry laboratory.

Examination of the CSF in the microbiology laboratory must be thorough, with meticulous attention to detail. Besides culture, it includes total white blood cell (including differential) and red blood cell counts, and estimation of protein. But the most critical investigation in patients with meningitis is the examination of a carefully prepared Gram-stained smear of the centrifuged deposit of CSF, because in most cases of bacterial meningitis the appropriate therapy is based on this result. Considerable caution should be exercised in the interpretation of the Gram-film, especially when the CSF has been obtained after antibiotic therapy, for the Gram-positive organisms may not only decolourize easily, but cocci may elongate and assume bacillary forms. When examined diligently and patiently by an experienced person the Gram-film may reveal the causative organism in 85 per cent of cases. Typical laboratory findings in bacterial and viral meningitis are given in Table 27.2.

Although there are a variety of other tests, e.g. countercurrent immunoelectrophoresis or latex particle agglutination for detecting specific bacterial antigens in the CSF, in most cases of bacterial meningitis the cell counts, chemistry, a prolonged search of a carefully prepared Gram-stain smear, and culture of CSF provide enough information for diagnosis and initial treatment.

If the patient is acutely ill with a short history suggestive of meningitis, or if the CSF appears cloudy, then empirical (based on age and clinical setting) high-dose intravenous antibiotics should be given

Table 27.2. Typical CSF changes in bacterial and viral meningitis

	Normal CSF	Bacterial meningitis*	Viral meningitis
Appearance	Clear; colourless	Purulent or cloudy	Clear or slightly opalescent
Cell count (per μl)	0–5	100s or 1000s	10s or 100s
Main cell type	(Lymphocytes)	Polymorphs†	Lymphocytes‡
Protein concentration	0.1–0.4 g/l	High (may be several g/l)	Normal or slightly raised
Glucose concentration	*c.* 60% of blood glucose	< 40% of blood glucose	Unchanged
Gram-film	Negative	Positive	Negative

* Excluding tuberculous meningitis.

† Exceptions; partially treated pyogenic meningitis; tuberculous, listeria, cryptococcal, or leptospiral meningitis, in which a lymphocytic response is common.

‡ In early cases an increased polymorph count may be seen.

immediately, without waiting for the Gram-film or clinical chemistry results. Mortality in these patients is high, and a delay of 30–60 min may worsen the prognosis.

Blood cultures

Since bacteraemia is present in a high proportion of patients and organisms may occasionally be isolated only from blood cultures (e.g. in patients with meningococcal disease who have not yet developed meningitis) it is crucial that at least two sets of blood cultures are taken before antimicrobial therapy is begun. Furthermore, when patients have to receive antibiotics before lumbar puncture, either because the patient is acutely ill or when lumbar puncture is contraindicated until CT scan has been performed (e.g. in the presence of focal neurological signs or papilloedema), blood culture may be the only investigation which might yield the causative agent.

Therapeutic considerations

Bacterial meningitis was difficult or impossible to treat before the advent of sulphonamides. Today, with a battery of potent antimicrobial agents, success rests on prompt initiation of treatment, started on the basis of Gram-film findings and on the appreciation of certain principles and guidelines.

Penetration of antibiotics into CSF

In bacterial meningitis, infection is located in a closed space within the CSF which represents an area of impaired host defence. Hence, it is imperative to ensure that the antimicrobial agent used is both lethal to the invading organism and able to penetrate into the CSF in therapeutic concentration. All organic compounds entering CSF must traverse the blood–brain barrier (a lipid membrane in the brain capillary), the epithelial layer of the choroid plexus, or both. The choroid epithelium is highly impermeable to lipid-insoluble molecules. For example, when the blood–brain barrier is normal all β-lactam antibiotics penetrate poorly (about 0.5 to 2 per cent of the peak serum concentration). The penetration of antibiotics into the CSF is enhanced by:

(1) high lipid solubility;

(2) low degree of ionization;

(3) low molecular weight;

(4) high serum concentration of the drug;

(5) low degree of protein binding;

(6) presence of meningeal inflammation.

The commonly used antimicrobial agents can be subdivided into three broad groups according to their ability to penetrate into CSF.

1. Those that penetrate inflamed and non-inflamed meninges, even when used in standard doses. These include chloramphenicol, sulphonamides, trimethoprim, metronidazole, the antituberculous agents isoniazid and pyrazinamide, and the antifungal agent fluconazole.

2. Those that penetrate when the meninges are inflamed, or when used in high doses. These include benzylpenicillin, ampicillin, flucloxacillin, extended-spectrum cephalosporins of the cefotaxime type, vancomycin, rifampicin, and the antifungal agents amphotericin B and flucytosine.

3. Those that penetrate poorly even when the meninges are inflamed. These include aminoglycosides, the earlier cephalosporins, erythromycin, tetracycline, and fusidic acid.

Choice of antimicrobial agent

The initial choice of an antimicrobial agent for patients with bacterial meningitis is based on the age of the patient, the clinical setting, the Gram-film results of the CSF, and prior knowledge of the local sensitivity patterns of the suspected organism. Since the CSF lacks intrinsic opsonic and bactericidal activity and, in the early stages of meningitis, the density of organism may reach high levels, a bactericidal rather than a bacteristatic agent is recommended for the treatment of meningitis. Both in experimental models and in clinical trials, rapid killing of bacteria in the CSF was seen only when the bactericidal titre of the CSF for the relevant bacteria was between 1 in 10 and 1 in 20.

Chloramphenicol, which in general is a bacteristatic agent, is bactericidal against *H. influenzae*, *N. meningitidis*, and most strains of *Str. pneumoniae*. Because of its excellent penetration into the CSF, it was until recently widely used for the three common meningeal pathogens and also, together with gentamicin, to treat Gram-negative bacillary meningitis in neonates and adults. However, chloramphenicol is bacteristatic *in vitro* against most bacteria belonging to the Enterobacteriaceae, and its use was frequently associated with failures. The development of the extended-spectrum cephalosporins of the cefotaxime type has revolutionized the treatment of Gram-negative bacillary meningitis. These agents exhibit excellent activity *in vitro* not only against all strains of *H. influenzae*, *Str. pneumoniae*, *N. meningitidis*, and group B streptococci, but also against *Esch. coli* and other members of the Enterobacteriaceae. Intravenous therapy with high doses of these agents usually results in CSF concentrations many times those necessary to kill the organisms. They are effective in meningitis due to the three common meningeal pathogens and in Gram-negative bacillary meningitis. Chloramphenicol has become a reserve agent for the treatment of selected patients who are allergic to penicillin, but it can no longer be recommended for Gram-negative bacillary meningitis.

Route and mode of administration

Intravenous administration of antibiotics is preferred in all cases of bacterial meningitis, for the essence of specific treatment is not merely to kill the organisms, but to kill them quickly. Since β-lactam antibiotics enter CSF reluctantly, it is essential to give these antibiotics parenterally in high intermittent bolus doses frequently rather than by continuous administration, to ensure that high peak levels are achieved in the CSF. The dosage interval is dependent upon the half-life of the drug used. For example for cefotaxime the interval is usually 4–6 hourly, but for ceftriaxone, which has a longer half-life, a 12–24 h interval is sufficient. In some patients the use of high-dose β-lactam antibiotics or vancomycin for prolonged periods may lead to bone marrow depression. Frequent monitoring of full blood counts is recommended.

When chloramphenicol is used for treating meningitis, the oral route can be used after the initial acute stages of illness, but oral penicillin V or amoxycillin have no place in the treatment of bacterial meningitis.

Duration of therapy

The duration of treatment in most cases of uncomplicated meningitis is short. Antibiotic treatment of meningococcal meningitis need last only 5 days, although in practice it is usually 7 days; *H. influenzae* is best treated for a minimum of 7–10 days to ensure complete eradication of the organism and prevent relapse. Antimicrobial treatment of pneumococcal meningitis should be continued for at least 10 days for most patients, and up to 2 weeks in young infants or in complicated cases. In neonatal meningitis and adult meningitis due to unusual organisms, more prolonged therapy may be indicated and each case should be reviewed in consultation with a microbiologist.

Adjunctive therapy

Despite the use of appropriate, effective, and bactericidal antibiotics in bacterial meningitis, the mortality and morbidity remain high. In an attempt to improve response to conventional antimicrobial therapy, attention in recent years has been focused on the possibility of modulating the complex inflammatory process within the subarachnoid space and meninges. This is a major factor contributing to mortality and morbidity, including sensorineural hearing loss.

Dexamethasone therapy in concert with antimicrobial agents appears to improve this inflammatory process in experimental models of meningitis and is associated with a decreased incidence of sensorineural hearing loss in children with meningitis. However, there was no reduction in the overall mortality rate, and gastrointestinal bleeding occurred in some patients who received dexamethasone. Hence its routine use as adjunctive treatment for bacterial meningitis remains controversial.

Meningococcal disease

Meningococcal disease, which represents a spectrum of illness caused by *N. meningitidis*, is a world-wide problem. Besides occurring in epidemics across the 'meningitis belt' in sub-Saharan Africa every 7–10 years, high or increased levels of endemic meningococcal disease have been reported from many other parts of the world. *N. meningitidis* primarily affects infants, children, and young adults. In Nottingham between 1980 and 1990, 54 per cent of 200 cases of meningococcal disease occurred in children less than 5 years and 11.5 per cent in adults over 40 years of age. The organism is carried asymptomatically in the nasopharynx of a small proportion of the population and this represents the reservoir of infection. The disease has a seasonal incidence; almost two-thirds of cases occur between December and May (winter and spring), and a co-existing or antecedent viral infection may play a part in invasive meningococcal disease.

The clinical presentation of meningococcal disease can vary widely and recognizing the symptoms can mean the difference between life and death. It is still not widely appreciated that life-threatening meningococcal disease does not present primarily as meningitis! The following broad clinical groups can be recognized in patients with meningococcal disease according to the presenting clinical features:

Transient bacteraemia. A mild, self-limiting febrile illness, seen occasionally in children, who usually recover quickly and spontaneously without the use of antibiotics. Diagnosis is made retrospectively because of positive blood cultures.

Septicaemia with or without meningitis. In about 15–20 per cent of cases of meningococcal disease, features of septicaemia predominate. It is characterized by the rapid development of a systemic illness over a period of 24 to 48 h. The symptoms include fever, chills, myalgias, and a widespread petechial rash. In a small proportion of these patients, headache, confusion, and neck stiffness may develop later, signifying the onset of meningitis following septicaemia. However, the onset of illness in those with fulminant meningococcal septicaemia is much more abrupt and dramatic. The duration of illness is often less than 24 h, and on admission the patient is gravely ill, shocked, and covered with a rapidly spreading purpuric rash which may coalesce in parts and become ecchymotic. Disseminated intravascular coagulation may soon follow and death can occur in a matter of hours. Blood cultures are invariably positive. There may be no signs of meningism, but it is not uncommon in some patients to culture *N. meningitidis* from an otherwise normal CSF, implying the onset of early meningitis. Mortality is 20–30 per cent in patients with septicaemic illness.

'Classical' meningitis with or without septicaemia. This is by far the commonest presentation. The clinical picture is usually dominated by signs and symptoms of meningitis which may occur rapidly or evolve more gradually over several days. The CSF is typically cloudy with pleocytosis, raised protein, and low glucose concentration. Typical petechial or purpuric rash is present in about 60 per cent of patients, but occasionally the rash may be maculopapular initially. Blood cultures are positive in approximately 40 per cent of cases and probably reflects secondary bacteraemia resulting from the local suppurative process within the subarachnoid space, rather than the ongoing primary bacteraemia following nasopharyngeal colonization. Mortality is 3–5 per cent.

Rarer forms of meningococcal disease. Occasionally *N. meningitidis* may localize in the joints or heart valves, producing acute septic arthritis or endocarditis, or the septicaemic illness may become chronic and indolent, producing chronic meningococcal septicaemia, which is characterized by intermittent pyrexia, rash, and arthralgias.

Treatment and prophylaxis
Before benzylpenicillin became widely available, sulphonamides (principally sulphadiazine) were used for the treatment of meningococcal

meningitis. They were also used for prophylaxis, since, unlike other agents used for treatment, such as benzylpenicillin or chloramphenicol, they are effective in eradicating *N. meningitidis* from the throat. However, sulphonamide-resistant strains now account for about 40 per cent of isolates in the UK and as many as 70 per cent in parts of the USA, and can therefore no longer be used for treatment or prophylaxis unless it is known that the isolate is sensitive.

The standard agent now used in the UK as prophylaxis for meningococcal disease is oral rifampicin for 2 days (adults, 600 mg twice daily; children, 10 mg/kg twice daily). Rifampicin-resistant strains do occur, but are presently very uncommon. A single intramuscular injection of ceftriaxone (adults, 250 mg; children, 125 mg) or a single oral dose of ciprofloxacin (adults, 500 mg) are alternative prophylactic agents. Ceftriaxone rather than rifampicin should be offered to pregnant women.

Benzylpenicillin in high (meningitic) doses is the drug of choice for the treatment of meningococcal disease. However, strains that are resistant or of reduced sensitivity to penicillin have been reported from several countries including the UK. Of 1266 isolates of *N. meningitidis* tested by the PHLS Meningococcal Reference Unit in 1993, 94 per cent were highly sensitive to penicillin (MIC <0.16 mg/l); for the remaining 6 per cent the MIC was in the range 0.16 to 1.28 mg/l. Benzylpenicillin can still be used for strains showing slightly reduced sensitivity to penicillin, but patients with isolates for which the MIC of penicillin exceeds 0.32 mg/l, or those who are allergic to penicillin, are best treated with either cefotaxime or chloramphenicol.

A report of β-lactamase-producing strains of *Neisseria meningitidis* from South Africa in 1988 is very disturbing, but no further report of this type of resistance has so far emerged. Since *N. meningitidis* can no longer be assumed to be sensitive to penicillin, all isolates must be tested for susceptibility.

Haemophilus meningitis

Almost all cases of meningitis due to *H. influenzae* are caused by the capsulate type b strains. Among 132 cases seen in Nottingham between 1980 and 1991, 126 (95 per cent) were due to *H. influenzae* (type b), and all but two were in children less than 6 years of age, probably reflecting the absence of anticapsular antibody in this age group. The mortality was 7.1 per cent. Six cases caused by non-capsulate strains of *H. influenzae* occurred in older children or adults with some predisposing factor, e.g. recent head trauma, neurosurgical procedure, or the presence of a shunt. The onset in patients with *H. influenzae* (type b) meningitis is often insidious, progressing over a period of 3–5 days. In some infants the illness may be limited to fever, vomiting, and diarrhoea in the early stages, making the diagnosis of meningitis difficult.

Treatment and prophylaxis

In the past virtually all strains of *H. influenzae* (type b) were sensitive to ampicillin, but this is no longer the case. In the UK 28 per cent of strains are ampicillin resistant usually, but not always, owing to the production of β-lactamase. Chloramphenicol resistance is rare in the UK, but in other parts of the world resistance to ampicillin and chloramphenicol or both is more common. In Spain resistance to both ampicillin and chloramphenicol appears to be particularly common.

It seems likely that, in countries in which conjugated *H. influenzae* (type b) vaccine is incorporated into the routine immunization schedule for infants, invasive disease will soon be eradicated.

Currently the antibiotic of choice is cefotaxime, which is active against both β-lactamase-producing and non-β-lactamase-producing strains of *H. influenzae*. In patients with a firm history of penicillin allergy, chloramphenicol can be used. Tests of sensitivity to ampicillin, chloramphenicol, cefotaxime, and rifampicin should be performed on all isolates. Tests for the detection of β-lactamase provide a rapid screening method for enzymic resistance, but will not exclude other forms of ampicillin resistance. Rifampicin is used as prophylaxis for close contacts when there is a sibling in the house aged 4 years or younger.

Pneumococcal meningitis

Str. pneumoniae is unique amongst the three common meningeal pathogens as being a threat throughout life. Of 120 cases of pneumococcal meningitis seen in Nottingham between 1980 and 1991, 40 per cent occurred in children. Most cases were in children up to the age of 6 years or adults over 40 years of age. The overall mortality in treated patients was 31 per cent; the mortality in children and adults was 19 and 37 per cent respectively. The outlook was exceptionally grim in those over the age of 60 years.

In contrast to meningococcal or haemophilus meningitis, in pneumococcal meningitis there is often either a pre-existing focus of infection elsewhere (e.g. pneumonia, acute otitis media or acute sinusitis) or the presence of an associated predisposing risk factor (e.g. recent or remote head trauma, recent neurosurgical procedure, CSF leak, sickle cell anaemia, various immunodeficiency states, alcoholism or an absent spleen). *Str. pneumoniae* is the commonest cause of recurrent or post-traumatic meningitis, when organisms may reach the meninges via abnormal communications between the nasopharynx and the subarachnoid space. Patients who have had splenectomy are permanently at risk of developing overwhelming pneumococcal infection. The onset may be sudden and the course rapid, with death within 12 h of admission to hospital. Alterations of consciousness and focal neurological defects are more frequent in pneumococcal meningitis than in meningitis caused by the other two meningeal pathogens. Furthermore, survivors often suffer significant neurological deficits.

Treatment

In places where there is still very little concern about penicillin-resistant strains of *Str. pneumoniae*, benzylpenicillin remains the drug of choice for the treatment of pneumococcal meningitis. But in areas where the incidence of reduced sensitivity to penicillin is not uncommon, antimicrobial therapy in all patients with suspected or proven pneumococcal meningitis should be commenced with cefotaxime and changed to benzylpenicillin only if the strain isolated is subsequently confirmed to be sensitive to penicillin. Penicillin-resistant strains of *Str. pneumoniae* have been reported from many countries of the world, including the USA and the UK, and penicillin sensitivity tests (with a 1 μg oxacillin disc to detect low-level resistance) should now be a routine procedure on all clinical isolates. Whereas high-dose benzylpenicillin may still be adequate for the treatment of pneumonia caused by strains showing intermediate resistance to penicillin, agents other than penicillin should be used in meningitis if any type of penicillin resistance is present. The antibiotic of choice for such strains is cefotaxime, but if a fully resistant strain is encountered then rifampicin should be considered as well. Vancomycin is a less attractive alternative because of its poor penetration into the CSF. Chloramphenicol is not an option in this situation, as half the strains have been reported to be resistant to chloramphenicol as well. Furthermore, failures have been recorded even when the strain appeared to be sensitive to chloramphenicol. Strains of pneumococci that are resistant to expanded-spectrum cephalosporins are being reported and recommendations may change in future years.

The duration of treatment for most patients is at least 10 days, but is extended up to 2 weeks in young infants or in complicated cases.

Neonatal meningitis

The neonate is at the highest risk of developing meningitis within the first 2 months of life, the incidence being about 0.3 per 1000 live births. Neonatal meningitis not only carries a high mortality, but the incidence of neurological deficits in those who survive is depressingly high. Although brain abscess rarely complicates meningitis, it should be considered as an associated possibility in Gram-negative bacillary meningitis in the neonate particularly if meningitis is due to *Citrobacter diversus*.

The predisposing factors include prematurity, low birth weight, prolonged and difficult labour, prolonged rupture of membranes, and maternal perinatal infection. Rarely, some cases are associated with congenital neurological defects.

The organisms responsible for neonatal meningitis are varied. They are usually acquired by vertical transfer from the mother *in utero* or during delivery through the birth canal, leading to early-onset (occurring within 7 days of delivery) septicaemia or meningitis; less commonly they are acquired from the environment, leading to late-onset (occurring after 7 days and occasionally up to 2 months after delivery) meningitis. This is classically illustrated with group B streptococci infection. The early-onset disease often presents as an overwhelming septicaemia with apnoea and shock. The pulmonary manifestations of this illness may be difficult to differentiate clinically or radiologically from respiratory distress syndrome. Meningitis will occur in 30 per cent of cases. It has been estimated that approximately 1 in 100 newborns colonized with group B streptococci may develop early-onset disease. Mortality with this type of disease is over 50 per cent. Late-onset disease usually presents as meningitis and mortality is around 20 per cent.

The early signs and symptoms of neonatal meningitis are frequently vague: lethargy, refusal of feeds, and fever. A bulging fontanelle is a relatively late sign. Therefore a high degree of suspicion and prompt investigation with lumbar puncture is essential. Of those who survive, about half will have some evidence of neurological damage.

Treatment of neonatal meningitis

Neonatal meningitis is particularly difficult to treat, since a wide variety of organisms may be involved; furthermore the susceptibility of the organisms (see below) involved is far from predictable. Traditionally, neonatal meningitis is usually managed with a combination of antibiotics. The chosen therapy should be backed up by appropriate laboratory tests.

Group B haemolytic streptococci. These are less sensitive to penicillin and are killed more slowly than are group A haemolytic streptococci. Penicillin and gentamicin act synergistically, causing accelerated killing of group B streptococci *in vitro*, and improving survival of animals with experimental group B streptococci infection compared with penicillin alone. The treatment of choice for meningitis caused by group B streptococci is high-dose benzylpenicillin for at least 2 weeks, together with gentamicin for the first 7–10 days.

Esch. coli and other enterobacteria. Before the extended-spectrum cephalosporins became available meningitis due to these organisms was a frequently fatal disease with mortality rates of 40–80 per cent. It was usually treated with chloramphenicol and gentamicin. But chloramphenicol, despite its excellent penetration into the CSF, is not bactericidal to *Esch. coli* and other enterobacteria and relapse has been recorded. Moreover, chloramphenicol may, on rare occasions, cause irreversible bone marrow aplasia and produce 'grey baby syndrome' in the neonate. Chloramphenicol can therefore no longer be recommended. In recent years, the most widely used regimen is high-dose cefotaxime in combination with gentamicin to provide synergistic bactericidal activity against *Esch. coli* or other enterobacteria. Ceftriaxone instead of cefotaxime, together with gentamicin, is recommended for meningitis caused by *Salmonella* spp., whereas ceftazidime plus gentamicin would be the treatment of choice for *Pseudomonas aeruginosa* meningitis. The duration of treatment for Gram-negative bacillary meningitis in neonates and adults should be at least 3 weeks. Since the use of the extended-spectrum cephalosporins became common for Gram-negative bacillary meningitis a significant reduction in mortality has been noted.

Listeria monocytogenes. This is a Gram-positive bacillus which is widespread in nature and exists as a soil saprophyte. It colonizes or infects a wide variety of domestic and wild animals and birds. Humans probably acquire *L. monocytogenes* by ingesting dairy or vegetable produce contaminated with listeria from animal sources. The organism may be carried asymptomatically in the gastrointestinal or the female genital tract. Infection in the neonatal period with *L. monocytogenes* may be acquired either by the transplacental route *in utero* or from the female genital tract during delivery. Bacteraemia with *L. monocytogenes* may occur in a pregnant woman following a flu-like illness, which might result in transplacental intrauterine infection of the fetus leading to abortion and stillbirth, or the neonate may develop symptoms of disseminated infection (granulomatosis infantiseptica) a few days after delivery. Neonatal mortality with intrauterine listeriosis is around 30 per cent. Most cases of late-onset infection present as meningitis in a previously normal neonate.

L. monocytogenes* also produces meningitis in adults, particularly in the elderly or in those who are immunocompromised or have some underlying disease. But occasionally the disease also occurs in previously healthy adults of all ages. Rarely, infection with *L. monocytogenes* is confined to the brain stem, producing multiple small abscesses. In such patients the organisms can only be isolated from blood cultures.

The organism is sensitive to a variety of agents, but the treatment of choice is high-dose ampicillin with gentamicin. *In vitro* and in the experimental rabbit model of meningitis a combination of the two drugs has a synergistic bactericidal effect. Moreover, gentamicin itself is bactericidal. In adults with a serious history of penicillin allergy, co-trimoxazole (which is bactericidal to *L. monocytogenes*) given intravenously or orally is the best alternative. Cephalosporins have no useful activity against *L. monocytogenes*.

The duration of therapy for *L. monocytogenes* meningitis should be 3 weeks for neonates or those who are immunocompromised and at least 2 weeks in normal hosts.

A summary of current recommendations for the initial therapy of the commoner forms of bacterial meningitis is outlined in Table 27.3.

Rarer forms of meningitis

Staph. aureus

Meningitis due to *Staph. aureus* may occur in patients with fulminating septicaemia secondary to pneumonia or endocarditis, or as a complication of penetrating head injury, recent neurosurgical procedures (including insertion of shunts), and ruptured cerebral or epidural abscess. The mortality rate in *Staph. aureus* meningitis is high, and the neurological sequelae are common in survivors.

The vast majority of *Staph. aureus* strains are resistant to penicillin, hence the choice of antibiotics is limited; for methicillin-sensitive strains high-dose flucloxacillin (at least 12 g daily) combined with oral rifampicin (600 mg daily) is recommended. In patients who are allergic to penicillin or in meningitis due to methicillin-resistant strains, treatment is even more problematic. Parenteral vancomycin (1 g every 12 h) combined with oral rifampicin is recommended. However, since penetration of vancomycin into the CSF is limited, daily intraventricular vancomycin (adult 20 mg; child 10 mg) for 7 to 10 days should also be considered. Daily intraventricular vancomycin is also warranted in patients with methicillin-sensitive *Staph. aureus* meningitis, when the CSF is persistently positive despite flucloxacillin and rifampicin, or in patients with shunt-associated meningitis. The duration of treatment for *Staph. aureus* meningitis should be at least 3 weeks.

Staph. epidermidis and shunt-associated meningitis

Patients with hydrocephalus due to any cause are treated by surgical decompression, whereby the CSF from the ventricular system is diverted to other compartments of the body (usually the peritoneal cavity or the right atrium) with a silastic catheter (shunt). Essentially, a typical CSF shunt is composed of three components: a ventricular catheter, a reservoir with a one-way valve, and a distal catheter directed into the peritoneum or the atrium. Unfortunately, 15–25 per cent of all patients with these shunts develop meningitis at some point in the life of the shunt. *Staph. epidermidis* accounts for 50 to 60 per cent and *Staph. aureus* for another 25 per cent of shunt infections. Other agents, amongst a great variety of micro-organisms associated with such infections, include *Propionibacterium acnes*, diphtheroids, enterococci, and Gram-negative bacilli. The vast majority of infections are believed to be due to colonization of the shunt at the time of surgery; occasionally

Table 27.3. Antibiotic treatment of the common types of bacterial meningitis (with normal renal and hepatic function)

Age of patient	CSF Gram-film findings	Presumptive organism	Treatment of choice			
			Antibiotic(s)	Total daily dose (Dosing interval)	Duration	Comments
<2 months	Gram-positive cocci in chains	Group B streptococci	Benzylpenicillin +gentamicin*	240 mg/kg/d (6h)	2 weeks	In selected patients, gentamicin may be discontinued after 7–10 d; Omit gentamicin if *Str. pneumoniae* (rare) is grown on culture
	Gram-negative bacilli	'Coliforms' (usually *Esch. coli*)	Cefotaxime + gentamicin*	200 mg/kg/d (6h)	3 weeks	Instead of cefotaxime, change to ceftriaxone if *Salmonella* spp. or ceftazidime if *Ps. aeruginosa* is grown on culture
	Gram-positive bacilli	*L. monocytogenes*	Ampicillin + gentamicin*	200 mg/kg/d (6h)	3 weeks	Relatively rare cause of neonatal meningitis
	No organisms seen	Any of the above 3	Cefotaxime + gentamicin* + (ampicillin)	200 mg/kg/d (6h) 200 mg/kg/d (6h)	variable†	Ampicillin may be added if *L. monocytogenes* infection is strongly suspected Change to appropriate combination according to culture result
2 months to 6 yrs	Gram-negative diplococci	*N. meningitidis*	Benzylpenicillin	300 mg/kg/d (4h)	7 days	Use cefotaxime or chloramphenicol if the patient is allergic to penicillin
	Gram-positive diplococci	*Str. pneumoniae*	Benzylpenicillin	300 mg/kg/d (4h)	10 days	Use cefotaxime if the patient is allergic to penicillin or the strain shows reduced sensitivity to penicillin or in areas where the incidence of reduced sensitivity to penicillin is not uncommon; In young infants or in complicated cases treatment may be extended up to 2 weeks

Table 27.3. cont.

Age of patient	CSF Gram-film findings	Presumptive organism	Treatment of choice			Comments
			Antibiotic(s)	Total daily dose (Dosing interval)	Duration	
2 months to 6 yrs	Gram-negative coccobacilli	*H. influenzae*	Cefotaxime	200 mg/kg/d (6h)	10 days	Chloramphenicol may be used in patients with a serious history of penicillin allergy
	No organisms seen	Any of the above 3	Cefotaxime	200 mg/kg/d (6h)	Variable†	Change to appropriate antibiotic according to culture result
>6 to 40 yrs	Gram-negative diplococci	*N. meningitidis*	Benzylpenicillin	Child—as above Adult-24 mega units or 14.4 g (4h)	7 days	As above
	Gram-positive diplococci	*Str. pneumoniae*	Benzylpenicillin	As above	10 days	As above
	No organisms seen	Any of the above 2	Benzylpenicillin	As above	Variable†	As above
>40 yrs	Gram-positive diplococci	*Str. pneumoniae*	Benzylpenicillin	24 mega units or 14.4 g (4h)	10 days	As above
	Gram-positive bacilli	*L. monocytogenes*	Ampicillin + gentamicin	12 g (4h)	2–3 weeks	Use co-trimoxazole if the patient is allergic to penicillin
	Gram-negative bacilli	'Coliforms' (*Esch. coli, K. aerogenes* etc.)	Cefotaxime+ gentamicin	12 g (4h)	3 weeks	
	No organisms seen	Pneumococci or listeria in most medical patients	Ampicillin	12 g (4h)	Variable†	Use cefotaxime and flucloxacillin for neurosurgical patients; Use cefotaxime for any medical patient with a complicated history; Change to appropriate antibiotic(s) according to culture result

Table 27.3. cont.

Age of patient	CSF Gram-film findings	Presumptive organism	Treatment of choice		Duration	Comments
			Antibiotic(s)	Total daily dose (Dosing interval)		
Any age	Gram-positive cocci in clusters	Staphylococci (usually *Staph. aureus*)	Flucloxacillin + rifampicin	Adult—12 g (4h) Child—200 mg/kg/d (4–6h) Adult—600 mg (12h) oral Child–10 mg/kg/d (12h) oral	3–4 weeks	Rare cause of meningitis, usually encountered after trauma or neurosurgical procedures; Removal of the shunt is essential for optimal therapy in most patients with shunt-associated meningitis; Vancomycin instead of flucloxacillin is recommended if: —the patient is allergic to penicillin; —*Staph. aureus* is methicillin resistant; —The organism isolated is *Staph. epidermidis* (see text)

* In neonates with normal renal function, the unit dose is based on the body weight (usually 2.5 mg/kg) but the interval between the doses varies with the gestational age and the postnatal age (Gestational age ≤28 weeks = 24 h; 29–35 weeks=18 h; 36–40 weeks = 12 h; ≥41 weeks = 8 h).

† Duration will depend upon the organism isolated or strongly suspected.

organisms may reach the CSF and shunt by haematogenous spread or travel in a retrograde fashion from the contaminated peritoneal end of the catheter. Examination of the CSF obtained by needle aspiration of the reservoir will yield an organism in over 90 per cent of cases of shunt-associated meningitis. It is not unusual to have a positive CSF culture in the presence of an otherwise normal CSF in some patients with shunt-associated meningitis. Blood cultures are positive only if meningitis is associated with a ventriculo-atrial shunt.

Most cases of shunt-associated meningitis are treated by complete removal of the shunt system followed by appropriate antibiotics. However, patients with CSF shunts who develop meningitis due to *N. meningitidis*, *H. influenzae* or *Str. pneumoniae* are treated with appropriate antibiotics, without shunt removal.

Since *Staph. epidermidis* is commonly resistant to flucloxacillin, antibiotic therapy should be commenced with parenteral vancomycin combined with oral rifampicin and daily intraventricular vancomycin. High-dose flucloxacillin should be substituted for parenteral vancomycin once it is confirmed that the *Staph. epidermidis* is sensitive to flucloxacillin.

Shunt-associated meningitis caused by *Staph. epidermidis* should be treated for 2 to 3 weeks before a new shunt is inserted.

Streptococcal meningitis

In addition to group B streptococci other streptococci may cause meningitis following head injury, neurosurgical procedures or rupture of cerebral abscess. High-dose benzylpenicillin is the drug of choice. Metronidazole should be added if meningitis is secondary to rupture of an intracranial abscess.

Cryptococcal meningitis

Cryptococcus neoformans is a saprophytic encapsulated fungus commonly found in soil and pigeon droppings. Until recently it was a rare cause of meningitis, occurring mainly in patients who were immunocompromised due to disease or drugs (e.g. lymphomas, leukaemias, organ transplant, sarcoidosis, or those on corticosteroids). The recent dramatic increase in the incidence of cryptococcal meningitis is mainly due to its association with AIDS. Cryptococcal meningitis is reported to occur in about 4 per cent of AIDS patients in the UK, but it can affect up to a third of African patients with AIDS. The most likely mode of transmission of *Cryptococcus* is via the respiratory tract. Most patients present with features of a subacute meningitis or meningo-encephalitis.

Amphotericin B (0.6 to 1.0 mg/kg per day up to a total dose of 2 to 3 g) has been the most common single agent used for the treatment of cryptococcal meningitis. The less toxic flucytosine can be used in combination with amphotericin B, but flucytosine should not be used alone since resistance may emerge during therapy. Addition of flucytosine (150 mg/kg/d) to amphotericin B is associated with fewer failures and relapses (at least in patients without AIDS) and sterilizes CSF more rapidly. Moreover the lower dose amphotericin used (0.3 mg/kg/d) is less nephrotoxic. The duration of treatment is usually 6 weeks. In patients with AIDS, flucytosine is frequently associated with bone marrow suppression and if flucytosine is to be used in these patients, a lower dose (75–100 mg/kg/d), given over a shorter period (2–4 weeks); frequent monitoring of serum levels is recommended.

The antifungal azole, fluconazole, is a welcome advance in the therapy of cryptococcal meningitis, since it is relatively non-toxic, penetrates well into CSF, and is well absorbed when administered orally. However, since relapse occurs in 50 to 60 per cent of patients with AIDS, the recommended therapeutic regimen consists of primary therapy with amphotericin B and flucytosine for 2–6 weeks, followed by long-term maintenance therapy with fluconazole (200–400 mg daily).

Mycobacterium tuberculosis

Tuberculous meningitis can affect any age after the neonatal period. It is uncommon in developed countries, but cases can be missed unless the physician is aware of the possibility and the laboratory is keen to exclude tuberculous meningitis in all cases where abnormal clinical or CSF findings (increased lymphocytes, raised protein, low CSF glucose) have not been satisfactorily explained.

The treatment of tuberculous meningitis is described in Chapter 26.

Culture-negative pyogenic meningitis

About 40 per cent of patients presenting with meningitis will already have received antimicrobial therapy prior to lumbar puncture. Antibiotics which penetrate CSF poorly should produce minimal changes, but those drugs which enter the CSF in significant amounts may cause failure to isolate the organism. Prior therapy does not seriously alter cell counts or protein and glucose concentrations and it is usually still possible to differentiate between bacterial and viral meningitis.

In approximately 10 per cent of cases the aetiology remains unknown. Although prior therapy may confuse the clinical picture it is not detrimental to the individual patient, who has as good a prognosis as those who are untreated. 'Best-guess' therapy should be aimed at all three common bacterial pathogens (see Table 27.3), and cefotaxime for a period of 7 to 10 days would be a reasonable choice, unless there is an obvious meningococcal rash, when benzylpenicillin would be more appropriate.

All patients with culture-negative pyogenic meningitis, especially those in whom there is no history of previous antibiotic to account for the negative results, must be investigated further to exclude other conditions such as tuberculous or cryptococcal meningitis, superficial brain abscess or other parameningeal infections.

BRAIN ABSCESS

Brain abscess is a localized collection of pus within the brain parenchyma. It is a life-threatening condition which used to carry a mortality of 40 per cent. This has now been reduced to less than 10 per cent by the introduction of computerized tomography (CT) and more recently magnetic resonance imaging (MRI), leading to earlier diagnosis and more precise localization, by improvements in surgical and bacteriological techniques, and by the use of appropriate antibiotics. Approximately 4–10 cases a year are seen in neurological units of developed countries.

Unlike bacterial meningitis, brain abscess in children accounts for less than 25 per cent of all cases and, other than in neonates, it is rare in those under 2 years of age.

Pathogenesis

Brain abscesses develop most commonly by spread of infection from an adjacent area (e.g. paranasal sinuses, middle ear, mastoid or dental site), following a penetrating cranial trauma or neurosurgery, or by haematogenous spread from a distant site (e.g. lung abscess, bronchiectasis or endocarditis). Blood-borne spread often causes multiple abscess formation. In about 20 per cent of cases of brain abscess the primary focus of infection remains unrecognized, the so-called 'cryptogenic abscess'. However, as the newer imaging techniques become more widely available, there may be further reduction in the prevalence of cryptogenic abscess.

The location of the predisposing condition has a direct bearing on the site of brain abscess, and on the organisms isolated, which usually reflect those found in the primary focus of infection. With proper attention to technique, the role of anaerobes and polymicrobial infection has become apparent. Brain abscess in association with sinusitis is usually located in the frontal lobe and is most commonly due to *Str. milleri* with or without anaerobes. In contrast, brain abscess following chronic suppurative otitis media or mastoiditis is usually located in the temporal lobe or cerebellum. The infection is invariably polymicrobial; the pus obtained may yield a variety of anaerobes including *Bacteroides* spp., anaerobic streptococci, *Fusobacterium* spp. or *Actinomyces* spp., together with other pathogens including *Str.*

milleri, Haemophilus spp., enterobacteria, or *Ps. aeruginosa. Staph. aureus* is usually isolated in pure culture from brain abscess which has followed trauma, neurosurgery or is secondary to a haematogenous spread from infective endocarditis, whereas *Str. milleri* together with anaerobes and other respiratory pathogens should be suspected in brain abscess complicating pyogenic lung abscess. Rare causes of brain abscess include *M. tuberculosis, L. monocytogenes, Nocardia asteroides, Toxoplasma gondii, Cryptococcus neoformans*, and other fungi.

Lumbar puncture is unhelpful in diagnosis and may be hazardous, but blood cultures may be positive and should be taken.

Treatment

Although a few selected patients with early cerebritis or small, deep or multiple abscesses have been treated successfully with antimicrobial therapy alone, most require surgical drainage of the abscess. This is usually achieved either by aspiration of the abscess after burr-hole placement or by complete surgical excision after craniotomy. Both have been advocated. More recently, CT-guided stereotaxic aspiration, which offers a more accurate drainage with minimal interference to the surrounding normal brain, is gaining popularity.

Pus obtained after any of the above procedures should be sent to the laboratory immediately for urgent microscopy and culture. Because mixtures of aerobic and anaerobic organisms are likely, antimicrobial therapy should cover both possibilities. In the past, benzylpenicillin plus chloramphenicol was widely advocated. Chloramphenicol penetrates well and its broad spectrum covers most anaerobes. However, chloramphenicol is not bactericidal against *B. fragilis* or enterobacteria, which are common in otogenic brain abscess, and its use in combination with β-lactam antibiotics has been associated with high mortality. The combination of chloramphenicol and gentamicin has been found to be antagonistic in experimental meningitis. Moreover, the potential toxicity of chloramphenicol puts it at a disadvantage, since therapy may need to be maintained for 4–6 weeks. For these reasons, cefotaxime and other similar agents (ceftriaxone, ceftazidime) are now recommended. When used in high doses these antibiotics penetrate well into brain abscess pus, and they are bactericidal against a variety of organisms commonly encountered including *Str. milleri, Actinomyces* spp., and enterobacteria. However, cefotaxime alone cannot be recommended in brain abscess for it is not reliably bactericidal against all anaerobes, and for this reason metronidazole should also be used. Although this agent is inactive against aerobes, it is bactericidal for almost all anaerobes and therapeutic concentrations are achieved in the brain even after oral administration.

The initial choice of empiric antimicrobial therapy in brain abscess depends upon the site of the abscess, any predisposing factors, and the results of the Gram-film on the pus, if available. Therapy may be modified, if required, once the culture results are available.

Frontal lobe abscess of sinus origin should be treated with high (meningitic) doses of benzylpenicillin in combination with metronidazole, since *Str. milleri*, with or without anaerobes, is the chief culprit. Temporal lobe or cerebellar abscess of otogenic origin is treated with a combination of high (meningitic) dose cefotaxime and metronidazole. Gentamicin may be added to this regimen if coliform organisms are seen on the Gram-film or are grown in culture. For brain abscesses secondary to trauma or a neurosurgical procedure, or when *Staph. aureus* is strongly suspected or grown, high-dose flucloxacillin in combination with oral rifampicin should be used.

The duration of antimicrobial therapy remains unsettled. It is our practice to administer antibiotics parenterally for at least 3 weeks to all surgically treated patients, often followed by appropriate oral therapy for 4–6 weeks.

28

Viral infections

W. L. Irving

Diseases caused by viruses are extremely common and range from trivial coughs and colds to life-threatening infections. Most viral infections are self limiting, although some that normally cause relatively minor problems can be serious in immunosuppressed patients, or neonates. Some viruses nearly always cause severe disease regardless of the initial status of the host. Rabies, HIV, and several of the viruses causing haemorrhagic fevers fall into this category.

Most success in the control of serious virus infections has been achieved by immunoprophylaxis and to a lesser extent immunotherapy, rather than by the use of specific antiviral chemotherapy. However, as knowledge of the molecular biology of viral replication increases, more potential targets for antiviral drugs are being identified, and several of the experimental compounds undergoing clinical trials hold great promise for the future.

Difficulties in developing drugs that are selectively toxic to the virus while being harmless to the host are explored in Chapter 6. Nevertheless, the advent of acyclovir, ganciclovir, foscarnet, tribavirin, amantadine, zidovudine (and its relatives), and the interferons has resulted in enormous benefit in the treatment of certain virus infections.

HERPESVIRUS INFECTIONS

All seven herpesviruses that infect humans (Table 28.1) exhibit the phenomenon of latency. Following acute infection, virus is not eliminated from the body, but viral DNA remains quiescent without causing any apparent damage to the latently infected cells. Later, virus may be reactivated, the virus replicates, and disease may re-emerge. Herpesvirus infections can therefore be classified as *primary*, the host's first encounter with the virus; or *secondary*, due to reactivation of latent virus, or occasionally to re-infection with exogenous virus. The clinical features of primary and secondary herpesvirus infections are often very different.

Acyclovir is very active against certain herpesviruses and is a truly selective antiviral agent (see Chapter 6). Not all herpesviruses are equally sensitive to the action of acyclovir (Table 28.1). CMV and HHV6 do not possess thymidine kinase, and cannot activate the drug. In practice,

Table 28.1. Human herpesviruses

Name (and usual abbreviation)	Sensitivity to acyclovir
Herpes simplex type 1 (HSV1)	Very sensitive
Herpes simplex type 2 (HSV2)	Very sensitive
Varicella-zoster virus (VZV)	Fairly sensitive
Epstein–Barr virus (EBV)	Poorly sensitive
Cytomegalovirus (CMV)	Insensitive
Human herpesvirus type 6 (HHV6)	Insensitive
Human herpesvirus type 7 (HHV7)	Not known

acyclovir is useful only in the treatment of disease due to the two types of HSV, in varicella-zoster virus infection, and in certain unusual manifestations of EBV infection.

Herpes simplex viruses

While most HSV infections are asymptomatic, there can be a wide range of clinical manifestations.

Primary orolabial HSV infection

Symptomatic primary infection, which usually occurs in children, presents with extensive painful blistering and ulceration of the lips, tongue and mucous membranes of the mouth, sometimes with marked cervical lymphadenopathy and fever. Left untreated, the infection is self limiting, with complete healing in 2–3 weeks. Oral acyclovir therapy significantly reduces the manifestations of systemic disease, the formation of new lesions, the period of virus excretion, and the time to healing; it is of unquestioned therapeutic benefit.

Recurrent orolabial HSV infection

Resolution of primary disease is followed by the establishment of latency of HSV within the trigeminal nerve ganglion. This virus can be reactivated in later life and track back down the nerve to reach the mouth.

The manifestations of reactivated disease in an immunocompetent host are usually mild: there is no systemic upset, only a few lesions (cold sores) localized to a small area on the lips; the inflammatory response is less, with less pain and swelling, and the lesions heal in about 5–6 days. Acyclovir therapy enhances resolution of lesions by about 24 h.

Given the mild nature of recurrent disease (as compared with primary infection), and the marginal benefit of acyclovir, routine systemic treatment of cold sores is not recommended. However, acyclovir cream is now available over the counter in the UK, and many patients with recurrent cold sores give eloquent testimony to the value of this therapy, whatever the results of double-blind placebo-controlled trials may say!

Eczema herpeticum

Intact skin is a very efficient barrier to the spread of viruses. However, in patients with chronic dermatitis or eczema, this barrier is not intact, and virus can spread freely. Eczema herpeticum is a severe complication of primary or secondary orolabial HSV infection in patients with eczema. Lesions extend for large areas on the face, neck, and upper chest. Virus may also gain access to the bloodstream through cracks in the skin, putting the patient at risk of death from disseminated HSV infection. Acyclovir therapy is mandatory. Patients should be given supplies of acyclovir so that they can initiate therapy themselves in the early stages of recurrent disease.

Ocular HSV infection

HSV is the commonest infectious cause of blindness in the UK. Children are particularly adept at self inoculating the eye with virus-infected oral secretions. Spread of virus on to the cornea results in keratitis and may lead to chronic ulceration and inflammatory changes. Management should include the early involvement of specialist ophthalmological advice, as well as acyclovir ointment.

Genital herpes

The clinical manifestations and management of primary and secondary genital herpes are analogous to those of orolabial disease. Thus primary infection results in extensive bilateral, painful ulceration with spread on to adjacent skin, inguinal adenopathy, and fever, lasting 2–3 weeks. Patients may experience difficulty in passing urine, and cervicitis with profuse discharge is common in women. Oral acyclovir is of proven benefit. Recurrent disease is much more localized, with no systemic upset, and shorter lasting; oral acyclovir is of marginal value.

Some unfortunate individuals may suffer severe recurrent attacks of genital herpes as frequently as once a month. The immunological basis for this debilitating and depressing condition is not understood. One approach to the management of these patients is to give them continuous prophylactic acyclovir. This results in a considerable decrease in the frequency of attacks, and many patients have now been on prophylaxis for many years without apparent side-effects.

Neonatal herpes

Pregnant women with genital herpes are at risk of passing on the infection during childbirth. Neonatal HSV infection is a potentially devastating disease, as virus may disseminate to internal organs very easily, and such babies may die of HSV hepatitis, pneumonitis, or encephalitis. Survivors are almost invariably left with severe neurological sequelae. Although mortality from neonatal herpes has improved with the use of intravenous acyclovir, overall morbidity has scarcely been affected, presumably because by the time the diagnosis is made, and therapy initiated, the damage has already been done.

Herpes simplex encephalitis

Herpes simplex encephalitis is the commonest form of sporadic viral encephalitis, with an annual incidence of about one case per million population. Most cases occur in individuals with evidence of prior infection with HSV. Thus the disease is usually a manifestation of secondary infection, although the route by which virus gains access to the brain is not clear.

Untreated, mortality is high, and survivors suffer severe long-term damage. Diagnosis is difficult. The CSF usually shows a pleocytosis, but it is very rare to succeed in isolating HSV from CSF. Specific viral DNA may be detected in CSF at the acute stage by the polymerase chain reaction, but this test is not universally available.

The use of intravenous acyclovir, in high dosage, has been shown to improve the prognosis of these patients dramatically, providing therapy is started as soon as the diagnosis is suspected, without waiting for laboratory confirmation. Vidarabine has also been used successfully in herpes encephalitis but trials have shown acyclovir to be at least as beneficial, considerably less toxic, and easier to administer.

Immunocompromised patients

Patients who are immunocompromised for whatever reason are at risk of severe primary or secondary HSV disease. All HSV infections in this group of patients should be treated promptly with acyclovir, if necessary by the intravenous route. In bone marrow transplant recipients, prophylactic acyclovir is recommended.

Varicella-zoster virus

Chicken-pox

The primary manifestation of infection with VZV is chicken-pox. This is usually a trivial disease of children, despite the dramatic rash. The most important complication of chicken-pox is varicella pneumonia, which can be life threatening. This is considerably more common in adults than in children, and seems to be more common in pregnant women who develop chicken-pox. Adults with chicken-pox should be referred to hospital for intravenous acyclovir therapy if evidence of respiratory involvement occurs.

It has been suggested that all adults, and even all children, with chicken-pox should be given acyclovir, and, indeed, the drug is now licensed in the UK for these purposes. The arguments in favour of this blanket approach are economic rather than medical. Acyclovir allows resolution of the disease 24–48 h earlier than would otherwise be the case, enabling adults, or carers of sick children, to return to work that much sooner. The frequency of complications in adults is so small that even large-scale clinical trials have failed to prove that acyclovir therapy will reduce their incidence.

Neonatal chicken-pox

Pregnant women who develop chicken-pox towards the end of their pregnancy may pass infection on to their baby if it is born within a week of onset of the maternal rash; i.e. before sufficient time has elapsed to allow the mother to generate protective antibodies which can be transferred across the placenta.

Neonatal chicken-pox is a feared disease, and babies at risk should be given passive immunization with hyperimmune zoster immune globulin. It is also reasonable to give such babies prophylactic acyclovir, although some would prefer to withhold the drug until the baby developed signs of disease.

Herpes zoster

The site of latency of VZV is the dorsal root ganglion. The systemic nature of the rash in chicken-pox means that dorsal root ganglia up and down the spinal cord become latently infected. Reactivation of infection thus results in virus travelling down the nerve in question, to reach the dermatome supplied by that nerve. This accounts for the characteristic rash of shingles, or herpes zoster, the clinical manifestation of reactivated infection. The onset of rash is often preceded by pain or abnormal sensation in the distribution of the dermatome. The rash usually heals uneventfully, but pain in the area of the rash may persist long after the rash itself has resolved. This *post-herpetic neuralgia* is more likely to occur in elderly patients, and can be extremely debilitating.

Other complications of secondary VZV infection occasionally occur: reactivation of virus in the ophthalmic branch of the trigeminal nerve may result in keratitis and damage to the cornea; facial nerve involvement may cause a form of Bell's palsy; involvement of sacral ganglia may result in urinary and anal retention.

A prolonged or atypical attack of herpes zoster may be the presenting feature of a number of diseases in which host immune responses are impaired. These include malignancy of the reticuloendothelial system, and HIV infection. In these patients dissemination of the reactivated VZV may occur with the appearance of lesions outside the initial dermatome. This may indicate that virus has disseminated to involve internal organs, and this can be life threatening.

The aims of antiviral therapy of reactivated VZV infection include alleviation of the pain and discomfort of the rash itself, and the prevention of complications, including post-herpetic neuralgia. Early acyclovir therapy may certainly achieve the former. Whether the natural history of post-herpetic neuralgia is affected by antiviral therapy is controversial. Evidence is emerging that acyclovir may alter the quality of the pain experienced by the patient from a continual burning with hyperaesthesia to a more manageable throbbing. The question remains as to which patients should receive acyclovir or famciclovir therapy. Most clinicians routinely treat all herpes zoster in elderly patients, but the definition of elderly varies, perhaps in relation to the age of the clinician concerned!

Other indications for acyclovir therapy of herpes zoster include zoster of the ophthalmic or facial nerves, sacral zoster, disseminated zoster, and any form of zoster in an immunocompromised host.

Epstein–Barr virus

Considerably larger doses of acyclovir are necessary to inhibit EBV replication *in vitro* than HSV or VZV. This presumably reflects the efficiency of the phosphorylation of the drug by the different viruses. The results of clinical trials of acyclovir in patients with infectious mononucleosis have been disappointing.

The only manifestation of EBV infection in which acyclovir is useful is that of oral hairy leukoplakia. This unusual disease arises only in immunocompromised patients, most commonly those with HIV infection. It presents as a whitish coating on the tongue and/or buccal mucosa, which may resemble candidiasis. The lesions are packed full of replicating EBV. The lesions may respond to acyclovir therapy, but reappear when treatment is stopped, so that long-term use of the drug may be necessary.

Cytomegalovirus

Primary infections

Primary CMV infections of immunocompetent individuals are usually asymptomatic, although a small minority result in glandular fever, the infectious mononucleosis syndrome. The site of virus latency is currently unknown, and reactivation fails to induce any recognizable disease in the individual concerned. There are two groups of patients, however, in whom CMV is a significant pathogen: babies infected *in utero*, and immunocompromised patients.

Congenital infection
Transfer of CMV across the placenta may arise from both primary and reactivated maternal CMV infection. Congenital CMV infection affects about 1 in 300 live births in the UK. Most of these babies develop normally, but about 5–10 per cent are born with so-called *cytomegalic inclusion disease*, which is often fatal. A further 5–10 per cent of infected babies are normal at birth, but later develop abnormalities such as deafness, impaired neurodevelopment, or learning difficulties.

There is presently no effective strategy for the prevention of congenital CMV infection. Antiviral therapy may be beneficial for normal babies who are destined to develop abnormalities, as there is evidence that some of the damage is mediated by replication of virus after birth. However, there is currently no way of prospectively identifying babies at risk, and, in any case, toxicity of the available anti-CMV drugs precludes their widespread use.

Immunocompromised patients
Symptomatic CMV disease may arise from primary or secondary infection in immunocompromised patients, including those infected with HIV and transplant recipients. The disease often presents with fever and leucopenia, together with hepatitis, retinitis, pneumonitis, encephalitis, oesophagitis, or colitis. Ganciclovir therapy is a useful advance, although it has to be administered intravenously, and treatment may be accompanied by a galaxy of toxic side-effects, particularly on the bone marrow. Not all complications of CMV infection respond equally well to ganciclovir.

Treatment of CMV pneumonitis is often unsuccessful because pathogenesis of the pneumonitis is not entirely due to the virus itself; aberrant host immune responses to the virus may also contribute to the disease process. Nevertheless ganciclovir can save the sight of patients with CMV retinitis, and CMV infections of the bowel and liver also respond well.

Therapy does not result in elimination of the virus, and, in patients who continue to be immunosuppressed, disease often recurs when therapy is stopped. Low-dose suppressive therapy, involving intravenous administration of ganciclovir on an outpatient basis, may prove to benefit such patients.

Prophylaxis of CMV disease
Prevention of serious CMV disease in transplant recipients can be achieved by avoiding transplantation of material from latently infected donors to uninfected recipients. Alternatively, the use of CMV immunoglobulin may be beneficial. Surprisingly, acyclovir prophylaxis reduces the frequency of serious CMV disease in renal and bone marrow

transplant recipients. Serum levels of acyclovir in these patients are well below the concentrations necessary to inhibit CMV replication, but sufficiently high levels are possibly achieved inside infected cells.

Foscarnet also exhibits anti-CMV activity, but is nephrotoxic and has to be given by the intravenous route.

Human herpesviruses 6 and 7

HHV6 is the causative agent of *roseola infantum*, one of the childhood rashes. Occasional cases are associated with a hepatitis or encephalitis. HHV6 is sensitive *in vitro* to ganciclovir, but not acyclovir; however, the value of treatment is unknown. No disease has yet been associated with either primary or secondary infection with HHV7.

RESPIRATORY TRACT INFECTIONS

Upper respiratory tract infections

Infections of the upper respiratory tract with rhinoviruses (of which there are over 100 serotypes), corona-, entero-, adeno-, respiratory syncytial, and parainfluenza viruses are extremely common, but, fortunately, result in very little serious morbidity or mortality. Despite considerable effort on the part of the pharmaceutical industry, no specific antiviral therapy has been successfully developed for treatment or prevention of these infections.

Intranasal interferon spray is effective in the treatment and prophylaxis of the types of common cold that are caused specifically by rhinoviruses, but patients using the interferon spray experience nasal stuffiness, irritation, and bleeding, which negates any possible therapeutic benefit. Thus for practical purposes this approach to the management of the common cold has now been abandoned.

Lower respiratory tract infections

Viral infection of the lower respiratory tract is potentially much more dangerous. The commonest viral infections giving rise to bronchiolitis and pneumonia are those due to respiratory syncytial and influenza viruses. Varicella pneumonia and CMV pneumonitis have been referred to above. In addition, giant-cell pneumonia is a rare and fatal complication of measles, usually in leukaemic children who escape vaccination.

RSV infection of infants

Bronchiolitis and pneumonia due to respiratory syncytial virus (RSV) infection are relatively common in infants under 1 year of age. Tribavirin (known as ribavirin outside the UK) is effective in achieving reduced viral shedding, faster resolution of fever, improved respiration, and a shorter stay in hospital. The main difficulty is that the drug needs to be administered as an aerosol by use of a small-particle aerosol generator. Furthermore, for maximum benefit, the patient must breathe nebulized drug for at least 12 h each day.

Untreated RSV infection is often fatal in babies with congenital immunodeficiency or heart or lung defects; in these patients, tribavirin therapy can be life saving. In immunocompetent babies, severe RSV infection may predispose to the later development of wheezing or asthma. Whether or not prompt treatment with tribavirin reduces this risk is under investigation.

Influenza

Influenza A (but not B) virus is susceptible to the action of amantadine. Clinical trials in boarding schools and other places in which large numbers of individuals are crowded together have shown that amantadine performs better than placebo in both treatment and prophylaxis of influenza A. Those treated with the drug have a milder, shorter-lasting infection. About 70 per cent of contacts given the drug are protected from infection. However, in the elderly, who suffer the brunt of serious influenza, amantadine is poorly tolerated, because of its stimulatory actions on the central nervous system. Patients become confused and agitated, and may be unable to sleep. As a result, the drug is unpopular. It may fare better as a prophylactic agent, to prevent spread in an institution where influenza infection has already occurred. Vaccination of non-infected individuals may take 2 weeks to induce protection, whereas protection with amantadine is demonstrable after a few hours. Amantadine is also an alternative for those in whom vaccination is contraindicated because of egg allergy or for other reasons.

Rimantadine, a derivative of amantadine, is said to be equipotent in its anti-influenzal properties while being less prone to side-effects. However, it is not currently licensed in the UK.

Influenza A and B viruses, as well as the parainfluenza viruses, are sensitive to tribavirin *in vitro*. The drug has been succesfully used in severe lower respiratory tract infection with these viruses, but experience is limited.

CHRONIC VIRAL HEPATITIS

Patients infected with hepatitis B or C viruses (HBV or HCV) may become chronic carriers. These patients are at risk of continuing inflammation in the liver, leading to chronic hepatitis, cirrhosis, and ultimately, hepatocellular carcinoma. So far, the only agents to have shown consistent therapeutic benefit in the treatment of chronic HBV or HCV hepatitis are the interferons.

All chronic carriers of HBV have detectable hepatitis B surface antigen (HBsAg) in their peripheral blood. However HBsAg-positive individuals can be subdivided further into those in whom HBeAg (a breakdown product of the viral core antigen) can be detected, and those with antibodies to this antigen, anti-HBe. HBeAg is a marker of active viral replication in hepatocytes. HBeAg-positive patients are considerably more infectious and are at much greater risk of the long-term deleterious consequences of HBV carriage, than are anti-HBe-positive patients. For these reasons, therapy for chronic HBV infection is targeted at those HBsAg carriers who are HBeAg positive.

It is the immunomodulatory activity of interferons which provides the basis for their action in reducing HBV replication in chronically infected patients. Interferon enhances the expression of human leucocyte antigen (HLA) class I molecules on the surface of HBV-infected hepatocytes, resulting in the efficient elimination of these cells by circulating cytotoxic T lymphocytes. This in turn reduces the amount of virus in the liver, and inhibits viral replication. The patient is now able to respond to the reduced amounts of HBeAg by generating anti-HBe.

A typical response of an HBV carrier to therapy with interferon is shown in Fig. 28.1. At the onset of therapy, the patient is HBsAg and HBeAg positive, and has a raised alanine aminotransferase level (ALT) which indicates continuing liver cell damage. Some weeks after the initiation of interferon therapy, there is a marked rise in ALT. Paradoxically, this indicates a good therapeutic response, since it shows that hepatocytes are now expressing sufficient HLA class I molecules to enable their recognition and destruction by cytotoxic lymphocytes. At the end of therapy, liver function returns to normal and the patient is now anti-HBe positive. Note that the patient remains HBsAg positive. Thus virus has not been completely eliminated, but the risk of ongoing liver damage is much reduced, and the patient is much less of an infection risk to sexual partners and family members. By following these patients for many years, it is possible to show that many of them eventually lose HBsAg.

Not all HBV carriers respond to interferon therapy. Those who have been carriers of the virus from birth (the vast majority of HBV carriers world-wide) and patients who are immunocompromised (including those with HIV infection, in whom HBV carriage is common, as the routes of transmission of the two viruses are similar) respond poorly. In other patients, response rates are over 50 per cent.

Most patients with chronic non-A non-B hepatitis are now known to be infected with hepatitis C virus (HCV). About 40-50 per cent of

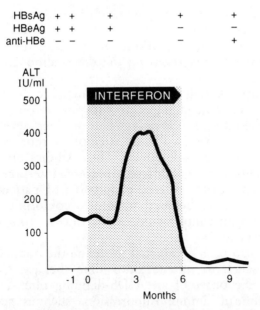

Fig. 28.1. Treatment of chronic hepatitis B infection with interferon showing the change in alanine aminotransferase (ALT) levels, loss of hepatitis B e antigen (HBeAg), and the appearance of antibody to HBe (anti-HBe). Hepatitis B surface antigen (HBsAg) is not eliminated.

such patients respond to a 6 month course of interferon, as judged by improvement in liver function, but about half relapse when therapy is stopped, indicating that virus is still active. Longer regimens of therapy or long-term low-dose maintenance therapy might reduce this relapse rate. Interferon does not cause a rise in ALT levels in patients with HCV, suggesting that the drug has a direct antiviral effect, rather than acting indirectly through its immunomodulatory activity.

Tribavirin therapy provides modest benefit in chronic HCV disease and may prove to be a useful adjunct to interferon therapy.

HIV INFECTION

Enormous effort is being expended in the development of potential anti-HIV agents, including exploration of viral protease inhibitors, anti-sense oligonucleotides, and inhibitors of the regulatory *tat* gene. However, the only drugs that have demonstrated clinically useful anti-HIV activity thus far are the reverse transcriptase inhibitors (see Chapter 6).

Double-blind, placebo-controlled clinical trials of zidovudine (AZT) in patients with end-stage HIV infection have demonstrated improved survival, reduced incidence of opportunistic infection, and partial restoration of laboratory markers of immune function (e.g. CD4 count) in those patients receiving the drug, although adverse effects were common.

Many subsequent trials have been conducted to define better the use of zidovudine. Combined regimens with interferon or acyclovir, and alternating schedules of zidovudine plus another reverse transcriptase inhibitor, have been assessed in an attempt to improve response rates and decrease unwanted side-effects. These studies often involve hundreds of patients in many different centres. Interpretation of results is not made any easier by the propensity of patients to exchange drugs, so that it may be hard to ensure conformity with the trial protocol. Not surprisingly, conclusions drawn from these trials are often controversial!

Trials have also been conducted to define the optimal stage of HIV infection at which to initiate zidovudine therapy. Options include waiting until the onset of an AIDS-defining illness, or of signs of clinically significant immunosuppression, such as severe zoster or oral candidiasis. Alternatively, the CD4 count can be monitored, and antiviral therapy considered when this falls below a critical level such as 500 per μl. There is conflicting evidence as to whether treatment of asymptomatic patients with normal CD4 counts is beneficial or not. The clinical significance of the emergence of zidovudine-resistant mutants in patients receiving long-term therapy (see Chapter 6) is not clear, but any possible benefits to be gained by the early treatment of asymptomatic patients have to be weighed against the possibility that early treatment with zidovudine may lead to correspondingly early emergence of drug-resistant mutants. The decision as to when to initiate antiviral therapy in an HIV-positive patient is one that can be taken only after informed discussion between clinician and patient.

HIV-positive patients are at risk of a wide range of serious infections. These are discussed in Chapter 29.

OTHER INFECTIONS

Warts

Papillomavirus infections (warts) are amenable to physical (cryotherapy, surgery) and chemical (podophyllin and derivatives, salicylic acid) therapies. Interferons may have a place in the management of recalcitrant warts. About 50 per cent of warts disappear following intralesional or intramuscular interferon, but they often recur.

Polyoma virus infections

Cytosine arabinoside (Ara C) is a cytotoxic drug which may be of benefit in the treatment of progressive multifocal leukoencephalopathy, a disease which occurs almost exclusively in HIV-positive and other immunosuppressed patients. It is a manifestation of reactivation of a polyoma virus in the brain.

Lassa fever

Tribavirin, taken orally, is very effective in the treatment and prophylaxis of lassa fever, a virus infection encountered in certain parts of West Africa.

Diarrhoea

The treatment of viral gastroenteritis is considered in Chapter 22.

29

Infection in immunocompromised patients

R. G. Finch

The care of the immunocompromised patient is an increasingly important and challenging aspect of medicine which encompasses individuals suffering from a variety of underlying disease states rendering them especially vulnerable to microbial challenge. The term *immunocompromised* describes patients with either immunodeficiency states or those who are immunosuppressed.

IMMUNODEFICIENCY

Immunodeficiency may be congenital or acquired and can affect particular aspects of humoral, cell-mediated or phagocytic cell function (Table 29.1). In general such states are relatively rare in medical practice. However, the advent of the HIV pandemic has altered this situation since it is now estimated that in excess of 10 million persons are infected world-wide, making it the commonest cause of acquired immunodeficiency. The primary deficiency in HIV infection is one of an inexorable decline in cell-mediated immune function as a result of the human immunodeficiency virus targeting a variety of cell lines, in particular the CD4 lymphocyte which has a central role in orchestrating the immune system.

IMMUNOSUPPRESSION

In contrast to immunodeficiency states, immunosuppression affects patients whose immune defences are impaired, either as a result of an underlying disease or its management by cytotoxic, immunosuppressive or radiation therapy. The immunosuppressed patient often has an underlying malignant disease, or has undergone organ or bone marrow transplantation. In both situations, part of the therapeutic strategy involves suppression or ablation of host immune functions.

In general the state of immunosuppression is finite, unlike immunodeficiency disorders which are generally permanent or progressive; once the immunosuppressive regimen is reduced or withdrawn the

Table 29.1. Examples of immunodeficiency states associated with an increased frequency of severity of infection

---

Primary immunodeficiency
  B cell deficiencies
    IgA deficiency
    X-linked agammaglobulinaemia
    Common variable immunodeficiency
    IgG subclass deficiency
  T cell deficiencies
    Severe combined immunodeficiency
    DiGeorge anomaly
    Wiskott–Aldrich syndrome
    Adenosine deaminase deficiency
    MHC class I deficiency
Secondary immunodeficiency
    Acquired immunodeficiency syndrome
    Genetic complement deficiencies
Congenital deficiency of phagocytosis
    Chronic granulomatous disease
    Leucocyte adhesion deficiency

MHC = major histocompatibility complex.

host's defences can recover. The compromised defences include not only the humoral, phagocytic, and cell-mediated components of the immune system, but also skin and mucous membranes, the integrity of which may be impaired by cytotoxic drugs. The vulnerability of the patient to infection may be compounded by the use of intravascular catheters, bladder catheters, and in the case of ventilated patients, endotracheal tubes.

The major features of immunosuppression associated with various malignant conditions are summarized in Table 29.2. Such patients are often cared for in high-dependency or intensive care facilities which provide opportunities for cross-infection and the acquisition of hospital-associated, and therefore more antibiotic-resistant, pathogens.

MICROBIAL COMPLICATIONS IN THE IMMUNOCOMPROMISED HOST

The variety of infections that may occur in the immunocompromised patient is extensive and arises from either exogenous or endogenous micro-organisms. The distinction between exogenous and endogenous

Table 29.2. Examples of immunosuppressive states associated with an increased frequency or severity of infection according to altered host defences

Disease	Mucosal surfaces	Phagocytosis	Humoral immunity	CMI
Acute lymphoblastic leukaemia	+	+ +	−	+
Acute myeloblastic leukaemia	+	+ +	−	+
Chronic lymphocytic leukaemia	−	−	+ +	+
Hodgkin's, non-Hodgkin's lymphoma	−	−	−	−
Solid tumours	+ +	−	−	+
Multiple myeloma	−	−	+ +	−

CMI cell-mediated immunity.
− = association absent; + = definite association; + + = marked association.

infections is not always clear cut, since in hospital the bacterial flora of the skin and mucous membranes often alters.

In the case of virus infections, the herpes group predominates and may represent primary infection or reactivation of latent virus; these infections are often more severe than those in the immunocompetent host and carry the risk of dissemination.

Fungal infections can be particularly severe. Candidosis of the mouth and upper gastrointestinal tract is particularly common and from time to time may be complicated by candidaemia, with spread to other organs. *Cryptococcus neoformans*, a yeast which was an uncommon cause of meningitis until the AIDS pandemic, occasionally complicates organ transplantation and malignant lymphoma.

Among the filamentous fungi, *Aspergillus* spp. are the most common pathogens. Their ubiquitous spores are normally harmless to the immunocompetent, but in the immunocompromised patient they can cause serious lung infection which may disseminate throughout the body. This risk is greatest in patients with profound neutropenia. Aspergillosis is not only difficult to treat but is also difficult to diagnose, especially in the early stages of infection.

The immunocompromised patient is also vulnerable to parasitic infections. Among these *Pneumocystis carinii* has emerged as the leading opportunistic infection complicating HIV infection. It primarily affects the lung where it produces a severe progressive pneumonia, which may be fatal unless treated early. Pneumocystosis may also occur in patients undergoing organ transplantation and in those with lymphoblastic leukaemia or malignant lymphoma; profound impairment of cell-mediated immunity characterizes all these conditions. *P. carinii* may be a fungus, although its pattern of susceptibility to chemotherapeutic agents is more in keeping with a protozoon. Other parasitic infections in the immunocompromised host include toxoplasmosis and a variety of gut infections such as giardiasis, cryptosporidiosis, microsporidiosis, and strongyloidiasis. The latter can progress to a state of hyperinfection with extensive larval invasion of the body.

PRINCIPLES OF CHEMOTHERAPEUTIC CONTROL

The vulnerability of the immunocompromised patient to infection has been emphasized. Not only is the range of possible infections broad, but, because of the state of immunosuppression, the presentation may be atypical and the course fulminant. A specific clinical and microbiological diagnosis can be difficult to establish; the therapeutic management of such patients is consequently based on a set of principles that has evolved to meet their particular needs.

It is essential that the patient is thoroughly examined at the earliest suspicion of infection. Particular attention should be paid to the skin, perineum, entry sites for catheters, the mouth, lungs, and abdomen. Appropriate microbiological samples should be collected and necessary radiographic investigations obtained. The approach to the chemotherapeutic management of the immunocompromised patient is particularly well demonstrated in:

(1) patients with haematological malignancies undergoing cytotoxic chemotherapy or bone marrow transplantation, especially during episodes of profound neutropenia;
(2) patients with the acquired immunodeficiency syndrome (AIDS);
(3) those with specific immunological defects such as hyposplenism.

Neutropenic patients

In the neutropenic patient infection can develop rapidly over a matter of hours, and if untreated can prove fatal. If fever of >38 °C persists for 2 h of more, it is now accepted that broad-spectrum antibiotic therapy should be administered promptly by the intravenous route. However, documentation of infection can be difficult: about 20 per cent of infections will be documented by blood culture, a further 20 per cent by other microbiological investigations, and a further 20 per cent by clinical criteria. In the remainder, infection may only be strongly suspected without supporting clinical or laboratory evidence, while non-microbial causes such as drug reactions, blood or platelet transfusions, or the underlying disease state may be responsible for the febrile episode.

Table 29.3. Distribution of bloodstream isolates complicating neutropenic states

Micro-organism	Approximate percentage
Gram-positive bacteria	
Staphylococcus epidermidis	28
Staph. aureus	10
Corynebacterium spp.	5
Streptococci	12
Gram-negative bacteria	
Gram-negative enteric bacilli	28
Pseudomonas aeruginosa	7
Others	7
Fungi	
Candida spp.	3

Treatment regimens

The variety and relative frequency of bloodstream pathogens in the neutropenic patient are summarized in Table 29.3. There has been a striking increase in Gram-positive infections in recent years, which in part relates to the widespread use of vascular catheters for drug administration, as well as the selective pressure arising from the use of broad-spectrum β-lactam antibiotics.

In general the antibiotic regimens have been based on a combination of a β-lactam antibiotic and an aminoglycoside, which together are active against most of the likely pathogens. Among the β-lactams, a broad-spectrum cephalosporin such as ceftazidime has been most widely used, although the ureidopenicillins, piperacillin and azlocillin are also popular. An aminoglycoside such as gentamicin or amikacin is administered simultaneously since both are active against Gram-negative bacilli, including *Pseudomonas aeruginosa*. The use of a single agent such as ceftazidime or imipenem has been adopted by some centres, but the combined regimen offers synergistic activity that may be useful, especially when dealing with serious *Ps. aeruginosa* bacteraemia. The recent increase in Gram-positive positive infections caused by staphylococci, enterococci, and viridans streptococci reflects a relative weakness in these regimens; as a result a glycopeptide, such as vancomycin or teicoplanin, may be needed, especially in patients who have recently undergone bone marrow transplantation in whom a neutropenic febrile episode can be particularly serious.

Systemic fungal infections need specific treatment. Yeasts may respond to azole derivatives, such as fluconazole or itraconazole. Failure to respond is an indication for intravenous amphotericin B, which is also the drug of choice for infections with filamentous fungi. This agent is very toxic and the drug is given in gradually increasing dosage. Administration of amphotericin B encapsulated within liposomes appears to be safer, and such a formulation is appropriate if toxicity problems preclude the use of the parent drug.

Chemoprophylaxis

The seriousness of infections in the severely immunosuppressed neutropenic patient has led to the use of chemoprophylactic drug regimens, particularly in patients undergoing cytotoxic chemotherapy for haematological malignancies and in bone marrow transplant recipients. Regimens are directed at those micro-organisms likely to result in bacteraemic disease.

The varied choice of prophylactic regimen reflects different views on the pathogenesis of infection in these patients. One view is that oral, non-absorbable antibiotics are desirable in that their effect is confined to the gastrointestinal tract, which is the major source of invasive micro-organisms. Regimens have included agents active against *Candida* spp. because of the frequency and severity of oral and upper gastrointestinal candidosis. A combination of framycetin, colistin, and nystatin was among the earliest of these oral, non-absorbable regimens. Other variations include neomycin, colistin, and nystatin; or gentamicin, vancomycin, and nystatin. One important problem with these regimens is that their bitter taste leads to poor patient compliance. Moreover, evidence that they reduce the frequency and severity of bacteraemic infections has been difficult to obtain.

As an alternative to these regimens, other agents have been adopted which have systemic antibiotic effects. Co-trimoxazole has been widely used for its activity against many Gram-negative enteric bacilli and Gram-positive pathogens. It is also active against *P. carinii*. However, the emergence of drug-resistant strains, poor activity against *Ps. aeruginosa*, and the danger of bone marrow suppression in bone marrow recipients make this antifolate compound less than ideal.

Fluoroquinolones provide broad-spectrum activity, high potency, and a systemic antibiotic effect, with substantial drug concentrations within the gut. There is strong evidence to indicate that these drugs achieve a reduction in serious Gram-negative bacteraemia, although the relative weakness of the quinolones against Gram-positive pathogens has also been clearly demonstrated. Ofloxacin and ciprofloxacin have been most widely used. When given by the oral route they appear to provide a cost-effective approach in high-risk patients, especially those undergoing bone marrow transplantation.

Selective decontamination of the digestive tract

As well as patients rendered neutropenic by chemotherapy or disease, the ventilated patient on the intensive care unit is at considerable risk of infection, in particular from pneumonia from aspiration of oropharyngeal flora. One experimental approach has been to use a topical antibiotic regimen, applied to the mouth in the form of paste and given in liquid form via a nasogastric tube into the stomach and hence the gastrointestinal tract. The aim is to suppress the flora of the gastrointestinal tract, which is largely made up of aerobic and anaerobic micro-organisms. One widely studied regimen is a combination of polymyxin, gentamicin, and amphotericin B, often supplemented for the first few days with intravenous cefotaxime. The pathogens targeted by this regimen include *Staphylococcus aureus, Escherichia coli, Proteus* spp., *Klebsiella* spp., and *Candida* spp., which are among the more common causes of infection in such patients. Studies have shown a reduction in bacterial counts in the mouth, stomach, and colon. There is also evidence that nosocomial pneumonia in young, relatively fit patients who have sustained major trauma may be reduced. However, the cost–benefit of this procedure in terms of reduced mortality and length of stay in hospital has proved more difficult to establish.

AIDS

The medical impact of HIV infection lies in its persistent nature and the progressive immunodeficiency which gives rise to a range of complicating infections and malignancies. These target many organs as well as producing systemic illness. Table 29.4 summarizes the more important complicating infections.

In contrast to their effects in the immunocompetent host, these infections often present atypically and with heightened severity. Furthermore, many of the infections recur after treatment. Thus, in the HIV-infected patient the initial course of treatment must be more intensive than in the immunocompetent host, and for many conditions long-term suppressive therapy is needed to prevent relapse. In addition, by controlling the underlying HIV infection, the frequency and severity of opportunistic infections can be reduced.

The chemotherapeutic approach to selective opportunistic infections is discussed in order to emphasize the principles and associated problems that arise. The chemotherapeutic options for control of HIV infection are discussed in Chapters 6 and 28. In brief, current antiretroviral chemotherapy relies on the nucleoside analogues—zidovudine, didanosine, and zalcitabine. All act in a suppressive manner to delay disease progression.

Table 29.4. Common opportunist pathogens complicating HIV disease

Site	Micro-organism
Gastrointestinal tract	*Cryptosporidium parvum*
	Giardia lamblia
	Salmonella spp.
	Mycobacterium avium complex
	Cytomegalovirus
	Herpes simplex
Respiratory tract	*Pneumocystis carinii*
	Streptococcus pneumoniae
	Mycobacterium tuberculosis
	Cytomegalovirus
Central nervous system	*Toxoplasma gondii*
	Cryptococcus neoformans
	Human immunodeficiency virus
	Herpes simplex

Pneumocystis carinii

Among the many opportunistic infections that complicate HIV infection, *P. carinii* predominates. The primary site of infection is the lung. Clinical disease represents reactivation of endogenous infection acquired in childhood. Typical symptoms include progressive shortness of breath, with or without a relatively unproductive cough, progressive hypoxaemia, and diffuse bilateral chest X-ray infiltrates. The diagnosis has been greatly facilitated by the availability of a fluorescent antibody to *P. carinii* which can be applied to expectorated sputum or to a saline lavage obtained by bronchoscopy. The treatment of choice is high-dose co-trimoxazole, by mouth or intravenously, for 3 weeks. The risk of hypersensitivity to the sulphonamide component is greatly increased in HIV disease and alternative regimens such as intravenous pentamidine or oral atovaquone may be necessary. Once the patient has recovered it is necessary to continue with life-long prophylaxis, either with low-dose co-trimoxazole, or nebulized pentamidine given once-monthly as an aerosol inhalation. Alternative agents that can be used in those intolerant to the standard regimens include dapsone, clindamycin, and primaquine. In view of the seriousness of *P. carinii* pneumonia, patients with HIV infection are now offered primary prophylaxis when their CD4 lymphocyte counts fall below $200/\mu l$ in order to prevent infection. The choice of agent is the same as for secondary prophylaxis.

Toxoplasmosis

The protozoon *Toxoplasma gondii* can cause serious disease in those with HIV infection. This may occur as a primary infection, although it more usually represents reactivation of dormant parasites. The disease presents most frequently as a space-occupying lesion of the brain with focal neurological features. The diagnosis is based on clinical suspicion and computed tomography (CT scan). Serodiagnosis is difficult. The presence of tachyzoites in brain biopsy is confirmatory. However, it is more usual to carry out a trial of chemotherapy in the first instance since this can avoid potentially dangerous neurosurgery.

Toxoplasmosis is treated with pyrimethamine and sulphadiazine in high dosage. This regimen often results in bone marrow suppression or is complicated by an allergic skin eruption. Alternative drugs include high-dose clindamycin or the azalide, azithromycin, which also exhibits useful activity. The principles of treatment are similar to those for controlling *P. carinii* pneumonia in that initial control is followed by lifelong maintenance therapy. There is evidence that co-trimoxazole given as prophylaxis for *P. carinii* may also be suppressive for toxoplasmosis.

Cytomegalovirus infection

Cytomegalovirus infection is extremely common. In those with HIV infection, reactivation is associated with a range of manifestations which may involve the gastrointestinal tract, lung, liver, and in particular the eye, where a progressive retinopathy may lead to loss of vision or total blindness. Treatment with ganciclovir or foscarnet is suppressive but not curative (see Chapter 28).

Mycobacteriosis

Patients with HIV infection are at increased risk of mycobacterial infection. This may be newly acquired but is more usually the result of endogenous reactivation as cell-mediated immunity steadily declines. *Mycobacterium tuberculosis* is the infecting organism, but disease may present atypically owing to altered host immunity. In many parts of the world drug-resistant tuberculosis has emerged as an important problem, and there have been instances of spread within prisons and hospitals. Where there is good evidence for previous tuberculosis, chemoprophylaxis with isoniazid is recommended for 1–2 years.

Infection with organisms of the *Mycobacterium avium* complex is a common problem in patients with AIDS. Disease presents with fever, sweats, weight loss, and diarrhoea. Patients are frequently bacillaemic and have high bacterial loads within the gut and bone marrow. The organisms are extremely resistant to conventional antituberculous agents and a number of experimental regimens, for example a combination of azithromycin with a quinolone, such as ciprofloxacin, and ethambutol are under trial. Response to treatment may be short lived. Attempts have therefore been directed at preventing disease with novel agents such as rifabutin, which controls bacillaemia and fever but does not prevent mortality.

Hyposplenism

The spleen is an important site of host defences, rich in lymphoid follicles and phagocytic cells. In its absence the patient is at increased risk of infection, including fulminating bacteraemia. Apart from splenectomy, a variety of medical conditions can cause hyposplenism. These include hereditary conditions such as sickle cell anaemia and hereditary spherocytosis. The risk of serious infections is greatest in early childhood but declines with age, although the risk remains throughout life. Among the fulminant infections are those caused by *Streptococcus pneumoniae*, *Haemophilus influenzae*, *Escherichia coli*, *Neisseria meningitidis*, and a rare pathogen of humans, *Capnocytophaga canimorsus*. Hyposplenic or asplenic patients should be alerted to their increased risk and recommended to seek early medical attention in the presence of symptoms suggestive of severe infection. Immunization against pneumococcal infections is possible in those over 2 years of age and is the best form of prevention. Long-term chemoprophylaxis with phenoxymethylpenicillin (penicillin V) is of proven benefit in children with sickle cell disease. However, the additional benefit of life-long prophylaxis in those who have been actively immunized is marginal. Compliance with lifelong penicillin V prophylaxis is a further problem, as is the steady increase in resistance to penicillin among pneumococci, especially in parts of Europe and North America.

30

Venereal diseases

R. C. B. Slack

Venus has a lot to answer for if she was responsible for the conditions that bear her name! These afflictions of love are a motley collection of microbial diseases (Table 30.1); some, like syphilis, are potentially very serious; others, like trichomonal vaginal discharge, are merely a nuisance. When two human beings are in close contact, their mucous membranes in apposition, transfer of microbes is facilitated. Not all cases of VD, however, are genital infections; varieties in sexual technique allow for many different parts, not necessarily private, to be in sufficient contact to lead to a clinical lesion. The preferred name for VD is now *sexually transmitted diseases* (STD) and the specialty dealing with them is genito-urinary medicine (GUM).

The explosive increase in STD world-wide makes it important for all doctors to have a knowledge of their treatment. In some parts of the world STDs are so common that their treatment constitutes

Table 30.1. Common venereal diseases and their treatment

Condition	Pathogen	Antimicrobial agent
Urethral discharges		
Gonorrhoea	*Neisseria gonorrhoeae*	Penicillin (amoxycillin)
Non-specific (NSU)	*Chlamydia or Ureaplasma*	Tetracycline (erythromycin)
Vaginal discharges		
Thrush	*Candida albicans*	Nystatin (clotrimazole)
Trichomoniasis	*Trichomonas vaginalis*	Metronidazole
Non-specific vaginosis	*Gardnerella vaginalis and Mobiluncus* spp.	Metronidazole
Genital sores		
Syphilis	*Treponema pallidum*	Penicillin (erythromycin)
Chancroid	*Haemophilus ducreyi*	Sulphonamides (tetracycline)
Lymphogranuloma venereum	LGV (chlamydia)	Tetracycline (erythromycin)
Herpes	Herpes simplex type 2	Acyclovir
Warts	Wart viruses (human papillomaviruses)	Local podophyllin (cryotherapy)

a disproportionate part of the total health care budget. Moreover, the recognition that the virus responsible for the acquired immune deficiency syndrome (AIDS) is usually spread sexually has greatly increased public awareness of these conditions.

LABORATORY DIAGNOSIS

Microscopy will give accurate rapid confirmation of a clinical diagnosis in many cases. The examination of exudate from a syphilitic chancre must be done by dark ground microscopy within a few minutes of collecting the specimen; the presence of motile spirochaetes makes the diagnosis as it is not possible to cultivate these organisms in artificial media. Typical Gram-negative intracellular diplococci in a Gram-stained film of a urethral discharge in the male is strongly supportive of the diagnosis of acute gonorrhoea. Culture of cervical swabs from women and from extragenital sites in both sexes is necessary because examination of Gram-stained smears is unreliable. The unstained 'wet' film of vaginal secretions is the most widely used method for the diagnosis of trichomoniasis and may also reveal *Candida* and cells suggestive of non-specific bacterial vaginosis.

Direct microscopic examination is of utmost importance in venereology as it confirms many clinical diagnoses and for this reason many GUM clinics have laboratory facilities on site. In the majority of cases a sufficiently accurate microbiological cause can be ascribed to the patient's complaints to enable specific chemotherapy to be given.

Few genital pathogens can be cultivated easily. The most commonly sought, *Neisseria gonorrhoeae*, is a fastidious organism requiring special media and growth conditions. Selective media containing antibiotics to inhibit commensal bacteria are used. Isolation of *Chlamydia trachomatis* requires cell culture. These obligate intracellular bacteria may also be seen by direct fluorescence microscopy; alternatively, the antigenic particles may be detected by enzyme immunoassay techniques, and gene probe methods are becoming available.

Serological investigation may also be valuable in STD, particularly in syphilis where it may be the only way of confirming the diagnosis. The Wassermann reaction, employing a non-spirochaetal antigen, was used for many years, but this test yields some false positive results. More specific treponemal antigens are available nowadays. One disadvantage of the newer tests [the *Treponema pallidum* haemagglutination antibody (TPHA) and the fluorescent treponemal antibody (FTA) tests] is that they often remain positive for life, even after effective treatment.

TREATMENT OF VENEREAL DISEASE

Many patients with STD default treatment. It is therefore important to render as many patients as possible non-infectious after a single visit to the clinic. Concomitant treatment of the sexual partner(s) is essential to prevent reinfection and contact tracing can help to keep the spread of the disease within bounds, particularly in the control of spread of antibiotic-resistant strains of *N. gonorrhoeae*.

Syphilis

Curing 'the pox' holds an important place in the history of chemotherapy. Heavy metals, in particular mercury, were used for many centuries and the development in the first decade of the twentieth century of arsenicals such as salvarsan heralded the start of modern chemotherapy. It is difficult to imagine nowadays the horror which was felt about the disease and the importance of finding a cure. It held something of the mystery and fear in the minds of laymen later occupied by cancer and now by AIDS. In its medieval heyday syphilis was apparently a more virulent infection than it is today and earned the adjective 'great', diminishing the importance of 'smallpox', a disease feared later in history. Syphilis is a chronic disease capable of involving nearly every organ of the body. The old student adage 'know syphilis and you will know medicine' indicates how widespread the disease may be and how it can mimic other conditions. The progression of the infection varies greatly; even in untreated cases, latent periods of many years frequently occur.

Penicillin has been the mainstay of therapy since 1943 when the drug was first used to treat syphilis. The primary sore (chancre) will respond to relatively low doses of many antimicrobials, but such treatment may only suppress the disease, which reappears in its later manifestations. This danger exists in treating a patient with non-syphilitic STD who may also be incubating syphilis. For this reason serological tests for syphilis should be done on all high-risk patients attending clinics and repeated after 6 weeks.

Animal work suggests that *T. pallidum* is exquisitely sensitive to penicillin: as little as 0.002 mg/l is bactericidal. There is no evidence of variation in sensitivity and resistance is not known to occur. Other antibiotics with treponemicidal activity include erythromycin, tetracyclines, chloramphenicol, and cephalosporins, but none is thought to be as active as penicillin, which is the drug of choice in all cases except those where there is definite evidence of allergy.

Even in the early stages of the disease, spirochaetes divide relatively slowly and in latent and tertiary syphilis division presumably occurs infrequently. Since β-lactam antibiotics require active growth to achieve a killing effect a low concentration of penicillin is required over a prolonged period. This is achieved by using forms of the drug which are released slowly from an intramuscular depot. Aqueous procaine penicillin (600 000 units) will give an adequate concentration for 24 h; Benzathine penicillin gives greatly prolonged release, but is no longer used in the UK. In tertiary syphilis treatment for several weeks is necessary. Slow-release penicillins do not achieve adequate CSF concentrations, and frequent high doses of benzylpenicillin are recommended in the treatment of neurosyphilis.

A common hazard of syphilis therapy is the Jarisch–Herxheimer reaction observed within a few hours of treatment with penicillin (or arsenicals). This is a hypersensitivity reaction due to spirochaetal endotoxin and is not related to penicillin allergy. The Herxheimer response is of little significance in primary cases, but may occasionally be fatal in some tertiary or late cases.

GONORRHOEA

In 1829 *The Lancet* published a series of lectures to students at St Bartholomew's Hospital, London, by Mr Lawrence. In his paragraph on how to cure a clap he proclaims 'If anyone could find a speedy and effectual mode of accomplishing this he would undoubtedly immortalise himself. The ladies of Fleet Street and the Strand would be inclined to erect a statue to his memory!'

Modern antibiotics have revolutionized the practice of genito-urinary medicine and no more so than in 'curing the clap'. Acute gonococcal urethritis occurs 2–10 days after contact and in the male is nearly always obvious, presenting as a visible thick yellow discharge accompanied by dysuria and itching. Asymptomatic cases represent less than 5 per cent of male infections, but about 50 per cent of female infections. Prompt treatment with appropriate antibiotics will cure the majority of patients with no residual effects: it is hard to imagine that only 60 years ago gonorrhoea was treated by weeks of local irrigation and many sufferers were left with urethral strictures. Nowadays, the major problems of the disease are seen in women, especially with disseminated gonococcaemia. It is one of the main causes of infertility in the world.

N. gonorrhoeae is sensitive to many antimicrobial agents, but penicillin has remained the drug of choice since it replaced sulphonamides in the later stages of the Second World War. Its value has been maintained by increasing the dose to keep ahead of bacterial resistance. This strategy worked successfully until the emergence of strains completely resistant to penicillin in 1976. In the late 1950s *in vitro* testing showed that some strains of *N. gonorrhoeae* were becoming less sensitive to penicillin. In one of the clearest demonstrations of the relevance of laboratory tests to clinical practice, Curtis and Wilkinson demonstrated that failure of penicillin was directly related to the MIC of penicillin for the infecting strain. In this study 300 000 units of penicillin were unable to cure any patient infected with gonococci for which the penicillin MIC was 0.5 units/ml (0.3 mg/l) whereas all those infected with strains displaying an MIC <0.015 units/ml were cured. Proportionately reduced cure rates were observed with organisms of intermediate susceptibility.

In the 1960s the widespread and increasing resistance of gonococci to penicillin became well recognized and standard therapy for acute gonorrhoea increased to 4.8 or 5 megaunits in some parts of the world. In countries where antibiotics can be purchased in the market place the prevalence of resistant gonococci is very high. For many of these strains the MIC of penicillin is greater than 1 mg/l, which makes treatment with that drug almost impossible and resistance to sulphonamides, tetracyclines, and newer drugs is common. Since the discovery of *N. gonorrhoeae* capable of producing β-lactamase, the position has worsened. These gonococci contain a transmissible plasmid (R-factor) from Enterobacteriaceae which renders them completely resistant to penicillin, ampicillin, and amoxycillin. In parts of the Far East and Africa over one-third of all strains are β-lactamase producers. Recommendations for the therapy of gonorrhoea must be tempered with a knowledge of the antimicrobial susceptibilities of local strains.

In the acute disease a single dose of penicillin giving high tissue concentrations for 12 h is sufficient. Procaine penicillin has been widely employed for this purpose together with oral probenecid to delay renal excretion. Where most strains are relatively sensitive, as in the UK, 2.4 megaunits is sufficient, but double or even larger intramuscular doses have been advised in other parts of the world. The size of the buttock becomes a critical factor and often these enormous doses have to be divided into two injections. A single oral dose of 2 or 3 g amoxycillin with probenecid has replaced injections in many clinics, but oral drugs are mistrusted by some patients who think they are not as good as the injection, and by doctors who worry that patients will not comply, especially if multiple doses have to be given without supervision. Patients with acute gonorrhoea are amongst the highest defaulters in VD clinics. There is therefore great importance in a single curative dose and more studies have been performed comparing different regimens of treating gonorrhoea than almost any other condition. Most give a greater than 90 per cent cure rate and many 'failures' may in fact be re-infections as patients do not always give accurate information.

For patients infected with β-lactamase-producing strains of *N. gonorrhoeae*, spectinomycin has been widely used. However, the newer cephalosporins, especially ceftriaxone, is commonly used. Co-amoxiclav and the newer quinolones, such as ciprofloxacin, are also effective. If there is known hypersensitivity to penicillin, cephalosporins may be used, but if the reaction was previously severe the danger of cross-allergy is too great and a non-β-lactam alternative (e.g. co-trimoxazole or ciprofloxacin) should be employed.

Antibiotics give a speedy and complete cure in most cases of acute gonorrhoea. Occasional complications such as epididymitis, arthritis, and pelvic infection in the female require admission to hospital and prolonged antibiotics. Non-genital gonococcal infection also requires more than a single dose of penicillin to effect a cure.

A more common complication following penicillin monotherapy is post-gonococcal urethritis, which is really a double infection with gonococci and the microbes causing non-gonococcal urethritis (NGU; see below). Many physicians prefer to treat all cases of gonorrhoea with amoxycillin plus a tetracycline to cover both infections. This is a good pragmatic public health method for disease control, but offends the principle of making a definitive diagnosis before prescribing antibiotics. If rapid, accurate tests for NGU become available, it may be possible to tailor treatment more scientifically.

Ophthalmia neonatorum

This occurs within a few days of birth in babies born to infected mothers. Gonococci in the female genital tract are implanted in the conjunctivae during delivery and the neonate develops a purulent discharge from one or both eyes. There may be considerable cellulitis and if untreated the infection may lead to destruction of the cornea. Treatment should be prompt with parenteral penicillin and frequent local instillations of chloramphenicol. The condition may be prevented by silver nitrate drops placed in the eyes immediately after birth. This therapy (Credé's method) is still used in areas where the risk of infection is high but does have a risk of inducing a chemical conjunctivitis especially if the concentration of $AgNO_3$ is too high.

NON-GONOCOCCAL URETHRITIS

In many men presenting with urethral discharge, gonococci cannot be demonstrated and a diagnosis of non-specific (NSU) or non-gonococcal urethritis (NGU) is made. Such cases are seen more frequently than gonorrhoea in the UK and are common everywhere. Although the primary disease is less severe and the complications fewer than with gonorrhoea, satisfactory treatment is more difficult. Thorough microbiological investigation has determined the aetiological role of *Chlamydia trachomatis* in nearly half these cases. Some are probably due to ureaplasma, a form of mycoplasma and a few to *Trichomonas vaginalis*, herpesvirus, urinary tract infection, and local causes such as trauma or tumours.

Even with elaborate microbiological study, the aetiology of many cases is unknown, but these infections appear to respond to treatment appropriate to chlamydial infection.

The most useful therapeutic agents are tetracyclines, especially doxycycline, but short courses are ineffective. The duration of therapy should be at least 7–10 days. In spite of this, failures are common; some are due to failure of compliance or re-infection, but many genuine relapses occur, confirming the view that chlamydial infections may have a latent phase. Since laboratory facilities for the diagnosis of chlamydial infection are not universally available (and even where they are, results take some time to obtain), 'blind' therapy is necessary. The new macrolide, azithromycin, appears, because of favourable pharmacological properties, to be effective in single dose treatment.

Complicated chlamydial infections

Women and their newborm babies are prone to infections that are more difficult to treat and have more serious complications. Chlamydiae are less often confined to the lower genital tract in women. Although most women who are culture positive are asymptomatic and are discovered only through contact tracing of a partner with NGU, they are able to pass infection to their offspring during delivery.

Neonatal conjunctivitis

Neonatal conjunctivitis due to chlamydia is a less severe form of ophthalmia neonatorum than that caused by gonococci. It may be so mild as to be unsuspected clinically and, like all the conditions due to chlamydia, it is underdiagnosed. In spite of its mild, self-limiting course it can cause permanent eye damage and, whenever suspected, chlamydial conjunctivitis should be treated. Without appropriate laboratory facilities an accurate diagnosis cannot be made, but an index of suspicion is an indication for using tetracycline eye ointment. Local treatment is often difficult to apply adequately and many clinicians advise giving erythromycin orally, in addition, to prevent the development of chlamydial pneumonia. Erythromycin is preferred in the infant because systemic tetracycline stains teeth and bones. Therapy needs to be for at least 3 weeks as with all complicated chlamydial infections. It is self-evident that the parents should be examined and treated as for non-specific urethritis.

Pelvic inflammatory disease

Upper genital tract infection with chlamydiae and other venereal pathogens commonly results in pelvic inflammatory disease (PID), which gives rise to serious complications of tubal blockage or dysfunction. Infertility, ectopic pregnancy or chronic PID, a condition with considerable morbidity, commonly occur.

Acute salpingitis may respond to treatment with tetracyclines for 7–10 days, but many authorities would advocate longer treatment. Because PID may be caused by a variety of microbes, especially strict anaerobes, combination therapy with metronidazole or co-amoxiclav is necessary. Chronic PID, although initiated by chlamydiae, is more often caused by commensal bacteria, and antimicrobial agents alone seldom have a curative effect.

Genital infection with chlamydiae is commonly undiagnosed and untreated. In the UK it has been estimated that there are about 20 000 untreated infections in women each year. Throughout the world, these organisms cause substantial morbidity in terms of pelvic infection and infertility as well as the blinding eye disease, trachoma, for which 1 per cent tetracycline eye ointment (applied twice daily for 6 weeks) is effective. In severe cases, oral erythromycin may also be used. There are indications that single-dose azithromycin may be useful in trachoma.

VAGINAL DISCHARGE

The normal bacteria flora of the adult vagina before the menopause consists of numerous lactobacilli, diphtheroids, and anaerobes. This maintains locally a pH between 4 and 5 which is inhibitory to coliforms. However, yeasts flourish in acid conditions, as wine-makers will know.

Candidiasis

Candida albicans, the commonest pathogenic yeast, may be found in up to a quarter of healthy women of child-bearing age and frequently the delicate balance between the resident flora and intruding *Candida* is disturbed to produce clinical 'thrush'. Oral antibiotics, in particular tetracyclines, are prone to produce this side-effect which is also more common in pregnancy. The male, especially if uncircumcised, may occasionally have clinical balanitis due to *Candida* and the organism is not infrequently carried by healthy individuals. Venereal transfer is probable in these circumstances, but thrush can occur without intimate contact. Local applications of nystatin or one of the imidazoles (clotrimazole, or miconazole) are sufficient, but prolonged and repeated courses are required in a few intransigent cases and oral ketoconazole or fluconazole is sometimes used. The partner must be concurrently treated, as with all venereally spread conditions.

Trichomonal infection

Trichomonas vaginalis is a flagellate protozoon commonly found throughout the world. It favours a more alkaline pH than does *Candida* and causes a foul-smelling yellow vaginal discharge often noticed because of staining of clothes and itching. It has been found in a high proportion of asymptomatic women in antenatal clinics, but may cause symptoms subsequently, especially after menstruation. In some patients the organism invades the anterior urethra and symptoms of dysuria and frequency may lead the clinician to make a tentative diagnosis of urinary tract infection. Some patients labelled as 'urethral syndrome' may be suffering from trichomoniasis. The organism is sometimes carried transiently and asymptomatically by the male, but a low-grade non-specific urethritis may occur.

The treatment of trichomonal infection has been revolutionized by the advent of metronidazole. Treatment is given orally. Metronidazole should not be used during pregnancy because of possible teratogenic effects; patients on metronidazole should also avoid taking alcohol because of a reaction similar to that caused by disulfiram (Antabuse). However, most patients under treatment for venereal diseases are asked to abstain from alcohol and sex: the former to reduce the willingness for the latter and so reduce spread.

Bacterial vaginosis

This is a term employed for a symptomatic discharge for which no obvious cause can be found. As with NSU there are likely to be many possible aetiological agents—not all microbial. There is evidence that a proportion of these cases are associated with a pleomorphic, Gram-variable rod previously named *Haemophilus vaginalis* or *Corynebacterium vaginale*, but now called *Gardnerella vaginalis*. Like many a potential pathogen it can be found in normal healthy individuals. Metronidazole appears to improve symptoms associated with this organism, but its role may be to inhibit associated anaerobic, curved bacteria, called *Mobiluncus*. Topical clindamycin may be useful, especially if metronidazole is contraindicated.

OTHER GENITAL LESIONS

Every genital sore thought to be venereal in origin must be considered potentially syphilitic. The long-term complications of treponemal infection are so serious that it is essential not to miss an early infection. Although with clinical experience it is possible to distinguish between the causes of such lesions, mixed infections are not rare in STD.

Herpes simplex type 2

This virus causes vesicles, usually on the penis or labia, similar to 'cold sores' found around the mouth. Proctitis is common in passive homosexuals. The painful vesicles burst to form superficial erosions which can be secondarily infected. Women may carry the virus in the cervix where there is a possible complication of infection of the newborn which may occasionally be fatal. Acyclovir is sometimes helpful (see Chapter 28).

Warts

Genital warts (*condylomata acuminata*) are similar to the common skin complaint and local therapy is palliative in many cases. A long course of chemical applications such as podophyllin, or burning the lesions with diathermy or liquid nitrogen is often required; in some patients the warts disappear spontaneously, giving rise to the myths of 'charmers'. There is a strong association between these warts, which are caused by some types of human papillomaviruses, and cancers of the cervix and penis. The treatment of genital warts occupies a good part of the work of GUM clinics and is often unrewarding.

Chancroid (soft sore)

This is caused by *Haemophilus ducreyi*. The genital lesions are painful and often multiple with large associated inguinal glands which may suppurate to form a 'bubo'. Sulphonamides and streptomycin alone or in combination for at least 10 days were the standard drugs. Tetracyclines work in the majority of cases except where bacterial resistance is common. Short courses of co-amoxiclav or fluoroquinolones have also been successfully used. Chancroid is rarely seen in the UK, but in warmer countries there have been several epidemics.

Lymphogranuloma venereum (LGV)

This is also a predominantly tropical condition, but caused by a chlamydial agent. It starts as a small ulcer which may be unnoticed until inguinal glands enlarge and become matted together. Associated inflammation may give the appearance of elephantiasis as a late complication and breakdown of abscesses may give recto-vaginal fistulae.

Tetracyclines, sulphonamides or erythromycin may be used but, as with other chlamydial infection, 2–3 weeks of therapy is required.

AIDS

The treatment of STD has been complicated by the AIDS pandemic. HIV infection, itself, may require (or demand) drug treatment (see Chapter 28); the opportunist infections associated with the syndrome also require specific therapy (see Chapter 29). Sexually transmitted diseases are an important link in the spread of the infection. Every occasion on which a patient presents with an STD should be used as an opportunity to reach the high-risk community with a health education message. In those already at risk of contracting HIV infection, counselling and advice should be available at the clinic. Those with 'full-blown' AIDS may also have intractable STDs such as herpes. This may, indeed, be the signal for the diagnosis, so that clinicians expert in the field may be alerted to deal with the patient.

31

Parasitic diseases

R. C. B. Slack

Examples of the more important parasites have been examined in Chapter 4 and this chapter will restrict itself to specific problems of the therapy of parasitic disease not dealt with in other chapters. The organisms considered as 'parasites'—that is the pathogenic protozoa and helminths—tend to cause chronic disease and many individuals, once infected, may become long-term carriers. This ensures that in the warmer countries of the world, where poorer standards of hygiene often prevail, there is a high prevalence of infection and a high incidence of new cases all the time. The areas with the highest parasitic burden tend to have the poorest medical care because of poverty, a legacy of inadequate facilities, and the logistics of reaching the majority of people living in scattered rural communities. In many countries the total annual health care budget would not be sufficient to treat a fraction of their population even if it were all spent on antiparasitic drugs.

HOST–PARASITE RELATIONSHIP

One of the peculiarities of treating parasitic infections is the varied relationship between man and microbe. The life cycles often ensure that at some stage the organism is not susceptible to a particular drug either because it is in a resting phase or in an inaccessible site. In many cases the host and parasite reach a steady state of coexistence with no symptoms at all. Parasites restricted to the gut lumen such as the protozoon *Giardia lamblia* (also known as *Giardia intestinalis*) or many helminths often reach this stage and the intruder is only discovered when stools are examined. In other cases, for example filariasis, the disease becomes 'burnt-out' after years. All these late asymptomatic cases may be diagnosed by chance during routine investigations or as part of mass screening campaigns. The contribution of the parasite burden to overall health is usually impossible to estimate and if the only available drug is potentially toxic the decision to treat an apparently healthy individual is difficult to make. Another factor in making such a decision is the likelihood of reinfection from the community or environmental reservoirs. Intestinal parasites are found in over 70 per cent of the population in some tropical countries and a child living in a rural environment will inevitably be quickly in contact with the parasite again. Treatment of an individual case without taking care to prevent reinfection is wasting resources and is not good practice. If the drug is non-toxic and inexpensive there is some justification in treating asymptomatic individuals, especially if the infection may at some stage cause further problems.

Some intestinal protozoa such as *Entamoeba coli* may be classed as true commensals for there is no evidence to incriminate them in human disease. Their only significance may be in misidentification in stool microscopy. Similarly, some helminths such as the whipworm, *Trichuris trichiura*, rarely cause problems in adults. However, many other parasites do clearly have a pathogenic role and in those cases an accurate laboratory diagnosis is essential if antiparasitic therapy is to be useful.

THERAPEUTIC DIFFICULTIES

In addition to the factors peculiar to treating parasitic infections, many of the general principles mentioned in Chapter 15 apply. Any therapy of extended duration in relatively healthy individuals in the community will be difficult to monitor and compliance may be a problem, especially if the drug is unpleasant to take and has conspicuous side-effects. This can occur even with well-educated travellers taking antimalarials.

Many of the remedies for the major parasitic infections are potentially toxic and it is always necessary to weigh the consequences of iatrogenic disease against the benefit of therapy which might not always be able to effect a complete cure. These considerations must still be borne in mind nowadays, even though less toxic compounds are gradually becoming available for some parasitic diseases.

PROTOZOAN INFECTIONS

Malaria

Fig. 31.1 shows the world-wide distribution of malaria, which is the most important of all parasitic diseases in terms of mortality. Although indigenous malaria is now virtually restricted to the tropics and subtropics, it is commonly imported into many temperate countries because of the rapid increase in world travel. The volume of international business travel continues to expand each year, and 'package' holidays to East and West Africa or other tropical destinations are becoming increasingly popular. It is therefore not surprising that the importance of imported malaria in non-malarious countries continues to grow. About 2000 cases of imported malaria are recorded in the UK each year; the figure is likely to be grossly underestimated because of considerable under-reporting. Each year there are fatalities from malaria reported and the tragedy is that these are all preventable. However, this is insignificant compared with the damage malaria inflicts on the populations of the tropical world; in parts of West Africa it is estimated that at least 10 per cent of children die of falciparum malaria before they reach the age of 5.

Acute malaria

Until recently the drug of choice in the treatment of acute malaria was always chloroquine, a 4-aminoquinoline derived from the traditional remedy, quinine. These agents are active against the blood forms of the parasite, which is important in the symptomatic stage of the disease when rapidly dividing schizonts cause red cell lysis; it is particularly important in falciparum malaria when infected erythrocytes block small cerebral blood vessels to give rise to the rapidly fatal form of cerebral malaria. In such a medical emergency parenteral therapy is necessary in spite of the hazards of infusion. In its time, chloroquine revolutionized the treatment and prophylaxis of malaria, but we are now beginning to pay the penalty for its extensive use by the appearance of resistant strains of *Plasmodium falciparum*. Although other species of *Plasmodium* usually retain susceptibility to the drug, chloroquine resistance in *P. falciparum* has become a major clinical problem in South East Asia, Central and South America, and Africa. The spread seems inexorable and it has become clear that resistance now has a firm foothold in tropical West Africa where falciparum malaria is hyperendemic and responsible for many thousands of deaths each year. Many chloroquine-resistant strains are also resistant to alternative drugs such as the combinations of pyrimethamine with sulphonamides (Fansidar) or dapsone (Maloprim). Indeed, quinine has returned to favour as the drug of first choice in severe falciparum malaria if chloroquine resistance is thought to be possible. Resistance to quinine is presently quite rare, but resistance to other antimalarials throughout the world has become such a problem that the need for new antimalarial compounds has become acute.

Mefloquine, a quinolinemethanol derivative developed by the Walter Reed Army Institute of Research in Washington, is active against resistant strains and has been successfully used for treatment. However, resistance to mefloquine is known to emerge readily and there are fears that widespread use will quickly negate its value. Moreover, mefloquine use has been associated with neuropsychiatric side-effects that may persist for some time owing to the very long plasma half-life of the drug. Halofantrine, another Walter Reed derivative, may have advantages over mefloquine since it has a shorter half-life and

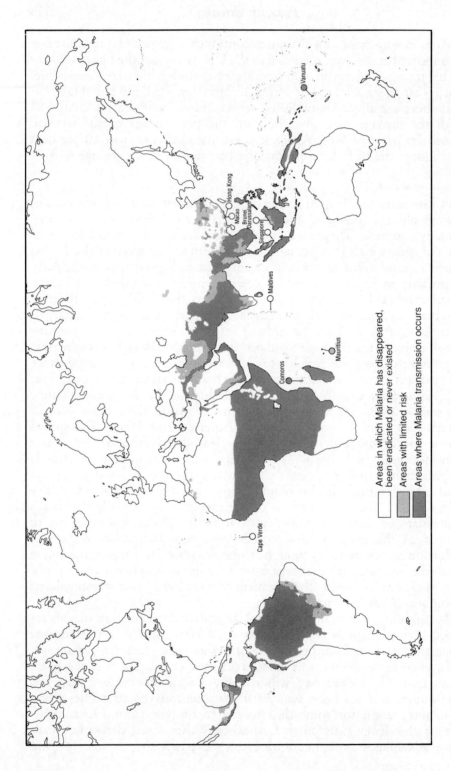

Fig. 31.1. Map showing distribution of malaria (situation in 1991). [Adapted, by permission, from: *WHO Weekly Epidemiological Record* 34, 246 (1993).]

Areas in which Malaria has disappeared, been eradicated or never existed

Areas with limited risk

Areas where Malaria transmission occurs

Vanuatu

Hong Kong

Macao
Brunei
Darussalam
Singapore

Maldives

Mauritius

Comoros

Cape Verde

fewer adverse reactions, but concern has been expressed over possible cardiotoxicity.

Derivatives of a Chinese herbal remedy, qinghaosu (artemisinin) are now in use in severe malaria in the Far East. Various formulations, including artesunic acid, arteether, and artemether (the ethyl and methyl ethers, respectively), are used for oral, intravenous, and intramuscular administration. A suppository formulation is also available and is particularly useful in children. Artemisinin derivatives have aroused considerable interest, since they are more rapidly effective than any other drug in severe malaria. Clinical trials have shown these compounds to be relatively non-toxic, but animal experiments have revealed a potential for neurotoxicity and their future as antimalarial agents is not yet secure.

Recurrent malaria

To effect a radical cure in recurrent malarias with a latent exoerythrocytic phase, such as 'benign tertian' malaria due to *Plasmodium vivax*, it is necessary to employ an 8-aminoquinoline. Primaquine is the most commonly used drug for this purpose. It is necessary first to make an accurate diagnosis by examining thin and thick blood films. Secondly, it is important to treat the acute erythrocytic attack with chloroquine before administering primaquine. Thirdly, patients must be screened for glucose-6-phosphate dehydrogenase (G-6-P D) deficiency. Low levels of this red blood cell enzyme occur in many populations in endemic areas and administration of primaquine to such individuals may lead to an acute haemolytic crisis worse than the original malaria. Iatrogenic reactions of this sort have given 8-aminoquinolines a bad name in India. Laboratory screening tests for G-6-P D deficiency are not difficult to perform and should be available widely in endemic areas. Primaquine should not be used during pregnancy.

Antimalarial prophylaxis

Advice on prophylaxis against malaria presents a great problem because of the difficulty in predicting drug resistance. Chloroquine has been widely used, but its usefulness has been seriously undermined by the spread of resistance in *P. falciparum*. Moreover, it has a bitter taste and more serious side-effects, such as skin photosensitization and retinal damage, may become apparent after prolonged use. For these reasons and because of the danger of further encouraging the emergence of chloroquine resistance, it is probably unwise to use the drug as a long-term prophylactic, even in areas known to be free of resistance. In general, it is preferable to use an antifolate agent (pyrimethamine or proguanil) whenever possible, but the unpredictability of resistance has led some authorities to recommend combinations of antifolates with chloroquine in an attempt to reduce the chances of breakthrough of protection. Mefloquine is a reliable prophylactic agent for short-term use in areas in which chloroquine resistance is prevalent, and is widely recommended despite its neurotoxicity.

Advice on the choice of prophylactic regimen has changed radically in the last few years and may alter again depending on drug resistance and the availability of new agents. Is is therefore wise for anyone counselling a traveller to a malarious area to seek advice from a specialist, or make use of the excellent databases held nationally by travel clinics and the expert tropical medicine institutes.

The most important aspect of chemoprophylaxis is regular medication and continuance of therapy for at least 4 weeks after the last possible exposure. Although it is not essential to premedicate patients before travelling it is advisable to start a routine a week prior in order to ensure acceptability and enable adequate drug concentrations to be achieved before exposure. In highly endemic areas where the risk of malaria is high a double dose may be given. With weekly drugs such as pyrimethamine or chloroquine a dose can be given in the middle of the week. This should not be continued long term with chloroquine due to chronic toxicity.

Sulphonamide and sulphone-containing mixtures should be avoided in persons known to be hypersensitive to these compounds. If antifolate agents are used during pregnancy, folic or folinic acid supplements should also be given. Of great importance, but often neglected, are practical hints to minimize exposure: wearing long clothes, using insect repellants, and sleeping under mosquito nets impregnated with insecticide. It is also important to stress to all travellers that prophylaxis may not be effective, so that any fever should be treated with suspicion until malaria has been excluded by examination of adequate blood slides.

Amoebiasis

Entamoeba histolytica may live harmlessly in the lumen of the gut, usually in the cyst form, or may invade the gut mucosa to cause amoebic dysentery. The factors that govern the transformation from harmless commensal to invasive pathogen are poorly understood although it is now clear that not all strains of *E. histolytica* have pathogenic potential. Secondary spread from the primary intestinal focus sometimes occurs to give rise to abscess formation in various parts of the body, usually the liver.

The treatment of symptomless cyst-passers, especially those living in endemic areas, is not worthwhile unless there is evidence of recurrent attacks of dysentery. Acute intestinal amoebiasis is characterized by bloody diarrhoeic stools. Motile amoebae with phagocytosed red cells are seen on direct microscopy of a freshly passed specimen. This is an indication for therapy to relieve symptoms and prevent possible complications: either local haemorrhage or invasion. Metronidazole is the agent of choice in a high initial dose which should be continued for 3–5 days. This drug gives a high cure rate; if there is a relapse and cysts are seen in the stool an agent more active against them such as diloxanide furoate should be given.

Invasion of trophozoites into tissues, especially into the liver, may occur without dysentery and the first indication of amoebiasis may be a hepatic abscess. Metronidazole has replaced emetine and older remedies in the treatment of invasive amoebiasis. Therapy needs to be of longer duration than with uncomplicated disease. There is no evidence of drug resistance in amoebae. Metronidazole is easy to administer and gives rise to few adverse reactions. The only drawback in the poorer countries of the world where amoebiasis is hyperendemic is cost and availability. In such situations emetine hydrochloride may be given parenterally. There is a severe risk of cardiac toxicity and treatment must be given in hospital with complete bed-rest, which nullifies any cost benefit. Exercise should be forbidden for 1 month after therapy. Oral di-iodohydroxyquinoline is a less effective alternative for amoebic colitis. Chloroquine may be used as an alternative for the treatment of amoebic liver abscesses.

Giardiasis

The flagellate protozoon *G. lamblia* is found only in the intestinal lumen. There is no invasion of the surface, the trophozoite being attached to the mucosa of the small intestine, especially the jejunum. Cysts are passed in the stools and infection is transmitted by contamination of food and water. *Giardia* is a frequent cause of chronic diarrhoea and is often underestimated as a pathogen. However, many infections are asymptomatic and, even with a heavy infestation in adults, the symptoms may be mild: nausea, flatulence, and steatorrhoea. In young children the condition may give rise to malabsorption. Although world-wide in distribution this intestinal infection, like most, is more common in less hygienic communities. Giardiasis is common in the UK as well as being the most frequently imported parasitic disease.

Metronidazole is the treatment of choice administered in a similar regimen to that used to treat amoebic dysentery although lower doses may suffice. Cases which do not respond to metronidazole require mepacrine after reinfection has been excluded.

Cryptosporidiosis

Cryptosporidium parvum is an intestinal zoonotic protozoon that is now recognized as a common cause of acute diarrhoea. The disease is generally mild and self limiting in otherwise healthy individuals, but in the immunosuppressed, especially those with AIDS, it causes a life-threatening prolonged enteritis. Many agents have been tried to combat infection, but none has been found to be reliably effective. Some success has been claimed with paromomycin, eflornithine, and the macrolide antibiotic, spiramycin.

African trypanosomiasis

Human trypanosomiasis due to *Trypanosoma brucei rhodesiense* is a sporadic disease in East and Central Africa although occasional outbreaks occur. The clinical course of the disease found in this area is more acute than that caused by *T. brucei gambiense*, which is a major health hazard in rural West Africa. Both parasites eventually infect the brain to give the clinical manifestations of 'sleeping sickness'. Before this stage a clinical diagnosis is difficult because of the non-specific nature of the symptoms. However, an early diagnosis is important as treatment is more effective and less toxic at this stage. Laboratory confirmation may be difficult to obtain except in specialized centres because the trypanosomes are often scanty in peripheral blood. Before CNS involvement suramin or pentamidine may be used in therapy but when a lumbar puncture indicates meningoencephalitis it is necessary to use an organic arsenical. Melarsoprol has replaced the more toxic tryparsamide for this purpose. All the antitrypanosomal drugs are toxic; treatment should be given in hospital and expert advice sought.

There are hopes that an important advance in the treatment of sleeping sickness caused by *T. brucei gambiense* has been achieved with the introduction of eflornithine. This drug appears to be effective even in the late meningoencephalitic stages of the disease, but, unfortunately, *T. brucei rhodesiense* appears to be refractory to treatment.

Chagas' disease

This form of trypanosomiasis is widespread in South America. The causative organism, *T. cruzi*, invades heart muscle causing myocardial damage which may be fatal. The condition had no known therapy until the nitrofuran, nifurtimox, appeared. This drug may succeed in eradicating parasites in the acute stage of the disease at the expense of some toxicity. Its value in established infection is more dubious. Similar considerations appear to apply to the nitroimidazole derivative, benznidazole.

Leishmaniasis

Kala-azar
Visceral leishmaniasis is a chronic, often fatal, condition characterized by fever, anaemia, and gross splenomegaly. Microscopy and culture of

bone marrow or splenic aspirate confirm the diagnosis. Pentavalent antimonials remain the agents of choice, although relapse possibly due to drug resistance or inadequate dosage and duration of treatment is not uncommon. Sodium stibogluconate (Pentostam) is given by the parenteral route in high dosage for at least 30 days and preferably longer. Drug resistance may be suppressed by use of high-dose antimonials for extended periods, but toxic effects such as cardiac irregularities are inevitable. Pentamidine has been used as an alternative for many years but patients fare little better on this toxic compound.

In an effort to reduce the toxicity of sodium stibogluconate, attempts have been made to package the drug in artificial liposomes—minute fat globules that are phagocytosed by cells of the reticuloendothelial system, where they release drug at the target site. Unfortunately, preparation of a suitable carrier that is stable in tropical conditions, and other problems, have militated against the success of this tactic. More success has been achieved with a liposome-encapsulated formulation of the antifungal agent, amphotericin B, which has also been found to be useful in kala-azar.

Treatment of kala-azar continues to evolve. Claims have been made for the efficacy of antifungal imidazoles, including itraconazole, ketoconazole, and fluconazole, and for the aminoglycoside antibiotic, paromomycin. Allopurinol has also been successfully used as an adjunct to therapy with antimonials.

Cutaneous and muco-cutaneous leishmaniasis

These forms of the disease are less serious and can be treated with lower total doses of pentavalent antimonial. Most respond to local excision.

Pneumocystis infection

Pneumonia is a common terminal event in patients with malignant disease. In those with immunodeficiencies a wide range of potential pathogens may give rise to respiratory disease (see Chapter 20). One particular opportunist parasite, *Pneumocystis carinii*, gives rise to an interstitial pneumonia in immunocompromised patients, especially those with AIDS. Prevention of this disease is possible using co-trimoxazole, and this is advocated in the USA where the condition is diagnosed more frequently than in the UK. Treatment of an established infection is more difficult, but co-trimoxazole is a safe alternative to pentamidine, which is also effective. It was increased demand for pentamidine which first alerted the Communicable Diseases Centers in Atlanta, Georgia, to the appearance of the AIDS problem in the USA.

Options for the treatment of *P. carinii* pneumonia are considered in Chapter 29.

NEMATODE INFECTIONS

Filariasis

In some areas of the tropics nearly the whole population is infected with filarial worms. Diagnosis is made by microscopical demonstration of the larval forms (microfilariae) in blood or, in the special case of *Onchocerca volvulus*, in superficial shavings of skin. Some of the blood microfilariae exhibit a curious periodicity in that they are found in peripheral blood during only the day (*Loa loa*) or the night (*Wuchereria bancrofti*). *Brugia malayi* usually exhibits a less complete nocturnal periodicity. *Wuchereria bancrofti* and *B. malayi* cause a clinically identical condition resulting in severe cases of elephantiasis due to blockage of the lymphatics of the lower trunk. This condition is seen in many parts of the tropics and probably over 250 million people are affected. The clinical syndrome is due to a variety of factors depending on degree of exposure and host reaction to the worms, and in any area a small proportion will have gross elephantiasis. Often by this stage the disease may be 'burnt out' and an anthelminthic may do little to improve the patient's condition, for which surgical and supportive measures are all that is left.

It is important to recognize *B. malayi* (which is restricted to South East Asia) because therapy with diethylcarbamazine (DEC) produces severer reactions than with Bancroftian filariasis. One of the factors limiting individual and mass therapy of filariasis is the frequent occurrence of hypersensitivity reactions to dead worms. This problem is seen particularly in the treatment of filariasis due to *O. volvulus*, the causative parasite of 'river blindness', which affects large numbers of people in West Africa and Central America. As with the other filariases, many infected persons exhibit only minor symptoms such as skin swelling and itching.

The decision to treat is tempered by a knowledge of the natural history of the disease, the patient's complaints, and the likelihood of reinfection in a hyperendemic community. The chances and severity of possible reactions must be balanced against any possible benefit. This was particularly true when DEC was the only effective microfilaricide. The introduction of ivermectin has changed the therapy of filariases. This relatively non-toxic drug is now the drug of choice for the treatment of onchocerciasis and lymphatic filariasis. One of the benefits of the use of ivermectin is that reactions to treatment are a good deal milder than with DEC. It is administered by a single oral dose which, in the control of onchocerciasis, is repeated annually in endemic areas. Mass treatment with ivermectin, together with vector control, has virtually eradicated onchocerciasis in some areas.

Toxocariasis

Infection with the dog roundworm, *Toxocara canis*, may cause a condition known as 'visceral larva migrans' which may result in serious eye infection usually presenting as a visual loss in childhood. Although not a common disease it is found world-wide and is probably under-recognized. The larvae of the worm migrate to the retina, setting up an inflammatory response. Treatment with DEC has been recommended but hypersensitivity reactions may require steroids to be given as well. There is some anecdotal evidence that thiabendazole or albendazole may offer an effective and less toxic alternative.

Intestinal helminth infections

Single doses of the common agents such as tetrachloroethylene, piperazine, and bephenium give acceptable cure rates. Table 31.1 shows the differential activity of these and the oral benzimidazole derivatives, which have a broader spectrum but are more expensive. Among benzimidazoles, albendazole exhibits the best broad-spectrum anthelminthic activity. In the warmer countries with poor water supplies and inadequate methods of sewage disposal, reinfection is almost inevitable, yet a few words of health education such as advice on wearing shoes to prevent hookworm may be extremely valuable.

TREMATODE (FLUKE) INFECTIONS

Schistosomiasis

Schistosomes (also known as bilharzia, or blood flukes) give rise to a chronic debilitating condition with hepatosplenomegaly and diarrhoea or haematuria. The adult worms adopt a more-or-less benign relationship with the host and it is fibrosis and tissue damage arising from the deposition of eggs which is responsible for most of the unpleasant manifestations of schistosomiasis.

In the days when trivalent antimonials were the only available agents for therapy of bilharzia, the decision to treat a specific case would depend on similar factors to those mentioned for filariasis: balancing the toxic effects of treatment with the severity of the patient's illness and the likelihood of rapid reinfection.

However, no area of antiparasitic chemotherapy has undergone such a transformation in recent years as has the treatment of schistosomiasis. As well as antimonials, a whole battery of drugs is now available, including one, praziquantel, which appears to offer the possibility of effective single-dose therapy for mass treatment campaigns. Available drugs are

Table 31.1. Spectrum of activity of drugs used in the treatment of intestinal helminthiasis

Drug	Ancylostoma duodenale	Necator americanus	Ascaris lumbricoides	Strongyloides stercoralis	Trichuris trichiura	Enterobius vermicularis
Tetrachloroethylene	+	+++	-	-	-	-
Piperazine	-	-	+++	-	-	+++
Bephenium	+++	+	+	-	-	-
Levamisole	++	++	+++	-	-	-
Pyrantel pamoate	++	++	+++	+	++	+++
Thiabendazole	++	++	+++	++	-	++
Mebendazole	++	++	+++	+	++	+++
Albendazole	+++	++	+++	++	++	+++

+++=Highly effective; +=poorly effective; - =no useful activity.

Table 31.2. Spectrum of activity of drugs used in the treatment of schistosomiasis

Drug	Schistosoma mansoni	Schistosoma haematobium	Schistosoma japonicum
Trivalent antimonials	+++	++	++
Niridazole	+	+++	+
Metriphonate	−	+++	−
Oxamniquine	+++	−	−
Praziquantel	+++	+++	+++

+++ = Highly effective; + = poorly effective; − = no useful activity.

not equally effective against all three types of schistosome infecting humans; their differential activity is summarized in Table 31.2.

With the advent of these relatively safe and cheap antischistosomal drugs, it has become possible to use chemotherapy as a means of control of the disease, in conjuction with the use of molluscicides to control the snail host and the provision of safe means of disposal of excreta. Unless there is development of drug resistance on a wide scale, such methods offer a good hope for the control of one of the major parasitic scourges of mankind.

Other trematode infections

Praziquantel has also transformed the treatment of most other trematode infections, including those caused by the Chinese liver fluke, *Clonorchis sinensis*, and the lung fluke, *Paragonimus westermani*. However, the liver fluke *Fasciola hepatica* does not usually respond to praziquantel. The treatment of fascioliasis is problematical, but the veterinary anthelminthic, triclabendazole, may be effective.

CESTODE INFECTIONS

Tapeworms

In addition to its use in trematode infections, praziquantel has emerged as an important agent in the treatment of tapeworm infections, including those caused by *Taenia saginata*, *T. solium*, *Diphyllobothrium latum*, and *Hymenolepis nana*. A single oral dose is usually effective, although more prolonged therapy is needed in cerebral cysticercosis caused by *T. solium*. In intestinal tapeworm infection, niclosamide is a suitable alternative. Older remedies including mepacrine and *filix mas* are effective, but have been superseded by the newer drugs.

Hydatid disease

Surgery to remove hydatid cysts after injection of a scolicide remains the treatment of choice in hydatid disease, but is not without risk. Therapy with benzimidazole derivatives, particularly albendazole, has been successful in some cases and may be the only option in inoperable conditions, including disease caused by *Echinococcus multilocularis*.

32

Topical use of antimicrobial agents

R. C. B. Slack

The concept of applying drugs directly to clinical lesions is appealing: problems of absorption and pharmacokinetics do not apply and agents too toxic for systemic use may be safely applied to skin or mucous membranes. The major drawback is that, even in the most superficial skin lesion, there may be areas inaccessible to a topical approach. Furthermore, collections of pus may prevent the agent reaching the infecting organisms and for this reason the management of any abscess includes drainage of pus.

Although skin, the largest and most accessible organ of the body, is the most obvious target for topical antimicrobials other sites are available for this approach to therapy: the mucous membranes of the mouth and vagina, and the external surfaces of eyes and ears. Direct application of antibiotics into normally sterile sites, such as joints, spinal fluid or the urinary bladder, or instillation into surgical wounds prior to suture may also be considered as a form of topical therapy, but will not be specifically dealt with in this chapter. Application of topical agents to mucous membranes or damaged skin may lead to considerable systemic absorption and the possibility of systemic toxicity should be borne in mind.

The chief reasons for using topical antimicrobial agents are:

(1) to achieve high drug concentrations at the site of infection;
(2) to treat trivial infections where use of a systemic drug is unjustified;
(3) to prevent infection in a susceptible site (e.g. burns);
(4) agents may be used that are too toxic for systemic use;
(5) cost: topical agents are generally cheaper than systemic drugs.

ANTISEPTICS

Disinfectant is a general term for chemicals which can destroy vegetative micro-organisms; those disinfectants that are sufficiently non-injurious to skin and exposed tissues to be used topically are called *antiseptics*. In order to achieve adequate antimicrobial activity, high concentrations of antiseptics are required and this serves to distinguish them from *antibiotics* in Waksman's original sense of 'substances produced by micro-organisms antagonistic to the growth or life of others in high dilution'. In many cases, true antibiotics are used topically in high concentration and might thus be classed as antiseptics. In fact, antiseptics and antibiotics are often used in exactly the same situations in dermatological practice and there has been some difference of opinion as to which class of agent to use in, for example, the treatment of infected ulcers or wounds. Antiseptics are usually cheaper and have the advantage that bacterial resistance rarely, if ever, develops. Preparations commonly employed include chlorhexidine, cetrimide, iodophors (non-irritant iodine complexes), triclosan and solutions liberating hypochlorite, such as Eusol or Dakin's solution.

Some concern has been expressed about the effect on tissue viability of many chemicals applied directly. There is some evidence *in vitro* of a direct toxic effect on epidermal cells and white blood cells of many antiseptics at concentrations well below those used topically.

METHODS OF APPLICATION

Drugs which are dissolved in aqueous solutions (*lotions*) have the disadvantage of running off the skin and cooling it by evaporation. This method of delivering antimicrobial agents to the site of infection is inefficient and not often used, except as ear or eye drops. For use in eye infections, frequent application on to the cornea and conjunctiva is necessary, because the drug is only in contact for a short time and much of the active component runs down the cheek as an expensive tear! The value of aqueous preparations resides mainly in their irrigant and cleansing action and much of the therapeutic success may be due to these properties.

It is usual to apply drugs to the skin in a fat base, either as an oil and water *cream*, or a largely lipid *ointment*. Drug solubility affects the achievable concentration in each component, while availability at the lesion depends on diffusion from the applicant and absorption from the skin. Antibiotics which are lipid soluble and freely diffusible, for example fusidic acid, are at an advantage in this respect.

Sticky ointments may remain in contact with the infected site for a considerable time and application may be needed only once daily, but this obviously depends on the frequency of washing.

Some of the commonly used topical preparations are listed in Table 32.1. Many of the formulations designed for topical use contain combinations of antimicrobials. Mixtures are intended to cover a wide antibacterial spectrum and to be compatible.

Table 32.1. Some of the most commonly used topical antimicrobial agents. The numerous topical antiseptics available are omitted

Agent	Application	Indication*	Comments
Antibiotics			
Chloramphenicol†	Drops/ointment	Eye/ear	Very broad spectrum
Fusidic acid†	Ointment/drops	Skin only	Best against *Staph. aureus*
Gentamicin†	Cream/ointment/drops	Ear/nose/eye	Should not be used in hospitals
Mupirocin	Ointment	Nose	Macrogol-based ointment unsuitable for nasal application
Neomycin (framycetin)	Cream/ointment/drops/powder	Ear/nose/eye	Often combined with gramicidin or bacitracin and/or polymyxin B
Nystatin (and other polyenes)	Cream/pessary/suspension/lozenges	Mouth/vagina	For thrush (candidiasis)
Tetracycline†	Ointment/cream/drops	Ear/eye	Broad-spectrum; resistance common
Other antimicrobial agents			
Silver sulphadiazine	Cream	Burns only	May cause sensitization
Acyclovir†	Ointment/cream	Eye/genitalia/mouth	Antiviral agents; for use on herpes lesions
Idoxuridine	Ointment/drops	Eye/genitalia/mouth	
Imidazoles (clotrimazole, etc.)	Cream/pessaries/gel/powder	Vagina	Antifungal; for use in skin infections and vaginal thrush
Metronidazole†	Gel	Skin only	Useful in rosacea
Norfloxacin†/ofloxacin†	Drops	Eyes	

* Indications other than skin, for which most are used.
† Compounds that are also used systemically.

CHOICE

The results of laboratory tests may be helpful if adequate specimens are sent to the laboratory, but frequently colonizing microbes are isolated from the surface of deep lesions while the true underlying pathogen remains undetected. The clinician must be careful not to use a battery of antimicrobials to treat harmless commensals colonizing an unoccupied niche.

Conventional antimicrobial sensitivity testing is often irrelevant because susceptibility of organisms to antiseptics can usually be assumed. Moreover, laboratory criteria of susceptibility to antibiotics usually apply to systemic use, not the high concentrations achievable by topical application. Nevertheless, complete resistance in laboratory tests is a contraindication to use of a particular agent. Regular monitoring of hospitalized patients with large skin lesions, such as ulcers and burns, is useful to determine the nature and prevalence of resistant organisms, as well as the extent of cross-infection.

Choice, if not based on microbiological evidence, must include agents active against all likely pathogens. Topical antiseptics and hydroxy-quinolines are to be preferred to antibiotics on microbiological grounds of avoidance of resistance, but many users prefer antibiotics because it is claimed that a quicker response is generally obtained. Tetracyclines are often recommended by clinicians, but not by microbiologists, who point to the prevalence of tetracycline resistance and the readiness with which such prevalence increases under selective pressure. Combinations of antibiotics, such as bacitracin and neomycin, or bacitracin, neomycin, and polymyxin are often used, and a corticosteroid is sometimes added for good measure. These antibiotics are not usually used for systemic therapy, so possible problems of compromising the activity of systemically useful agents by encouraging the emergence of resistance are minimized (see below). Nevertheless, it should be remembered that the topical use of neomycin might generate strains of bacteria cross-resistant to other aminoglycosides such as gentamicin.

One antibiotic, mupirocin (pseudomonic acid), has been marketed solely for topical use. The spectrum of activity of this agent is virtually restricted to Gram-positive cocci. Mupirocin is unsuitable for systemic use since it is quickly metabolized in the body. It has a unique mode of action (on protein synthesis) and cross-resistance is not a problem.

In practice, one of the most important limitations to choice is the availability of a particular drug as a topical product. Manufacturers are well aware that it makes little commercial sense to market a relatively cheap topical formulation if it is going to encourage resistance which diminishes the usefulness of more expensive parenteral forms of the drug. Here, at least, the interests of industry and the consumer coincide.

BACTERIAL SKIN INFECTIONS

Trivial skin sepsis, often due to staphylococci, is common, but usually self limiting in healthy individuals. Impetigo is frequently a more severe and widespread condition which may involve both *Streptococcus pyogenes* and *Staphylococcus aureus*. In general, mild infections of the skin respond to local measures involving cleansing of the crusted areas and application of topical agents, such as fusidic acid or mupirocin, to the raw surfaces. More severe staphylococcal and streptococcal skin lesions may require systemic therapy and this is discussed in Chapter 24.

Nasal carriage

In recurrent sepsis with *Staph. aureus* it may be necessary to attempt to eradicate the organism from the body. This is also desirable in patients and staff colonized with antibiotic-resistant strains, particularly methicillin-resistant *Staph. aureus* (MRSA) which can cause serious cross-infection problems. The external surface of the skin can be washed in antiseptics, but nasal carriage of staphylococci is often resistant to this treatment. For this purpose, nasal creams should be applied at least twice a day for 5 days. Chlorhexidine/neomycin cream (Naseptin) has been widely used, but does not appear to be as effective as mupirocin in the eradication of nasal carriage of MRSA. The normal dermatological preparation of mupirocin, which is in a macrogol (polyethylene glycol) excipient, is unsuitable for nasal application and a paraffin-based ointment should be used for this purpose.

ACNE

The role of bacteria in the pathogenesis of acne vulgaris is still under debate, although commensal diphtheroids, such as *Propionibacterium acnes*, are thought to play some part. Systemic antibiotics, including tetracycline and erythromycin, do improve severe intractable cases and success has also been claimed for topical antimicrobials, in particular for clindamycin. Treatment with any of these agents needs to be prolonged and is an adjunct to other measures aimed at improving the condition.

BURNS

The treatment of burns is an enormous specialized topic that cannot be covered adequately in this chapter. However, topical agents do have definite value in the prevention of infection in patients with burns so it is appropriate that their use should be mentioned.

Initially, a thermal burn renders the skin sterile, but bacterial colonization is inevitable, even with scrupulous aseptic technique. Indeed, infection, usually with *Str. pyogenes, Staph. aureus*, or *Pseudomonas aeruginosa*, is an important determinant in the outcome of extensive burns, since it is a major cause of delay in skin healing and of death.

Prophylaxis with topical antibiotics and antiseptics has been shown significantly to reduce colonization and sepsis. Mafenide, a sulphonamide derivative, was widely used, but has been largely replaced by silver sulphadiazine or chlorhexidine in the UK. None of these agents will reliably prevent infection by multiply resistant Gram-negative rods, especially *Ps. aeruginosa* (an organism that has replaced *Str. pyogenes* as the major scourge of burns units), or fungi. Aggressive surgical approaches of early wound closure by skin grafting after debridement has reduced the requirement for topical applications to burned surfaces.

In cases where infection becomes established, systemic drugs will often have to be employed, the choice being dictated by laboratory tests. However, since the penetration of antibiotics to surface lesions with a poor blood supply may be inadequate, topical dressings are additionally required.

Urinary and respiratory infections are commonly encountered in the burned patient, as is septicaemia, which has a poor prognosis. These infections require, of course, systemic therapy, but choice may be limited by bacterial resistance since many burns units are notorious for the prevalence of highly resistant strains, especially of *Ps. aeruginosa*.

SKIN ULCERS

Ulceration of the skin of the leg or the area overlying the sacrum may arise from a variety of pathological states and infection is usually a sequela, not an initiating event. Disorders of the circulation, including obliterative arterial disease, small-vessel damage consequent on diabetes mellitus, and varicose veins are the most common underlying conditions and correction of the underlying cause is essential to the healing of any ulcer. Continuous pressure is another common factor in the formation of a break in the skin, particularly in the bed-ridden. Such bed sores are difficult to prevent without scrupulous nursing care. This problem has led to the development of special air beds and cushions to minimize local vascular occlusion to the skin overlying bony areas such as the sacrum.

The presence of infection in a skin ulcer may be detected by odour, local cellulitis, and appearance of pus, which in the case of pseudomonas infection may be characteristically green. Gas in the tissues, detected as crepitus on palpation, may indicate anaerobic infection. Swab reports showing the presence of potential pathogens do not prove infection since colonization of a large raw skin area is inevitable. *Staph. aureus*, environmental and gut bacteria are the organisms most commonly found in these sites. *Ps. aeruginosa* is frequently found in long-standing ulcers because of its intrinsic resistance to many antibiotics and chemical agents used as antiseptics. In some cases infection is sufficiently invasive to warrant systemic treatment and metronidazole should be given to patients in whom *Bacteroides fragilis* infection is suspected.

Local therapy with antiseptics, combined with measures to improve the nutrition of the site, are the mainstays of management of skin ulcers. Chlorine- or iodine-containing compounds (especially *iodophors*, which are iodine complexes that do not stain the skin and are less irritant) are often used, but older remedies such as honey, sugar, and vinegar may be as effective as modern antiseptics. In addition, topical antibiotics such as tetracycline are often used in severe infected ulcers which do not respond to conservative management. Many weeks of regular dressing combined with bed rest may be required to heal large ulcers; admission to hospital often speeds up the process. Skin grafting is frequently used for the most recalcitrant cases.

SUPERFICIAL FUNGAL INFECTIONS

Confirmation of the diagnosis of superficial fungal infections such as ringworm and tinea pedis of the skin, or thrush of the mouth or vagina, depends on laboratory investigation of appropriate specimens from the affected area (nail, hair, skin scrapings, swabs of lesions of mucous membranes). Microscopy alone will be sufficient to establish a fungal cause in most cases, but culture is necessary to identify the aetiological agent. Susceptibility testing presents technical difficulties, but dermatophytes may usually be assumed to be susceptible to appropriate agents (see Chapter 4, Table 4.1). *Candida albicans* may acquire resistance to some drugs, but this is only of great importance in invasive candidiasis.

The limiting factor in treating dermatophyte infections is penetration of the agent. For superficial skin infections old-fashioned remedies, such as benzoic acid-containing ointments (e.g. Whitfield's ointment) are perfectly effective, but for hair and nail infections agents which penetrate into keratinized tissue are needed. Oral griseofulvin is uniquely suited to this purpose, since it is absorbed from the gastrointestinal tract and is perferentially concentrated in keratin. Because of the slow turnover of nail and hair, treatment for several months may be required; indeed, fungal infections of toenails may not completely clear even after a year's treatment with griseofulvin, despite susceptibility of the infecting fungus. In such cases terbinafine may be successful.

Thrush responds in most cases to an appropriate antifungal agent, applied topically (e.g. nystatin or an imidazole), but precipitating factors, such as diabetes or antibiotic therapy, must also be corrected if they are present. If there is clinical evidence for invasive infection, as, for example, *Candida* oesophagitis, appropriate systemic drugs, such as amphotericin B, 5-fluorocytosine, fluconazole or ketoconazole, must be added.

DISADVANTAGES OF TOPICAL THERAPY

Topical therapy is not without its hazards. Although the direct toxic effects of drugs given systemically are reduced, exposed tissues and mucous membranes offer a fairly efficient site for drug absorption. For example, aminoglycoside ototoxicity has been reported following local application of neomycin, especially in the newborn. A more frequently observed effect is sensitization to the agent so that subsequent use of the drug, either topically or parenterally, produces a hypersensitivity reaction. Penicillin, in particular, is prone to sensitize the host and because of possible anaphylactic reactions it is not advisable to use any β-lactam antibiotic on the skin. A further hazard of topical therapy is that local irritation may lead to a delay in wound healing, even though the actual infection is controlled.

Superinfection with resistant bacteria or with fungi is a common consequence of using any topical antibiotic for a prolonged period. Widespread use of one particular agent will lead to a larger reservoir of resistant organisms and the possibility of cross-infection. This is particularly likely to occur in burns units and dermatology wards, where there are many patients with large open skin lesions. Prevention of infection and cross-infection by aseptic methods is desirable, but often difficult in practice.

Of equal concern is the development of bacterial resistance during therapy. It has been shown that topical neomycin can select resistant *Staphylococcus epidermidis* strains, which can transfer resistance to *Staph. aureus* on the skin. The emergence of gentamicin-resistant *Ps. aeruginosa* and coliforms has been associated with topical use of that aminoglycoside, particularly on leg ulcers. In some instances the resistance is plasmid mediated. In this manner, topical agents select multi-resistant organisms which may subsequently cause systemic infection in the patient or, by cross-infection, others. This is the most powerful argument against the indiscriminate use of topical antibiotics, and since antiseptics lack this disadvantage they are to be preferred wherever possible.

33

Postscript: The development and marketing of antimicrobial drugs

D. Greenwood

Most new antimicrobial agents emerge by a process of chemical modification of existing compounds, although a few novel substances continue to be described.

In the past, most effort has been expended on the discovery and development of antibacterial drugs, but the emphasis may be shifting. Of 23 new antimicrobial agents released on to the UK market between 1990 and 1993 (Table 33.1), nine were not antibacterial agents.

The progress of a new antibiotic from discovery to marketing is outlined in Fig 33.1. When a new antimicrobial drug is discovered or invented, the first indications of its activity and spectrum are usually gleaned from fairly crude *in vitro* inhibition tests against a few common representative organisms. *In vitro* screening tests will not

Table 33.1. New antimicrobial agents 1990–93 (UK)

Antibacterial compounds	Other antimicrobial agents
Azithromycin	Albendazole (anthelminthic)
Cefixime	Amorolfine (topical antifungal)
Cefodizime	Foscarnet (antiviral)
Cefpodoxime	Halofantrine (antimalarial)
Ceftriaxone	Itraconazole (antifungal)
Clarithromycin	Liposomal amphotericin B (antifungal)
Enoxacin*	Mefloquine (antimalarial)
Norfloxacin	Terbinafine (antifungal)
Ofloxacin	Tioconazole (topical antifungal)
Sulbactam†	
Tazobactam†	
Teicoplanin	
Temafloxacin*	
Temocillin	

† β-lactamase inhibitors marketed as combination products.
* Later withdrawn.

detect potentially useful activity if *in vivo* metabolism of the compound is a prerequisite for the antimicrobial effect (e.g. Prontosil; see Historical Introduction); nor will such tests reveal agents which might modify microbial cells sufficiently to render them non-virulent or susceptible to host defences, without actually preventing their growth. Furthermore, conventional laboratory culture media occasionally contain substances which interfere with the activity of certain antimicrobial compounds, which may consequently go undetected.

Despite these difficulties, *in vitro* screening offers an extremely simple and generally effective way of detecting antimicrobial activity which has yielded a rich harvest of therapeutically useful compounds over the years. In contrast, the rational design of new antimicrobial agents by targeting potentially vulnerable stages of microbial development has not been very fruitful, although advances in molecular modelling based on computer graphics may help to facilitate this in the future.

DEVELOPMENT OF NEW COMPOUNDS

Those compounds that pass the initial screening tests must be made available in sufficient quantities and in sufficiently pure form to enable preliminary tests of toxicity and efficacy to be carried out in laboratory animals, and more extensive and precise *in vitro* tests to be performed. Pilot-stage production usually presents little problem, although considerable difficulties may be experienced in scaling up production at a later date, when relatively large quantities are needed for clinical trials and subsequent marketing.

Animal tests of toxicity, pharmacology, and efficacy are an indispensable part of the development of any new drug, but they also have considerable limitations. Idiosyncratic reactions may suggest toxicity in a compound that would be safe for human use or, more importantly, adverse reactions peculiar to the human subject may go undetected. The pharmacological handling of the drug may be vastly different from that encountered in the human subject. As regards efficacy testing, animals have important limitations in that experimental infections seldom correspond to the supposedly analogous condition in humans, either anatomically or in the relationship of treatment to the natural history of the disease process.

If preliminary tests of toxicity and efficacy indicate that the compound is worth advancing further, full-scale acute and chronic toxicity tests are carried out in animals. These include long-term tests of mutagenic or carcinogenic potential, effects on fertility, and teratogenicity. Mutagenicity tests may also be performed in microbial systems (*Ames test*).

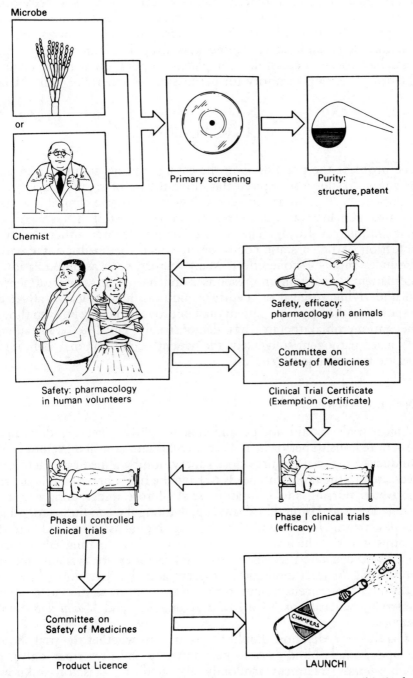

Fig. 33.1. Diagrammatic representation of the progress of a new antibiotic from discovery to marketing.

Provided the animal toxicity studies reveal no serious toxicity problems, the first tentative trials are undertaken in healthy human volunteers (usually employees of the company involved) to investigate the pharmacology and safety of the new drug in humans. Once these tests have been successfully completed, application may be made to the drug-licensing authority for permission to undertake clinical trials.

CLINICAL TRIALS

The proof of the pudding is in the eating, and no amount of *in vitro* or animal testing can replace the ultimate test of safety and efficacy: therapeutic use in human infection. Nevertheless, the clinical trial stage remains, in many ways, the least satisfactory aspect of the testing of any new antimicrobial drug. The reasons for this are not difficult to find: 'infection' is not a static condition in which therapeutic intervention produces an all-or-none effect. Many factors, such as mobilization of the patient's own immune response, drainage of pus, or treatment of an underlying surgical or medical condition, may crucially affect the response to therapy. The patient may improve subjectively, even though the antimicrobial therapy has demonstrably failed to eradicate the supposed pathogen; conversely, the patient's condition may deteriorate despite bacteriological 'success'.

Design of trials

Clinical trials should not be undertaken lightly. They are difficult to design, tedious to perform, and are fraught with ethical difficulties. The conduct of the trial requires close supervision by a medical practitioner dedicated to the task, who needs to have the full support of reliable and motivated nursing and laboratory staff. Before undertaking a trial, a detailed protocol should be drawn up, defining the conditions for which the new treatment is intended, the dosage regimens to be used, and the treatment with which it is to be compared. Participating laboratories should be consulted to ensure that full facilities are available for the monitoring of microbiological progress and the detection of adverse reactions. Most licensing authorities now require studies to conform to strict standards of 'Good clinical practice' and 'Good laboratory practice'.

Careful consideration should be given as to whether the trial should be open, single-blind (treatment known to the prescriber only), or double-blind (treatment randomly allocated in a fashion unknown to prescriber or recipient). In general, uncontrolled, open trials are unsatisfactory, except as preliminary indicators of safety and efficacy.

Controlled, double-blind trials are the most desirable scientifically, but are subject to ethical difficulties in that the prescribing doctor does not have full control over the patient's treatment.

Ethical requirements

Ethical considerations need to be taken fully into account. The basic principles which should govern all research involving human subjects are embodied in the *Declaration of Helsinki*, which was adopted by the 18th World Medical Assembly in 1964 with subsequent revisions. In the UK and many other countries, health authorities have ethical committees which monitor clinical trial protocols. The committee will need assurance that the safety of the new compound has been satisfactorily established and will wish to know what form of patient consent is to be obtained. It will also require adequate safeguards to be built in for the detection of unexpected adverse reactions and may have views as to whether a double-blind format, or a placebo control, are acceptable.

Statistical considerations

Many ambitious trials fail because insufficient numbers of patients are found to fulfil the criteria required for the study. Alternatively, the condition may be one (acute cystitis is a good example) in which the natural cure rate is so high, and the efficacy of standard treatment so good, that huge numbers would have to be examined to establish the superiority of a new agent, although it may be possible to establish efficacy. It is essential to be reasonably sure, before the trial starts, that sufficient patients can be accumulated to satisfy statistical requirements. During the conduct of the trial, regular checks of relevant microbiological, haematological, chemical, and radiological parameters should be made. All findings should be fully documented as soon as the information is available, rather than attempting to glean information from the patients' notes retrospectively, after the trial is completed.

DRUG LICENSING

Most countries have enacted some sort of legislation aimed at controlling the marketing of pharmaceutical products. In the USA, Federal regulations are administered by the Food and Drug Administration (FDA). Within the European Union, a Committee on Proprietary Medical Products issues guidelines for harmonizing regulatory requirements among member nations. From 1995, a European Medicines Evaluation Agency, based in London, will co-ordinate drug licensing and safety throughout the European Union, although companies will still be able to seek registration of their products by national regulatory authorities.

In the UK, the Medicines Act of 1968 (implemented on 1 September 1971) invested executive powers in the government health and agriculture ministers, who constitute the British Drug Licensing Authority. Ministers are advised by a statutory body, the Medicines Commission, which, through its specialist advisory committees, reviews all pharmaceutical products intended for medical or veterinary use. The manufacture, promotion, and distribution of all medicines in the UK is supervised by the Medicines Control Agency.

Before clinical trials can be performed on a new drug in the UK, full toxicological data must be submitted to the Licensing Authority together with a full trial protocol and the names of the proposed investigators. Such applications are scrutinized by the Committee on Safety of Medicines (CSM), who must satisy themselves that all reasonable criteria are met before recommending that a *Clinical Trial Certificate*, valid for 2 years, be issued.

Pharmaceutical manufactures have long complained about the delays inherent in processing applications for a Clinical Trial Certificate and firms in the UK may now be granted a *Clinical Trial Exemption Certificate*, provided certain criteria are met. In particular, the holder of the exemption certificate must undertake to notify any adverse reaction arising during the trial, or any other matter which might reasonably cause the Licensing Authority to doubt the safety or quality of the product.

When clinical trial data have been accumulated, an application for a *Product Licence* may be made. All valid applications are again passed to the CSM for scrutiny. In some countries, licensing authorities require that new compounds should be shown to be superior to existing products, in an effort to reduce so-called 'me-too' products. However, in the UK the CSM judge new applications only on the grounds of safety, efficacy, and quality. If the CSM recommends refusal of a Product Licence, the application may be withdrawn or the applicant may elect to answer the objections raised, either in writing or in person before the CSM. Should the application still be refused, the applicant has the right of appeal to the Medicines Commission. Product Licences, once issued, are valid for 5 years.

Over the years, the requirements of licensing authorities world-wide (particularly for toxicological testing) have become progressively more stringent. Consequently, the cost of developing a new drug has escalated enormously. Attempts are being made to harmonize the drug registration requirements of Europe, the USA, and Japan, but progress so far has been modest. The period between the discovery and marketing of a new product is seldom less than 5 years and may be substantially longer. Shortening this period is important to the company marketing the new drug, since it maximizes the time during which it can recoup the cost of research and development (which may exceed £100 million) and profit from the discovery while enjoying patent protection.

DRUG MARKETING

Data sheets

Under the 1968 Medicines Act, all companies marketing products provided for the use of medical practitioners in the UK are required to produce a data sheet giving a summary of relevant information about the drug, including the conditions for which its use is licensed, contraindications and known side-effects. Most pharmaceutical firms collaborate in producing an annual *Data Sheet Compendium*, which is distributed free to registered medical practitioners.

Post-marketing surveillance

Issue of a Product Licence is no guarantee that a compound is 100 per cent safe, nor even that all adverse reactions have been detected before marketing. Because of this, the CSM issue to all practitioners postage-paid 'yellow cards' for the notification of adverse reactions. Although the scheme is voluntary, it is important that prescribers collaborate fully with it. Such notifications are particularly important in the first few years in which a new compound is marketed. Copies of the notification form are routinely included with each issue of the *British National Formulary*, and compounds under particular scrutiny are flagged with a black triangle ▼.

Relationship with the medical profession

The conduct of pharmaceutical companies in marketing their products is governed by a voluntary Code of Practice agreed between the members of the Association of the British Pharmaceutical Industry in consultation with the British Medical Association and the Department of Health. The Code of Practice is published in the *Data Sheet Compendium*. It covers, among other things, the content and distribution of advertisements and other promotional literature; hospitality, gifts, and inducements to the medical and allied professions; marketing research; and relationships with the general public and lay communications media.

Advertisements

The subject of advertising is a perennial bone of contention between doctors and the pharmaceutical industry. The former complain that the industry tries to cloud their professional judgement under a deluge of irrelevant, mendacious, and uninterpretable gobbledegook; the latter claim their commercial right to exploit their products to their best advantage in the market place, and point to the factual data sheets and other information services that they place at the disposal of the medical profession.

The truth, as usual, inhabits the middle ground. Advertisements are subject to the usual advertising regulations and may not tell overt lies. None the less, they are intended to sway the prescriber in favour of a particular product. Doctors cannot ignore advertisements and should be wary of claiming that they are uninfluenced by them. If they were not influenced, advertisements would not be so cost effective as they clearly are.

Prescribers should therefore make a conscious effect to separate fact from fantasy in advertisements and cultivate a healthy critical attitude, especially towards new products. In particular, doctors should learn to distinguish between genuine advances and new products which, though effective, are no better than older, well-tried, and cheaper remedies. They should also be wary of impressive claims ostensibly based on published independent assessments which turn out, in the small print, to refer to 'data on file' or dubious publications in obscure sources.

Sources of independent advice

In the UK the *British National Formulary* and *Drug and Therapeutics Bulletin*, published by the Consumers' Association, offer reliable sources of objective information to the medical practitioner. In the USA, the *National Formulary* and the *Medical Letter* provide a similar service. Many hospitals now produce therapeutic guides for use by medical staff. Pharmacies often offer a formal 'drug information service' to which general practitioners also have access, and most medical microbiology laboratories are able to offer accurate up-to-date advice on antimicrobial therapy.

It should be emphasized that, although the marketing of drugs is fairly well regulated throughout the industrially developed world, the same is not true of less favoured countries; in many nations of the world the standards of advertising and marketing often appear to overstep the bounds of what would be considered ethical in more developed countries.

DRUG NAMES

When a new antibiotic is first described in the scientific literature it usually appears under a number representing the manufacturer's

Table 33.2. Antimicrobial agents (excluding topical agents) on the WHO list of essential drugs (seventh list, 1992)

Antibacterial agents	Antimycobacterial agents	Antifungal agents	Antiprotozoal agents	Anthelminthic agents
Amoxycillin*	Clofazimine	Amphotericin B	Benznidazole	Albendazole
Ampicillin*	Dapsone	Griseofulvin	Chloroquine*	Ivermectin
Benzathine penicillin	Ethambutol	Ketoconazole	Diloxanide*	Levamisole
Benzylpenicillin	Isoniazid	Nystatin	Meglumine antimonate*	Mebendazole*
Chloramphenicol*	Pyrazinamide	(Flucytosine)	Melarsoprol	Metriphonate
Cloxacillin*	Rifampicin		Metronidazole*	Niclosamide
Co-trimoxazole*	Streptomycin		Nifurtimox	Oxamniquine
Erythromycin*	Thiacetazone + isoniazid		Pentamidine	Piperazine
Gentamicin*			Primaquine	Praziquantel
Metronidazole*			Proguanil	Pyrantel
Phenoxymethylpenicillin			Quinine*	Suramin
Piperacillin*			Suramin	Thiabendazole
Procaine penicillin			(Eflornithine)	
Spectinomyin			(Mefloquine)	
Sulphadimidine*			(Sulfadoxine + pyrimethamine)*	
Tetracycline*			(Tetracycline)*	
(Ciprofloxacin)				
(Clindamycin)				
(Doxycycline)				
(Nitrofurantoin)				
(Trimethoprim)				

Drugs listed are on the main list, except those in brackets, which are on the complementary list of reserve drugs.
* Examples of a therapeutic group for which acceptable alternatives exist.

laboratory code for the compound. This practice is to be discouraged, since the code is forgotten once a drug is named and, in later years, source references become difficult to locate. The reason for using a code is that names proposed by the manufacturer are not always subsequently accepted by the bodies controlling drug nomenclature. These are the British Pharmacopoeia Commission in the UK who recommend a *British Approved Name* (BAN) to the Medicines Commission and the United States Adopted Name (USAN) Council in the USA. International agreement is co-ordinated by the World Health Organization who specify or recommend an *International Non-proprietary Name* (INN). Once the Approved Name is introduced into the national Pharmacopoeia of a country, it becomes the *Official Name*. In addition to the Approved or Official Name, the drug may have various *proprietary names* under which it is marketed by the manufacturer(s) or his agents.

Approved Names try to avoid close nomenclatural similarities, but the profusion of 'sulpha-s', 'cefa-s', and '-cillins' still produces some confusion; when the same compound is marketed under different proprietary names, bewilderment is often complete.

Generic prescribing

There has been a good deal of debate as to whether doctors should use proprietary names in writing prescriptions. On the one hand, it is pointed out that formulations differ so that the pharmacological properties of a drug may vary from product to product. Moreover, adverse reactions caused by a particular formulation may be more easily detected if the product is specified. On the other hand, non-proprietary names are less likely to cause confusion; they remove the necessity of pharmacies keeping a large and varied stock of similar products, and enable the pharmacist to dispense the cheapest version of a particular drug.

The *British National Formulary* sensibly recommends prescribers to use non-proprietary names in all but those few instances where bioavailability problems are so important that the patient should always receive the same brand.

WHITHER ANTIBIOTICS?

The number of antimicrobial drugs available to the prescriber is now enormous and, at least as far as antibacterial compounds are concerned, the undoubted value of having a wide and varied choice has been overtaken by the confusion that is caused by the conflicting claims of so many agents with similar or overlapping indications. There is no dispute about the fact that we currently possess more antibacterial drugs than we need; most of the common infections can be adequately dealt with using a few well-tried agents. Indeed, most general practitioners rely on a few favourite antibiotics which they use to cover most bacterial infections. The WHO includes only a handful of antibacterial agents in its list of essential drugs (Table 33.2). The availability of antimicrobial drugs varies widely among different countries for reasons that must be commercial rather than therapeutic: for example, in Norway, where a restrictive licensing policy is in operation, the number of β-lactam antibiotics available represents only about a quarter of those marketed in Japan, while the WHO essential drug list has a mere eight, all of which are penicillins.

Apart from the financial attractions of a share in a huge market, the main impetus for continuing research into antibacterial agents is the ever-present spectre of resistance. Seldom has this reached the point where effective antibacterial treatment has become impossible, but it is difficult to assess how the continuing influx of new drugs has influenced the course of events (see Chapter 11).

The situation with the chemotherapy of non-bacterial infection is much less satisfactory. Although great strides have been made in the prevention of viral infection by immunization, chemotherapy for viral disease is extremely limited (see Chapters 6 and 28). Some sort of effective chemotherapy is available for most fungal, protozoal, and helminth infections, but the choice is very limited and, in many ways, unsatisfactory (see Chapters 4, 5, and 31). On a global scale, it is these conditions, rather than the traditional bacterial infectious diseases, which are responsible for the great majority of morbidity and mortality among humankind. The greatest challenge for the future is to provide for these diseases the same sort of safe, effective chemotherapy that is now available for most bacterial infections, and to make effective therapy for all infections readily available for those who need it most.

Recommendations for further reading

A large number of books are available dealing with the practicalities of the use of antimicrobial agents. Since availability and usage differ considerably in different countries, no one book has universal applicability. The following are among the most authoritative texts in the English language.

Conte, J. E. and Barriere, S. L. (1992) *Manual of antibiotics and infectious diseases*. Lea and Febiger, Malvern, USA.

Kucers, A. and Bennett, N. McK. (1987). *The use of antibiotics*, 4th edn. Heinemann, London.

Lambert, H. P. and O'Grady, F.W. (1992). *Antibiotic and chemotherapy*, 6th edn. Churchill Livingstone, Edinburgh.

Simon, C., Stille, W., and Wilkinson, P.J. (1993). *Antibiotic therapy in clinical practice*, 2nd edn. Schattauer, Stuttgart.

Books specifically dealing with the treatment of diseases caused by protozoa and helminths include:

Bruce-Chwatt, L. J. (ed.) (1986). *Chemotherapy of malaria*. WHO, Geneva.

Campbell, W. C. and Rew, R. S. (eds.) (1986). *Chemotherapy of parasitic diseases*. Plenum Press, New York.

James, D. M. and Gilles, H. M. (1985). *Human antiparasitic drugs: pharmacology and usage*. John Wiley & Sons, Chichester.

Report (1990). *Practical chemotherapy of malaria*. WHO Technical Report Series 805. WHO, Geneva.

WHO Model Prescribing Information (1991). *Drugs used in parasitic diseases*. WHO, Geneva.

Books dealing with the mode of action of antimicrobial agents and the principles underlying their use include:

Franklin, T. J. and Snow, G. A. (1989). *Biochemistry of antimicrobial action*, 4 edn. Chapman and Hall, London.

Gale, E. F., Cundliffe, E., Reynolds, P. E., Richmond, M. H., and Waring, M. J. (1981). *The molecular basis of antibiotic action*, 2nd edn. John Wiley & Sons, Chichester.

Greenwood, D. and O'Grady, F. (eds.) (1985). *The scientific basis of antimicrobial chemotherapy*. Cambridge University Press, Cambridge.

Pratt, W. B. and Fekety, R. (1986). *The antimicrobial drugs*. Oxford University Press, Oxford.

Russell, A. D. and Chopra, I. (1990). *Understanding antibacterial action and resistance*. Ellis Horwood, London.

Laboratory aspects of antimicrobial therapy are dealt with in:

Lorian, V. (ed.) (1991). *Antibiotics in laboratory medicine*, 3rd edn. Williams & Wilkins, Baltimore.
Reeves, D. S., Phillips, I., Williams, J. D., and Wise, R. (1978). *Laboratory methods in antimicrobial chemotherapy*. Churchill Livingstone, Edinburgh. (New edition in preparation.)

An indispensable guide to the use of all therapeutic drugs for practitioners in the UK is provided by:

British National Formulary. British Medical Association and the Royal Pharmaceutical Society of Great Britain. (Revised at intervals of about 6 months.)

Comprehensive monographs on antimicrobial agents are to be found in large reference texts on drugs including:

Dollery, C. (ed.) (1991). *Therapeutic drugs*. Churchill Livingstone, Edinburgh. (Two volumes, plus supplements issued 1992 and 1994.)
Reynolds, J. E. F. (ed.) (1993). *Martindale: the extra pharmacopoeia*, 30th edn. The Pharmaceutical Press, London.

An excellent guide to the use of drugs specifically designed for the East African situation, but having a much wider applicability to developing nations of the world, is provided by:

Upunda, G., Yudkin, J., and Brown, G. (1980). *Therapeutic guidelines*. African Medical and Research Foundation, Nairobi. Also published in the Macmillan Tropical Community Health Manuals series as: *Guidelines to Drug Usage* (1983). Macmillan, London.

Books providing a valuable insight into the use and abuse of antimicrobial agents in the Third World include:

Chetley, A. (1990). *A healthy business? World health and the pharmaceutical industry*. Zed books, London.
Melrose, D. (1982). *Bitter pills: medicines and the Third World poor*. Oxfam, Oxford.
World Health Organization (1988). *The world drug situation*. WHO, Geneva.
World Health Organization (1992). *The use of essential drugs*. 5th report of WHO Expert Committee. WHO Technical Report Series, No. 825. WHO, Geneva.

Antimicrobial drugs are used so widely that papers dealing with aspects of their use appear in numerous journals. English language journals specifically devoted to antibiotics and antimicrobial therapy include:

Antibiotics and Chemotherapy
Antimicrobial Agents and Chemotherapy
Antiviral Chemistry and Chemotherapy
Antiviral research
Chemotherapy
International Journal of Antimicrobial Agents
Journal of Antibiotics
Journal of Antimicrobial Chemotherapy

The *British Society for Antimicrobial Chemotherapy* periodically publishes authoritative reviews of aspects of antimicrobial therapy. Articles that have appeared so far are:

The antibiotic prophylaxis of infective endocarditis. *Lancet* 1982; **ii**, 1323–6. (Updated: *Lancet* 1986; **i**: 1267; 1990; **i**: 88–9; and 1992; **i**: 1292–3.)

Antibiotic treatment of streptococcal and staphylococcal endocarditis. *Lancet* 1985; **ii**: 815–17.

Guidelines for the control of epidemic methicillin-resistant *Staphylococcus aureus* (Joint report with the Hospital Infection Society). *Journal of Hospital Infection* 1986; **7**: 193–201. (Revised guidelines: *Journal of Hospital Infection* 1990; **16**: 351–77.)

Diagnosis and management of peritonitis in continuous ambulatory peritoneal dialysis. *Lancet* 1987; **i**: 845–9.

Breakpoints in in-vitro antibiotic sensitivity testing. *Journal of Antimicrobial Chemotherapy* 1988; **21**: 701–10.

The clinical evaluation of antibacterial drugs. *Journal of Antimicrobial Chemotherapy* 1989; **23** (Suppl. B): 1–42.

A guide to sensitivity testing. *Journal of Antimicrobial Chemotherapy* 1991; **27** (Suppl. D): 1–50.

Laboratory monitoring of antifungal chemotherapy. *Lancet* 1991; **337**: 1577–80.

Antifungal chemotherapy in patients with acquired immunodeficiency syndrome. *Lancet* 1992; **340**: 648–51.

A survey of undergraduate and continuing medical education about antimicrobial chemotherapy in the United Kingdom. *British Journal of Clinical Pharmacology* 1993; **36**: 511–19.

Chemoprophylaxis for candidosis and aspergillosis in neutropenia and transplantation: a review and recommendations. *Journal of Antimicrobial Chemotherapy* 1993; **32**: 5–21.

Management of deep *Candida* infection in surgical and intensive care unit patients. *Intensive Care Medicine* 1994; **20**: 522–8.

Antimicrobial prophylaxis in neurosurgery and after head injury. *Lancet* 1994; **344**: 1547–51.

Index